Pediatric and Adolescent Gynecology

Guest Editor

S. PAIGE HERTWECK, MD

OBSTETRICS AND GYNECOLOGY CLINICS OF NORTH AMERICA

www.obgyn.theclinics.com

Consulting Editor
WILLIAM F. RAYBURN, MD, MBA

March 2009 • Volume 36 • Number 1

SAUNDERS an imprint of ELSEVIER, Inc.

W.B. SAUNDERS COMPANY

A Division of Elsevier Inc.

Elsevier, Inc. ● 1600 John F. Kennedy Blvd. ● Suite 1800 ● Philadelphia, PA 19103-2899

http://www.theclinics.com

OBSTETRICS AND GYNECOLOGY CLINICS OF NORTH AMERICA Volume 36, Number 1
March 2009 ISSN 0889-8545, ISBN-13: 978-1-4377-0510-2, ISBN-10: 1-4377-0510-3

Editor: Carla Holloway
Developmental Editor: Theresa Collier

Obstetrics and Gynecology Clinics (ISSN 0889-8545) is published quarterly by Elsevier Inc., 360 Park Avenue South, New York, NY 10010-1710. Months of issue are March, June, September, and December. Business and Editorial Offices: 1600 John F. Kennedy Blvd., Suite 1800, Philadelphia, PA 19103-2899. Customer Service Office: 11830 Westline Industrial Drive, St. Louis, MO 63146. Periodicals postage paid at New York, NY, and additional mailing offices. Subscription price per year is $234.00 (US individuals), $399.00 (US institutions), $118.00 (US students), $281.00 (Canadian individuals), $504.00 (Canadian institutions), $174.00 (Canadian students), $342.00 (foreign individuals), $504.00 (foreign institutions), and $174.00 (foreign students). To receive student/resident rate, orders must be accompanied by name of affiliated institution, date of term, and the signature of program/residency coordinator on institution letterhead. Orders will be billed at individual rate until proof of status is received. Foreign air speed delivery is included in all *Clinics* subscription prices. All prices are subject to change without notice. POSTMASTER: Send address changes to *Obstetrics and Gynecology Clinics*, Elsevier Periodicals Customer Service, 11830 Westline Industrial Drive, St. Louis, MO 63146. **Customer Service: 1-800-654-2452 (US). From outside of the United States, call 314-453-7041. Fax: 314-453-5170. E-mail: JournalsCustomerService-usa@elsevier.com (for print support); JournalsOnlineSupport-usa@elsevier.com (for online support).**

Reprints. For copies of 100 or more of articles in this publication, please contact the Commercial Reprints Department, Elsevier Inc., 360 Park Avenue South, New York, New York 10010-1710. Tel.: 212-633-3818; Fax: 212-462-1935; E-mail: reprints@elsevier.com.

Obstetrics and Gynecology Clinics of North America is also published in Spanish by McGraw-Hill Interamericana Editores S.A., P.O. Box 5-237, 06500, Mexico; in Portuguese by Reichmann and Affonso Editores, Rio de Janeiro, Brazil; and in Greek by Paschalidis Medical Publications, Athens, Greece.

Obstetrics and Gynecology Clinics of North America is covered in MEDLINE/PubMed (Index Medicus), Excerpta Medica, Current Concepts/Clinical Medicine, Science Citation Index, BIOSIS, CINAHL, and ISI/BIOMED.

Printed and bound by CPI Group (UK) Ltd, Croydon, CR0 4YY

Transferred to Digital Print 2011

GOAL STATEMENT

The goal of *Obstetrics and Gynecology Clinics of North America* is to keep practicing physicians up to date with current clinical practice in OB/GYN by providing timely articles reviewing the state of the art in patient care.

ACCREDITATION

The *Obstetrics and Gynecology Clinics of North America* is planned and implemented in accordance with the Essential Areas and Policies of the Accreditation Council for Continuing Medical Education (ACCME) through the joint sponsorship of the University of Virginia School of Medicine and Elsevier. The University of Virginia School of Medicine is accredited by the ACCME to provide continuing medical education for physicians.

The University of Virginia School of Medicine designates this educational activity for a maximum of 15 *AMA PRA Category 1 Credits*™. Physicians should only claim credit commensurate with the extent of their participation in the activity.

The American Medical Association has determined that physicians not licensed in the US who participate in this CME activity are eligible for *AMA PRA Category 1 Credits*™.

Category 1 credit can be earned by reading the text material, taking the CME examination online at: http://www.theclinics.com/home/cme, and completing the evaluation. After taking the test, you will be required to review any and all incorrect answers. Following completion of the test and evaluation, your credit will be awarded and you may print your certificate.

FACULTY DISCLOSURE/CONFLICT OF INTEREST

The University of Virginia School of Medicine, as an ACCME accredited provider, endorses and strives to comply with the Accreditation Council for Continuing Medical Education (ACCME) Standards of Commercial Support, Commonwealth of Virginia statutes, University of Virginia policies and procedures, and associated federal and private regulations and guidelines on the need for disclosure and monitoring of proprietary and financial interests that may affect the scientific integrity and balance of content delivered in continuing medical education activities under our auspices.

The University of Virginia School of Medicine requires that all CME activities accredited through this institution be developed independently and be scientifically rigorous, balanced and objective in the presentation/discussion of its content, theories and practices.

All authors/editors participating in an accredited CME activity are expected to disclose to the readers relevant financial relationships with commercial entities occurring within the past 12 months (such as grants or research support, employee, consultant, stock holder, member of speakers bureau, etc.). The University of Virginia School of Medicine will employ appropriate mechanisms to resolve potential conflicts of interest to maintain the standards of fair and balanced education to the reader. Questions about specific strategies can be directed to the Office of Continuing Medical Education, University of Virginia School of Medicine, Charlottesville, Virginia.

The faculty and staff of the University of Virginia Office of Continuing Medical Education have no financial affiliations to disclose.

The authors/editors listed below have identified no professional or financial affiliations for themselves or their spouse/partner:

Carla Holloway (Acquisitions Editor); William Irvin, MD (Test Author); Mary Anne Jamieson, MD, FRCSC; Sari Leanne Kives, MD, FRCSC; Marc R. Laufer, MD; Diane F. Merritt, MD; Samantha M. Pfeifer, MD; William F. Rayburn, MD, MBA (Consulting Editor); Taraneh Shafii, MD, MPH; Claire Templeman, MD; and Elizabeth B. Yerkes, MD.

The authors/editors listed below identified the following professional or financial affiliations for themselves or their spouse/partner:

Lisa Allen, MD is an industry funded research/investigator for Organon.

Lesley L. Breech, MD and spouse both serve on the Speakers Bureau for Merck Pharmaceuticals.

Gale R. Burstein, MD, MPH, FAAP serves on the Speakers Bureau for Merck, Inc. and GlaxoSmithKline and serves on the Advisory Committee for Merck, Inc.

Jennifer E. Dietrich, MD, MSc serves on the Speakers Bureau for Merck and CSL Behring.

S. Paige Hertweck, MD (Guest Editor) is an industry funded research/investigator for Merck and Barr/Duramed, serves on the Speakers Bureau and Advisory Committee for Merck, and has a financial relationship with Ethicon.

Andra H. James, MD, MPH is an industry funded research/investigator and serves on the Advisory Board for CSL Behring.

Eduardo Lara-Torre, MD, FACOG serves on the Speakers Bureau for Merck, Organon, and Wener-Chilcott.

Joel Palefsky, MD is an industry funded research/investigator for Merck and Co, and is on the Advisory Committee/Board of GlaxoSmithKline.

Mary M. Rubin, PhD, NP, RNC, CRNP serves on the Advisory Committee for Merck, Inc., GlaxoSmithKline, and PharmaDem.

Donald L. Yee, MD, MS is a consultant for Bristol-Myers Squibb.

Disclosure of Discussion of non-FDA approved uses for pharmaceutical products and/or medical devices:

The University of Virginia School of Medicine, as an ACCME provider, requires that all faculty presenters identify and disclose any off-label uses for pharmaceutical and medical device products. The University of Virginia School of Medicine recommends that each physician fully review all the available data on new products or procedures prior to clinical use.

TO ENROLL

To enroll in the Obstetrics and Gynecology Clinics of North America Continuing Medical Education program, call customer service at 1-800-654-2452 or visit us online at: www.theclinics.com/home/cme. The CME program is available to subscribers for an additional fee of $195.00.

Contributors

CONSULTING EDITOR

WILLIAM F. RAYBURN, MD, MBA
Seligman Professor and Chair, Department of Obstetrics and Gynecology; Chief of Staff, University Hospital, University of New Mexico Health Science Center, Albuquerque, New Mexico

GUEST EDITOR

S. PAIGE HERTWECK, MD
Director, Division of Pediatric and Adolescent Gynecology; Associate Professor, Department of Obstetrics, Gynecology, and Women's Health, University of Louisville School of Medicine, Louisville, Kentucky

AUTHORS

LISA ALLEN, MD, FRCSC
Assistant Professor, Department of Obstetrics and Gynecology and Pediatrics, University of Toronto, Toronto, Ontario, Canada

LESLEY L. BREECH, MD
Associate Professor, Pediatric and Adolescent Gynecology, Department of Pediatrics, University of Cincinnati College of Medicine, Cincinnati Children's Hospital Medical Center, Cincinnati, Ohio

GALE R. BURSTEIN, MD, MPH
Clinical Assistant Professor, Department of Pediatrics, SUNY at Buffalo School of Medicine and Biomedical Sciences, and Medical Director, Epidemiology and Surveillance, Erie County Department of Health, Buffalo, New York

JENNIFER E. DIETRICH, MD, MSc
Assistant Professor, Department of Obstetrics and Gynecology, Department of Pediatrics, Baylor College of Medicine, Houston, Texas

ANDRA H. JAMES, MD, MPH
Associate Professor, Department of Obstetrics and Gynecology, Division of Maternal-Fetal Medicine, Duke Unviersity Medical Center, Durham, North Carolina

MARY ANNE JAMIESON, MD, FRCSC
Director, Pediatric and Adolescent Gynecology; Associate Professor of Obstetrics and Gynecology, and Pediatrics, Department of Obstetrics and Gynecology, Queen's University, Kingston General Hospital, Kingston, Ontario, Canada

SARI KIVES, MD
Hospital for Sick Children, Toronto, Ontario, Canada

EDUARDO LARA-TORRE, MD, FACOG
Associate Residency Program Director, Director of Ambulatory Gynecology and Pediatric and Adolescent Gynecology, Department of Obstetrics and Gynecology, Carilion Clinic, Virginia Tech-Carilion School of Medicine, Roanoke, Virginia

MARC R. LAUFER, MD
Chief of Gynecology, Children's Hospital Boston; Associate Professor of Obstetrics, Gynecology and Reproductive Biology, Harvard Medical School, Boston, Massachusetts

DIANE F. MERRITT, MD
Professor of Obstetrics and Gynecology; Director of Pediatric and Adolescent Gynecology, Washington University School of Medicine, Barnes-Jewish Hospital, Saint Louis Children's Hospital, Missouri Baptist Medical Center, Saint Louis, Missouri

JOEL M. PALEFSKY, MD
Professor of Medicine, Division of Infectious Disease, University of California, San Francisco; Director, of Anal Neoplasia Clinic, University of California Helen Diller Family Comprehensive Cancer Center, San Francisco; Associate Dean for Clinical and Translational Research School of Medicine, San Francisco, California

SAMANTHA M. PFEIFER, MD
Associate Professor Obstetrics and Gynecology, Division of Reproductive Endocrinology and Infertility, University of Pennsylvania Medical Center, Philadelphia, Pennsylvania

MARY RUBIN, PhD, NP
Associate Clinical Professor, School of Nursing, University of California, San Francisco; and Nurse Practitioner, Anal Neoplasia Clinic, University of California San Francisco, Helen Diller Family Comprehensive Cancer Center, San Francisco, California

TARANEH SHAFII, MD, MPH
Assistant Professor of Pediatrics, Section of Adolescent Medicine, Department of Pediatrics, University of Washington School of Medicine; Director of Teen Health Services, Harborview Medical Center; and Deputy Medical Director, STD Clinic, Public Health Seattle and King County, Seattle, Washington

CLAIRE TEMPLEMAN, MD
Assistant Professor, Department of Obstetrics and Gynecology, Keck School of Medicine, University of Southern California, Los Angeles; and Division of Pediatric Surgery, Children's Hospital, Los Angeles, California

DONALD L. YEE, MD, MS
Assistant Professor, Department of Pediatrics, Baylor College of Medicine, Houston, Texas

ELIZABETH B. YERKES, MD
Assistant Professor of Urology, Northwestern University's Feinberg School of Medicine, Division of Urology, Children's Memorial Hospital, Chicago Illinois

Contents

> Although dysmenorrhea, pelvic mass or pain, genital irritation, and amen-
> orrhea are relatively common complaints, the astute clinician needs
> a broad differential diagnosis to avoid missing uncommon underlying
> etiologies such as Müllerian anomalies and cryptomenorrhea, ovarian
> teratomas and torsion, labial hypertrophy, vaginal foreign bodies, dermo-
> pathies, genital ulcers, imperforate hymen, and the absent vagina. This
> article discusses and illustrates uncommon pediatric and adolescent gy-
> necologic conditions that present with these common complaints.

> Disorders of sex development are medical conditions in which the devel-
> opment of chromosomal, gonadal, or anatomic sex varies from normal
> and may be incongruent with each other. This article primarily addresses
> the medical conditions where infants may be born with ambiguous genita-
> lia leading to decisions with regard to gender assignment. The approach to
> investigations and diagnosis in the newborn period will be stressed within
> an interprofessional team. Policies with regard to surgery have developed,
> with techniques evolving and data emerging from long-term outcome
> studies. Current medical and surgical management are reviewed. Finally,
> a developmental approach to disclosure is presented.

> The development of the Müllerian system and the female reproductive
> tract is a complex process involving an integrated series of events with sig-
> nificant potential for abnormal development and anomalies. Structural
> anomalies of the female reproductive tract may be isolated or occur in as-
> sociation with other congenital anomalies, including renal or bladder
> anomalies and anorectal malformations. Although rare in occurrence, it
> is important to be familiar with these conditions for appropriate diagnosis,
> management, and possible referral. The diagnosis, management, and

surgical treatments of female reproductive tract anomalies in girls and young women have advanced with improvements in diagnostic imaging techniques, surgical and nonsurgical techniques and innovative instrumentation and developments.

This article lends the urologist's perspective on complaints commonly seen in a pediatric and adolescent gynecology practice, such as perineal pain, repetitive posturing, vulvovaginitis and interlabial masses. Evaluation and management of urinary tract infections and daytime incontinence is discussed. The role of constipation and pelvic floor dysfunction in many of these complaints is emphasized.

Genital injuries in female children and adolescents may occur accidentally or as the result of an act of violence. This article discusses the etiologies and management of genital trauma. Awareness needs to be heightened among individual providers of medical care, as well as in the international community, to protect young girls from becoming victims of violence and to provide avenues for recovery.

Addressing sexual health, screening, and counseling to prevent sequelae of risky sexual behavior are essential components of the adolescent visit to the gynecologist. Discussing sexuality and taking a sexual history may cause feelings of discomfort for the provider and adolescent patient alike. Taking the time to build rapport and trust and the guarantee of confidentiality are key to engaging adolescent patients to discuss their personal health concerns with their provider. This article offers recommendations to facilitate dialog with the adolescent patient, addresses special considerations for the adolescent examination, discusses the use of some of the newly available tests for sexually transmitted infections (STIs), and suggests the recommended approach to management of STIs in adolescents.

Pregnancy rates in the United States seem to have stabilized in the past decade but continue to be higher than those in other industrialized nations. Although abstinence and barrier methods are available and efficient in preventing pregnancy, a comprehensive approach is a better choice when counseling patients on available options. The new approach to old contraceptive methods provides new alternatives to adolescents seeking safe and reliable methods. The availability and proved safety with longterm reversible contraceptive methods, such as the intrauterine system and subdermal implant, may allow adolescents to make better choices in preventing pregnancy. Future efforts in research should concentrate on finding the reasons why adolescents are at increased risk for unplanned pregnancy and solutions for this problem. Future contraceptive technology continues to focus on safety and convenience to facilitate the use of contraceptives in adolescents.

Polycystic ovary syndrome (PCOS) is now recognized as a heterogeneous disorder that results in overproduction of androgens, primarily from the ovary, leading to anovulation and hirsutism and is associated with insulin resistance. Long-term sequellae of PCOS include higher risk for diabetes, obesity, metabolic syndrome, endometrial hyperplasia, and anovulatory infertility. Symptoms in the adolescent include oligomenorrhea, hirsutism, acne, and weight gain. Insulin resistance, impaired glucose tolerance, and diabetes have also been demonstrated in adolescents who have PCOS. Treatment should be instituted early to decrease symptoms and long term sequellae of PCOS. Weight loss, oral contraceptives, and antiandrogens are effective in treating the symptoms of this disorder. Insulin-sensitizing medications have been shown to be effective but should be used with caution until larger randomized trials have shown short- and long term benefits and efficacy over traditional therapies in the adolescent population.

Adolescents who have bleeding disorders are more likely to experience abnormal reproductive tract bleeding, particularly menorrhagia or heavy menstrual bleeding. Even though most abnormal reproductive tract bleeding in adolescents is not attributable to a bleeding disorder, adolescents with abnormal reproductive tract bleeding are more likely to have an underlying bleeding disorder. After proper evaluation, most abnormal reproductive tract bleeding in adolescents can be managed hormonally, with the addition of hemostatic therapies when necessary.

As Virchow's triad suggests, a fine balance exists between the vascular wall, intravascular contents, and dynamic blood flow, such that a shift in this balance predisposes to thrombosis. Although thromboembolic events (TEs) are relatively infrequent in adolescents, the morbidity and mortality associated with TEs can be significant. Over the past 15 years, TEs and inherited and acquired thrombophilic conditions underlying them have become increasingly recognized in teens at risk, with combined hormonal contraception constituting one of the most significant of these risk factors.

Therefore, managing gynecologic problems in teens who have thrombophilic conditions can be challenging. It is important to have a clear understanding about safe options available to help address adolescent gynecologic concerns in this setting and to manage situations collaboratively with a hematologist.

The presence of endometrial glands and stroma outside the uterus, typically in the pelvis, is known as endometriosis. An adolescent with this diagnosis usually presents with chronic pelvic pain, and she and her family are anxious for an explanation of her symptoms. Traditionally, endometriosis had been thought to occur only rarely in adolescence, but with an increasing awareness of the disease among the medical community, it is being diagnosed more frequently. An outline of the disease and the issues surrounding its diagnosis and management in adolescents is the focus of this article.

Postscript: The following article is an addition to Colposcopy, Cervical Screening, and HPV, the December 2008 issue of *Obstetrics and Gynecology Clinics of North America* (Voume 35, Issue 4)

The relationship between cervical cancer and human papillomavirus (HPV) is well known. Like cervical cancer, anal cancer is preceded by a series of precancerous changes, raising the possibility that like cervical cancer, anal cancer can be prevented. Further, given the known risk factors for anal cancer, prevention efforts could be targeted to high-risk groups, providing a unique example of a screening program targeted to high-risk individuals. This article describes the epidemiology of anal HPV infection, anal intraepithelial neoplasia, and anal cancer among men and women, as well as current efforts to prevent anal cancers.

THE CLINICS ARE NOW AVAILABLE ONLINE!

Access your subscription at:
www.theclinics.com

Foreword

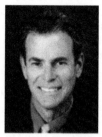

William F. Rayburn, MD, MBA
Consulting Editor

This issue pertaining to Pediatric and Adolescent Gynecology (PAG), edited by S. Paige Hertweck, MD, provides expert perspectives from a multidisciplinary team, many of whom helped define pediatric and adolescent gynecology as a specialty. An important clinical reference, this issue combines contemporary approaches to diagnoses with the latest management advice to address gynecologic problems in infants, children, and adolescents.

Gynecologic problems encountered in infants and children (genital trauma, intersex disorders, mullerian anomalies) are unique to these age groups and involve physician skills differing from those utilized for adults. Because of these unique circumstances, practicing obstetrician-gynecologists are often uncomfortable in evaluating and managing these children. For this reason, pediatric gynecology was created as a new specialty incorporating the expertise of gynecologists, pediatricians, urologists, pediatric surgeons, endocrinologists, and geneticists.

The American College of Obstetricians and Gynecologists recommends that the initial reproductive health visit to the obstetrician-gynecologist occurs as early as age 13. This initial visit would not include a pelvic examination unless indicated by the medical history. Instead, this encounter would provide an opportunity for the obstetrician-gynecologist to begin a physician-patient relationship, counsel patients and parents or guardians regarding health behaviors and dispel myths and fears. It also will assist an adolescent in building trust into the health care system when she has a specific need.

Health care of the adolescent female should include a review of normal menstruation, diet and exercise, healthy sexual decision-making, relationships, immunizations, and injury prevention. Preventive counseling is beneficial for parents, guardians, or other supportive adults, and can include discussions about physical, sexual, and emotional development; signs and symptoms of common conditions affecting adolescents; and encouragement of lifelong health choice behaviors.

This issue highlights differences between adolescents and adults about certain gynecologic disorders (endometriosis, polycystic ovarian syndrome, abnormal cervical cytology, menstrual disorders, contraception and intrauterine devices). Several articles cover topics emphasized by the American College of Obstetricians and Gynecologists

Obstet Gynecol Clin N Am 36 (2009) xiii–xiv
doi:10.1016/j.ogc.2009.01.002
0889-8545/09/$ – see front matter © 2009 Elsevier Inc. All rights reserved.

Committee on Adolescent Health Care. The risks of exposure to violence, substance use, sexually transmitted disease, and unintended pregnancy threaten the health and well-being of adolescents. Additional research is needed to determine the best care for adolescents, especially in defining optimal treatment. Unfortunately, there exists confusion about adolescents participating in research because of uncertainty about the need for parental permission and what constitutes appropriate protection as research subjects. We look to the distinguished group of contributors in this issue to carry this agenda forward.

William F. Rayburn, MD, MBA
Department of Obstetrics and Gynecology
University of New Mexico School of Medicine
MSC10 5580; 1 University of New Mexico
Albuquerque, NM 87131-0001, USA

E-mail address:
wrayburn@salud.unm.edu

Preface

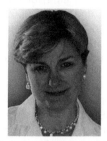

S. Paige Hertweck, MD
Guest Editor

Pediatric and adolescent gynecology (PAG) is a unique subspecialty of gynecology that encompasses reproductive healthcare of young women under the age of 22. The spectrum of conditions that a gynecologist may see present in young women between the newborn period and adolescence is wide and varied. Many conditions are an overlap between the fields of gynecology and pediatrics, pediatric endocrinology, hematology, urology, pediatric surgery, dermatology, psychiatry, public health medicine and genetics.

As past president of the North American Society for Pediatric and Adolescent Gynecology (NASPAG), I have had the opportunity to interact with PAG experts across the United States and Canada. This issue of *Obstetrics and Gynecology Clinics* provides a collection of PAG topics presented by some of those physicians who have been recognized as experts in each chosen area. These authors have been hand-selected based on their expertise, their history, and their ability to make a complex topic understandable by all health care providers.

I am pleased to begin this issue with a written summary of one of my favorite lectures given at NASPAG: *My PAG Photo Album* by Dr. Mary Anne Jamieson. In this article, Dr. Jamieson provides a wonderful visual overview of PAG cases with nuances and clinical "pearls" to assist the reader in providing the best treatment for the presenting condition. This should stir the readers' interest and enhance the reading of the rest of the issue.

In this issue, PAG issues addressed range from disorders of sexual development, including müllerian anomalies, to those of genital trauma and urologic conditions that may present to the gynecologist. A helpful and practical article, "The Adolescent Sexual Health Visit," begins the latter half of this issue, and like the articles on updates of polycystic ovarian syndrome and contraception in the adolescent, it has an overlap with public health issues facing teens and our society today. The issue closes with a look at hematologic conditions (both thrombophilias and bleeding disorders) that present to the gynecologist, and dysmenorrhea and endometriosis in the adolescent. Each author, as mentioned, was selected because of their expertise in their topic, and by reading their articles, you should glean practical information for those young women whom you encounter who have PAG conditions.

Obstet Gynecol Clin N Am 36 (2009) xv–xvi
doi:10.1016/j.ogc.2009.02.004
0889-8545/09/$ – see front matter © 2009 Elsevier Inc. All rights reserved.

obgyn.theclinics.com

Let me close with a thank you to Drs. Jamieson, Allen, Breech, Laufer, Yerkes, Merritt, Shafi, Burstein, Lara-Torre, Pfeifer, Kives, James, Dietrich, Yee, and Templeman for their timely adherence to a tight deadline to facilitate publication in time for the 2009 Annual Clinical Meeting of NASPAG in San Antonio, Texas, and for the 2009 Annual Clinical Meeting of the American College of Obstetricians and Gynecologists.

I would also like to acknowledge the noteworthy assistance of Carla Holloway whose kind persistence and patient but firm demeanor has kept us on track. She is a credit to her field. Thank you.

For those readers with further interest in PAG, please consider membership to the North American Society for Pediatric and Adolescent Gynecology (NASPAG) or attendance at one of NASPAG's annual meetings. The mission of NASPAG is to provide a forum for education, research, and communication among healthcare professionals who provide gynecologic care to children and adolescents. NASPAG is a small society of approximately 400 to 500 members making it a very collegial and interactive group. Membership includes a subscription to the *Journal for Pediatric and Adolescent Gynecology* and access to a list serve to assist you with the ability to ask experts for advice in the care of PAG patients.

I hope that you find this issue not only enjoyable, but helpful as you care for this unique type of gynecologic patient. We have a unique role as healthcare providers to this special population as their interaction with us is often their introduction to gynecology. A proper diagnosis, management, and positive interaction with us can empower these young women to take charge of their own healthcare and best care for themselves.

S. Paige Hertweck, MD
Department of Obstetrics and Gynecology
University of Louisville School of Medicine
550 South Jackson Street
Louisville, KY 40202, USA

E-mail address:
phertweck@louisville.edu

A Photo Album of Pediatric and Adolescent Gynecology

Mary Anne Jamieson, MD, FRCSC

KEYWORDS

- Images • Cases • Dysmenorrhea • Amenorrhea
- Vulvar diseases • Pelvic neoplasms • Pelvic mass
- Mullerian ducts • Pelvic pain

During the past decade as the sole pediatric and adolescent gynecology subspecialist in a tertiary care academic center, the author has had the privilege of caring for many patients with many problems, some common and some unique or challenging. Often these patients and their families have allowed the author to take photographs (protecting their anonymity) with the understanding that educating health care providers is an essential part of ensuring that other young girls who have similar conditions will receive the care that they need. This article presents a selection of images depicting pediatric and adolescent gynecologic conditions that, although not particularly common, present with a relatively common complaint such as dysmenorrhea, pelvic mass or pain, genital irritation, and amenorrhea. Health care providers who recognize the unusual underlying condition will save patients and their families days, weeks, or even years of misdiagnoses, frustration, fear, or even pain and suffering. When possible, references to useful publications/articles about the particular conditions are provided. Textbooks on pediatric and adolescent gynecology also devote full chapters to each of these four topics.[1–3]

DYSMENORRHEA

Most cases of dysmenorrhea in adolescents represent primary dysmenorrhea; that is, prostaglandin-mediated physiologic menstrual cramping associated with ovulatory cycles. Because perimenarchal girls are not always ovulatory, early menstrual cycles often are irregular and painless. Girls who do experience primary dysmenorrhea should get relief from properly administered non-steroidal anti-inflammatory drugs (NSAIDS), and for those who still suffer, the combined use of oral contraceptives and NSAIDS usually suffices. When these strategies fail, or when severe pain accompanies early cycles, other underlying conditions, such as obstructive Müllerian congenital anomalies (see the article by Breech in this issue), endometriosis (see

Pediatric & Adolescent Gynecology, Obstetrics & Gynecology (and Pediatrics), Queen's University, Victory 4, Kingston General Hospital, 76 Stuart Street, Kingston, Ontario, Canada
E-mail address: maj3@queensu.ca

the article by Templeman in this issue), constipation, and pelvic adhesions, should be considered.[4–18]

Case 1: Obstructed Non-Communicating Uterine Horn (Figs. 1A, 2)

A 12-year-old complained of predominantly right-sided dysmenorrhea beginning with menarche. She visited the emergency department with each of her first three menstrual cycles. A routine ultrasound did not identify any abnormality, but the MRI was classic for a non-communicating right-sided obstructed uterine horn adjacent to a normal left hemi-uterus with patent outflow tract. After excision of the non-communicating horn, the patient experienced only mild central dysmenorrhea that responded well to NSAIDS. Although this horn was removed by laparotomy, laparo-scopic excision is possible, depending on the junction and the surgeon's comfort and skill. Removal of the horn did leave a bed of myometrium on the left uterus that required layered closure. Although the recommendation is controversial, the patient was advised to discuss elective cesarean with any future obstetrics care provider (see Case 4 and references listed regarding myomectomy and future obstetric uterine rupture). (For a list of useful references, see the discussion of dysmenorrhea in the previous paragraph.)

Case 2: Obstructed Hemi-Vagina with Right Hematocolpos (Figs. 1B, 3–6)

A precoital 17-year-old girl did not experience dysmenorrhea until 3 years after she began menstruating. She was thought to have primary dysmenorrhea, but instead of improving with treatment with NSAIDS and an oral contraceptive pill, the problem seemed to be worsening. The patient began to notice intermenstrual

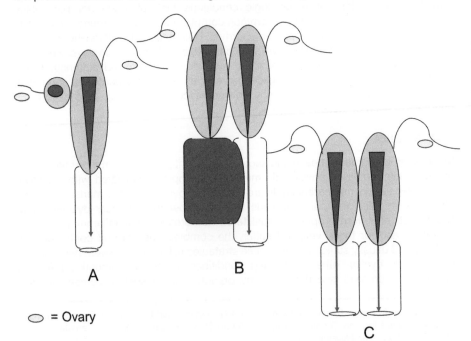

○ = Ovary

Fig. 1. (A) Noncommunicating R uterine horn (Case 1). (B) Obstructed R Hemivagina (Case 2)–often associated with Ipsilateral Renal Agenesis (OHVIRA). (C) Uterine Didelphys with complete longitudinal vaginal septum (Case 3).

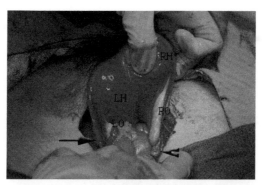

Fig. 2. (Case 1) Non-communicating right uterine horn (RH) with unobstructed left hemi-uterus (LH) with right and left ovaries (RO and LO, respectively) and normal left tube (*long arrow*) with attenuated hypoplastic right tube (*short arrow*) to fibria remnant.

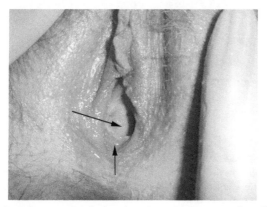

Fig. 3. (Case 2) Bulging obstructed right hemi-vagina with hematocolpos (*long arrow*). Short arrow indicates the hymen.

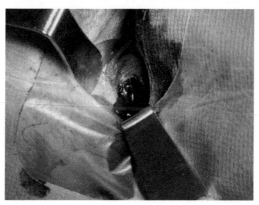

Fig. 4. (Case 2) Evacuation of clotted hematocolpos from obstructed right-sided hemi-vagina.

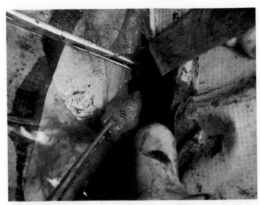

Fig. 5. (Case 2) Septum (*S*) excision in progress.

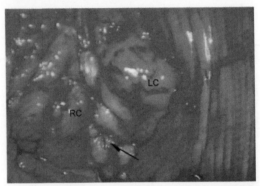

Fig. 6. (Case 2) Two cervices (left, LC, and right, RC) at the apex of the vagina. Often at least one cervix looks a little atypical. Note the excision suture line (*arrow*) is taken up as high as possible between the two cervices.

pelvic pressure and new-onset difficulty with tampon insertion. Although an MRI was performed, the pelvic ultrasound (done transabdominally) and gentle single-digit vaginal examination were enough to make the diagnosis of non-communicating right-sided hemi-vagina. The vagina has a capacity to expand with the slow accumulation of menstrual blood, and symptoms and therefore diagnosis can be delayed several months to a couple of years. Especially because the left side of this uterine didelphys and duplicated vagina are not obstructed, early menstrual cycles can seem quite normal. The vaginal septum was excised in the operating room under regional or general anesthetic (**Figs. 3–6**), and every effort was made to wedge out the base to avoid leaving a ridge of uncomfortable remnant. The lines of excision need to be oversewn with absorbable suture in a hemostatic fashion. After this outpatient procedure the patient had no menstrual or coital complaints, and a single tampon sufficed. (For a list of useful references, see the earlier discussion of dysmenorrhea.)

Case 3: Uterine Didelphys with Complete Longitudinal Vaginal Septum (Figs. 1C, 7)

In contrast to the patient in Case 2, the patient shown in **Fig. 7** has a complete longitudinal vaginal septum and must wear a tampon in both sides unless she chooses to

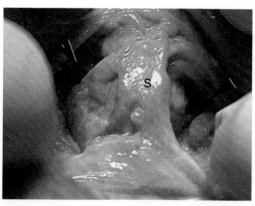

Fig. 7. (Case 3) Introital image of complete longitudinal vaginal septum (*S*) with right and left vaginas identified by arrows.

have the septum removed (performed in the same fashion as that described in Case 2). Patients who have this condition can have obstructed hemi-vagina and ipsilateral renal anomaly (OHVIRA) syndrome.[13]

Patients who have a complete longitudinal vaginal septum most often have duplication of their Müllerian anatomy. Unless they have some type obstruction of menstrual outflow at the uterine/cervix level, they experience only primary dysmenorrhea. They may be asymptomatic or may present with perceived tampon overflow, perceived menorrhagia, difficulty with tampon insertion, or difficulty with intercourse. Sometimes they present to the emergency department after intercourse has resulted in tearing of the septum, which can bleed quite briskly and require urgent surgical repair (or removal). It often takes an astute clinician to find the septum during the gynecologic examination, but for patients in whom Pap smears and cervix swabs are indicated, both cervices need to be sampled. This particular patient had two separate Müllerian systems and had a total of two pregnancies, one in each horn. Each uterus will have an ipsilateral fallopian tube and ovary. (For a list of useful references, see the earlier discussion of dysmenorrhea.)

Case 4: Leiomyoma (Rare in This Age Group) (Figs. 8, 9)

A precoital 15-year-old presented with worsening dysmenorrhea that did not respond to standard medical therapies. A single-digit gynecologic examination was limited, and a rectal examination was "normal." The transabdominal pelvic ultrasound identified an isolated 4- to 5-cm intramural fibroid, but in her age group this finding was completely unexpected. After the myomectomy menstrual cycles were much more tolerable. This surgery was performed by laparotomy, based on surgeon's comfort and skill, with meticulous hemostasis, layered closure, and minimal use of cautery. Some surgeons would have chosen a laparoscopic approach. Although the recommendation is controversial, the patient was advised that future childbirth probably should be by elective cesarean section. The medical literature has several case reports and case series regarding laparoscopic myomectomy and the risk of uterine rupture during subsequent pregnancies. The reported rates of rupture are low, but they tend to be rates of prelabor uterine rupture, because many patients in the series do undergo elective cesarean section.[19–29]

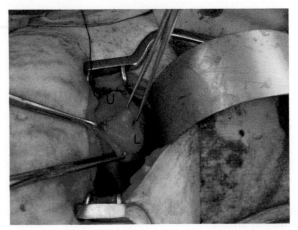

Fig. 8. (Case 4) Open myomectomy in 15-year-old girl. L, leiomyoma; U, uterus.

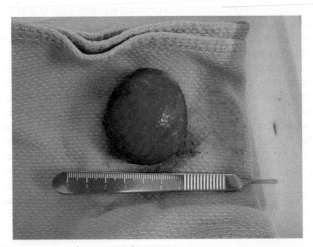

Fig. 9. (Case 4) Leiomyoma after removal.

PELVIC MASS/PAIN

Children and teenaged girls can present with abdominal pain and abdominal masses **(Fig. 10)**. Ovarian masses are relatively common in this context, and the differential diagnosis of an ovarian mass is quite broad. Most often, in this age group, the ovarian mass represents a functional ovarian cyst (with our without hemorrhage), benign teratoma, cystadenoma, or even an unrecognized pregnancy; malignancy is far less common.[30–34] When surgery is necessary, laparoscopy should be considered, and efforts should be made to salvage/preserve ovarian tissue, even when the mass is quite large (assuming that it is benign). The following two cases were chosen because the first represents a relatively common cause of ovarian enlargement/mass/pain, and the second is far rarer. They can be difficult to distinguish, but the treatment is different.

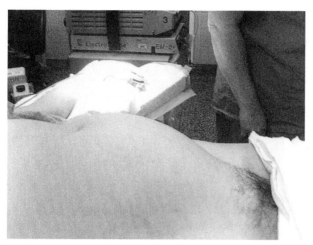

Fig. 10. Abdomen distended by ovarian dermoid in an adolescent.

Case 5: Benign Dermoid (Teratoma) (Figs. 11–14)

A peripubertal girl presented with an abdominal mass and worsening pain. An ultrasound reported a large "complex" mass arising out of the pelvis. One ovary was identified, but the other was not. Although removal of small dermoids is controversial, and the surgical approach to large dermoids (laparoscopy versus laparotomy) is similarly controversial, this patient was taken to laparotomy for dermoid cystectomy. She did, in fact, have ovarian torsion as well (**Fig. 11**). The pedicle was untwisted, and the ovarian tissue surrounding the mass and the ipsilateral fallopian tube were preserved (**Fig. 12**). The ovarian bed was closed in layers with a final result similar to the image in **Fig. 13**.[35] **Fig. 14** depicts typical contents of a benign ovarian teratoma, including skin, hair, and a tooth.

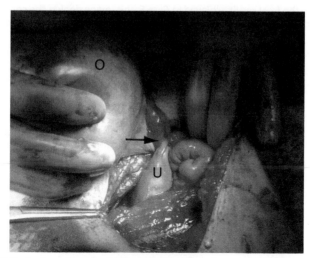

Fig. 11. (Case 5) Peripubertal child with large left ovarian dermoid (O) at laparotomy. Uterus (U) and torted ovarian pedicle and fallopian tube (*arrow*).

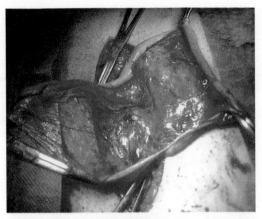

Fig. 12. (Case 5) Ovarian cystectomy salvaging ovarian cortex in progress.

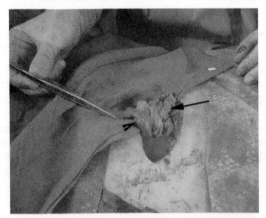

Fig. 13. Similar to the final result achieved in Case 5, this image depicts the completion of the ovarian cortex preservation. Closure was performed in layers (*long arrow*). Short arrow indicates Fallopian tube.

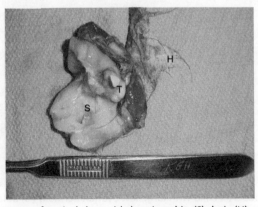

Fig. 14. (Case 5) Contents of typical dermoid showing skin (S), hair (H), and a tooth (T).

Case 6: Massive Ovarian Edema (Fig. 15)

A perimenarchal 11-year-old presented with abdominal pain, but she was overweight and, in the office, no mass was appreciated. The ultrasound reported a solid-appearing mass arising out of the pelvis. Only one distinct ovary could be identified, and the impression was that the mass represented some type of atypical ovarian neoplasm/tumor. Under that assumption the patient was taken to laparotomy. Tumor markers (alpha fetoprotein, lactate dehydrogenase, human chorionic gonadotropin) were all negative.[31,32] When a linear incision was made in the outer layer of this ovarian mass and no distinct inner cyst or tumor could be identified, a small wedge excision was made, and tissue was sent for frozen section. The report was of very edematous but otherwise normal ovarian stroma. There was no sign of torsion. The other ovary was entirely normal. The ovarian defect was closed, and the "massive ovary" was returned to the pelvis. The child was followed, and within 6 weeks an ultrasound revealed entirely normal ovaries bilaterally. A review the medical literature found several publications describing massive ovarian edema.[36–44] Although some have postulated intermitted torsion with only lymphatic and venous (not arterial) obstruction, no definite cause or etiology is known. The treatment, however, is conservative, and efforts should be made to avoid the natural instinct to remove the gonad. This patient did have irregular and subjectively heavy menstrual periods and was given a combined contraceptive pill postoperatively. Whether the relative ovarian suppression aided in the regression of the edema is unclear.

GENITAL IRRITATION

Genital irritation from contact irritants/allergens, agglutination, infections, dermopathy, and other causes is quite common in childhood and adolescence. The following cases depict less common causes of genital pain or irritation. For a review of vulvovaginal irritation in childhood, the reader can refer to any of the pediatric and adolescent gynecology texts listed at the beginning of this article. (Although *Candida* is a common cause of vulvovaginitis in women of reproductive age, it does not tend to be the culprit for genital irritation in children. There are exceptions, such as children who have diabetes, who are immunocompromised, who have been treated recently with antibiotics, or who are in diapers. Topical antifungals can cause further irritation to the child's vulnerable genital skin.)[45,46]

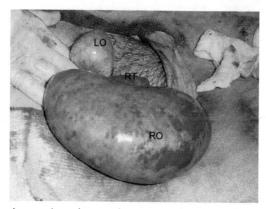

Fig. 15. (Case 6) Massive ovarian edema at laparotomy showing right ovary (RO), right tube (RT), and left ovary (LO).

Case 7: Labial Hypertrophy (Figs. 16A, 16B. See also Case 13 Figs. 23, 24)

In North America today, gynecologists and plastic surgeons are seeing more and more young females concerned about and dissatisfied with the appearance of their external genitalia and in particular with the size of their labia minora. The natural history is for the labia minora to enlarge and become more pigmented at puberty. There is quite a large variation of normal size. In a small number of cases, this process is extreme, and the redundant skin tends to trap secretions and cause pruritus or soreness. The skin can be problematic in certain athletic activities, tampon insertion, intercourse, and in wearing some styles of clothing. The indications for labial reduction are controversial, but when deemed necessary the procedure involves either simple linear excision with oversewing of the cut edge (**Fig. 16**Aii), or segmental excision and a pull-down swing repair (**Figs. 16**Ai, **16**B). With the latter technique, it is extremely

A   Labial Hypertrophy (Case #7)
     Surgical techniques (schematics)

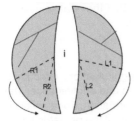
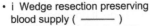
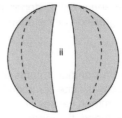

- i Wedge resection preserving blood supply (————)
- Edge 1 reapproximated with edge 2 sewing medial surfaces and lateral surfaces separately

- ii Redundant Edges trimmed oversewing cut edge (- - - - ·) in a hemostatic fashion

B

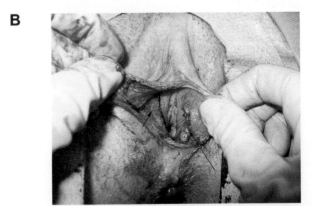

Fig. 16. (Case 7) (*A*) Schematics showing labial hypertrophy surgical techniques. (*B*) Planned right-sided V-shaped wedge excision for surgical management of symptomatic labial hypertrophy (*short arrow*) and completed left-sided medial suture line (*long arrow*). (Note: **Figs. 23** and **24** depict unilateral labial hypertrophy in conjunction with imperforate hymen.)

important to retain the blood supply by transilluminating a section before removal and also to reapproximate medial surface to medial surface and lateral surface to lateral surface with good hemostasis of the labial core tissue.[47] If the closure imbricates the outer labial surfaces, the repair will not take. (Note: In Case 13, **Figs. 23, 24** depict unilateral right-sided labial hypertrophy in a peripubertal, premenarchal patient. This patient also had an imperforate hymen, but since becoming menstrual and as puberty has progressed, she has become more symptomatic from the redundant labial tissue. Labial reduction is being deferred until pubertal labial growth is complete, presumably after Tanner 5 thelarche/pubarche.)

Case 8: Vaginal Foreign Body (Figs. 17, 18)

This child's presenting complaint was of vulvar burning with associated vulvar excoriation (**Fig. 17**). Upon questioning, there had in fact been foul-smelling vaginal discharge for the past 4 months. Well-intentioned but somewhat misguided health care providers had prescribed repeated courses of topical antifungals. The child also had been given a single course of a broad-spectrum antibiotic and, although the discharge did improve during the course of therapy, it returned quickly thereafter. There was no history to support victimization. The child did undergo an office vaginal lavage using a pediatric feeding tube and warm saline, but nothing was retrieved. She gave no history of inserting anything into her vagina, and an index finger rectal examination was negative. The child was taken for examination under anesthetic, and an old fragment that was assumed to be paper towel was removed (**Fig. 18**). All her symptoms resolved very quickly.

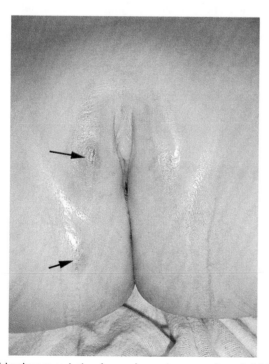

Fig. 17. (Case 8) Mild vulvar excoriation (*arrows*) seen in a prepubertal child who had genital burning and foul-smelling vaginal discharge refractive to conservative strategies.

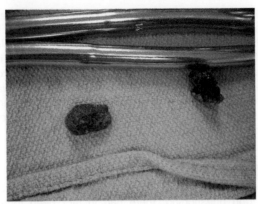

Fig. 18. (Case 8) Old fragment of presumed paper towel retrieved from the vagina of the child pictured in **Fig. 17.**

Case 9: Psoriasis of the Vulva (Fig. 19)

A prepubertal child complained of chronic external vulvar itching. Good vulvar hygiene with daily soaks, avoidance of irritants, and other conservative measures had been instituted, but the problem persisted. Again, antifungals were of no benefit. A trial of over-the-counter, low-potency corticosteroid had reduced the symptoms, but treatment was sporadic. Although the child would not agree to a photograph of the vulva, she gladly agreed to this anonymous photograph of the skin lesion behind her ear, which was instrumental in making the diagnosis of vulvar psoriasis. The vulvar dermopathy was not quite as obvious, with less marked scaling and a shinier appearance, but upon close examination there was patchy texturing to the labia majora. Higher-potency corticosteroid tapered to a lower-potency product for maintenance, along with bland emollients, has eliminated her symptoms. Werlinger's[48] review article and Casey's[45] textbook chapter provide more information on vulvar psoriasis and other dermatologic conditions.

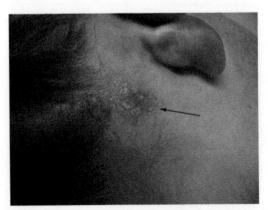

Fig. 19. (Case 9) Psoriasis discovered during assessment of child who had chronic vulvar pruritus who ultimately was found to have vulvar psoriasis.

GENITAL ULCERS

Genital ulcers in children and teens tend to cause a great deal of anxiety among the patients, their families, and the health care providers who are called upon to assess, diagnose, and treat the condition. Certainly Herpes simplex type I and II come to mind, as do other sexually transmitted infections (eg, chancroid) and autoimmune conditions (eg, Behcet's disease).[49–55] The following three cases depict ulcers caused by vulvar apthosis, Varicella, and Crohn's disease.

Case 10: Vulvar Apthosis (Fig. 20)

In recent years a nonspecific, non–sexually transmitted condition referred to as "vulvar apthosis" has been reported in children and teens. This condition probably represents a condition reported almost a century ago and referred to as "Lipchutz ulcers." A variety of viral infections have been blamed, such as Epstein-Barr virus, Cytomegalovirus, and influenza A. This peripubertal child presented with extreme genital pain, vulvar ulcers with associated edema, and erythema of the labia minora (**Fig. 20**). She was premenarchal, precoital, and there was no history of victimization. The outbreak was preceded by fever and malaise. The ulcers lasted 2 to 3 weeks, and the severe pain was present for the first 10 to 14 days. She was treated with analgesics, topical xylocaine jelly, and regular tub soaks. Initially ice packs were soothing and were thought to reduce swelling. Urinary retention was avoided by having the patient void while soaking in warm water. Despite the look of cellulitis, antibiotics were not used in this particular patient. It remains to be seen whether antivirals or corticosteroids will prove helpful, because current reports of their use are anecdotal and case based.[49–51,54–57]

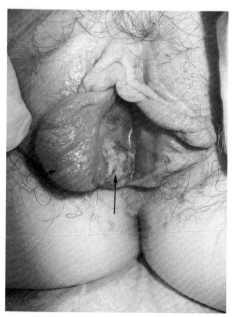

Fig. 20. (Case 10) Vulvar apthosis of about 5 days' duration showing early eschar (*long arrow*) associated labial edema and erythema (*short arrow*).

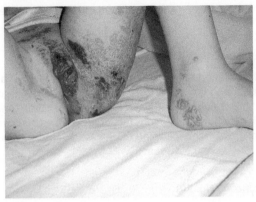

Fig. 21. (Case 11) Varicella zoster infection in an 8-year-old girl who had no history of chicken pox. Note the left-sided dermatome distribution.

Case 11: Vulvar Varicella (Fig. 21)

An 8-year-old girl presented with a 5-day history of increasing pain and pruritus involving her left vulva, buttock, and lower left limb. Her symptoms were accompanied by fever, lethargy, and decreased appetite. Examination revealed a vesiculobulbous rash in the left-sided vulvar and sacral dermatomes. A diagnosis of Herpes zoster/ shingles was made.

She was treated with intravenous antivirals, analgesics, and local care strategies (as described earlier in Case 10) and was well enough for discharge 4 days later. History revealed that the patient had never had chicken pox, but her mother had had primary chicken pox at 36 weeks during the pregnancy. Although Herpes zoster infections are well known, and management, as for recurrent Herpes simplex, is well described, the medical literature contains little information summarizing strategies for treating children who have such a severe case of genital zoster.[52,53,58–60]

Case 12: Crohn's Disease Fistula (Fig. 22)

An 18-year-old had been unwell for more than 3 years. She had had biopsy-proven classic ulcerative colitis and had undergone colectomy. She did have

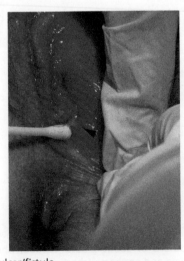

Fig. 22. (Case 12) Crohn's ulcer/fistula.

a rectal stump, and re-anastomosis was planned in the future. Unfortunately, she continued to suffer intermittent abdominal pain and weight loss despite the colectomy and presented with a painful introital swelling that initially resembled a Bartholin's abscess. The abscess began to drain spontaneously, and the site became more ulcerated. She has subsequently been diagnosed with a Crohn's rectovaginal (introital) fistula. Crohn's disease is a recognized cause of genital ulcers and fistulas. The management of these fistulas usually involves antibiotics, immunomodulators, and biologic agents before consideration of conservative surgical repair.[61–64]

Case 13: Imperforate Hymen (Figs. 23–25)

Although imperforate hymen is not usually a cause of genital irritation, it can present with the sensation of a vulvar or introital uncomfortable pressure or bulge (**Fig. 23**). If the condition is not identified with a mini-genital examination during the newborn or childhood period, teens tend to present with the symptoms of mucocolpos or hematocolpos (ie, pelvic pressure or pain, an abdominal mass, or urinary retention). In this case, an astute clinician noticed that the girl had begun puberty but had not experienced her first menstrual bleed. Hymenotomy was performed in the operating room under anesthetic. This patient presented in urinary retention because of a very large liquefied mucocolpos (**Fig. 24**), but old menstrual blood is found more often. **Fig. 25** depicts completion of the hymenal resection. As mentioned in the discussion of Case 7, this patient had unilateral right-sided labial hypertrophy.

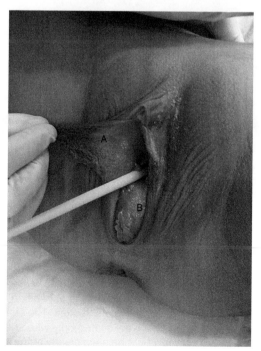

Fig. 23. (Case 13) (A) Right labial hypertrophy and (B) imperforate hymen.

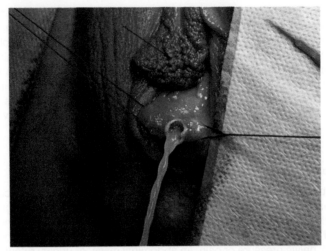

Fig. 24. (Case 13) Draining liquefied mucocolpos. Stay sutures on imperforate hymen. Hypertrophied right labia minora (*arrow*).

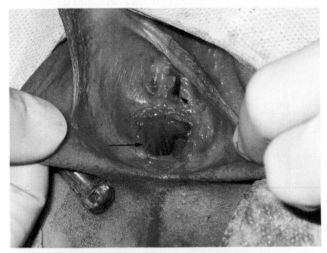

Fig. 25. (Case 13) After hymenotomy with excision of imperforate hymen, leaving a square-shaped rim and oversewing the edge with absorbable suture for hemostasis (*long arrow*). Short arrow indicates urethral meatus.

AMENORRHEA
Case 14: Acquired Colpoclesis (Fig. 26)

Unfortunately, an 16-year-old female who had factitious disorder and self-harm demonstrated escalating behaviors and douched her vagina with a bathroom cleaning product.[65,66] Because of her mental illness, she was treated as an inpatient with daily vaginal irrigation, estrogen vaginal cream, and a soft stent. The entire vaginal mucosa sloughed, and she was discharged (2–3 weeks later) only when new, healthy vaginal surfaces were present and the cervix could be seen clearly at the apex of the vagina. Unfortunately she did the same thing within 24 hours of discharge and ultimately had

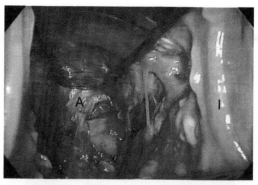

Fig. 26. (Case 14) Caustic vaginal douche injury with sloughing of vaginal mucosa. A, apex; I, introitus.

a complete mid-vaginal colpoclesis similar to that performed in patients who have graft-versus-host disease of the vagina.[67] This patient was a type I diabetic and died at age 18 years.

Case 15: Complete Androgen Insensitivity (Figs. 27, 28; Table 1)

A 16-year-old presented with primary amenorrhea. She gave no history to suggest an endocrinopathy and gave no history of lower abdominal pain. She claimed that secondary sexual characteristics had occurred normally, and she admitted to past intercourse. The physical examination revealed a female with a height of 5'8" and a weight of 200 pounds with Tanner 5 breasts (**Fig. 27**). Surprisingly, she had no pubic hair and no axillary hair. When asked, she claimed to shave, but later recanted this statement. The labia majora and minora were normal bilaterally, and the urethral meatus was at 12 o'clock in the vestibule under a very normal appearing "clitoris" (**Fig. 28**). Palpation of the inguinal areas was negative; no masses were present. There was a distensible vaginal pouch with no sign of genital ambiguity, but no cervix and no uterus were present on either speculum examination or bimanual examination. A presumptive diagnosis of complete androgen insensitivity was made. As expected, her genotype was 46XY, and her testosterone level was in the normal male range.

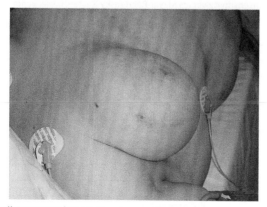

Fig. 27. (Case 15) Full Tanner V breast development.

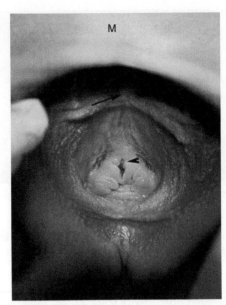

Fig. 28. (Case 15) Introitus of a patient who had complete androgen insensitivity. Note mons with no pubic hair (M), no sign of clitoromegaly (*large arrow*), and normal female positioning of urethral meatus (*small arrow*).

Several visits took place thereafter to educate both the patient and her family about her condition and the implications. Ultimately full disclosure took place. She was offered counseling for the emotional, sexual, and psychologic ramifications and was educated about the fertility/reproductive implications. She underwent laparoscopic bilateral gonadectomy and, at least for a while, took exogenous estrogen therapy. The patient was seen informally approximately 5 years later. She was married, comfortably coital, and planned to adopt a child. She seemed quite well adjusted.[68–78] **Table 1** presents a very basic comparison of complete androgen insensitivity and Mayer-Rokitansky-Kuster-Hauser syndrome (presented in Case 16), two

Table 1
Complete androgen insensitivity versus Mayer-Rokitansky-Kuster-Hauser syndrome

Feature	Complete Androgen Insensitivity	Mayer-Rokitansky-Kuster-Hauser Syndrome
Thelarche	Tanner 5	Tanner 5
Pubarche	Tanner 1	Tanner 5
Vagina (dilator or vaginoplasty)	Blind pouch or absent (often)	Absent (often)
Uterus	Absent	Variable
Gonads (gonadectomy)	Testes – Leydig cell replete Sertoli-cell only (yes, after puberty)	Normal ovaries (No)
Testosterone level	Normal male	Normal female
Karyotype	46XY	46XX
Associated anomalies	No	Yes: vertebral/renal
Fertility implications	No childbearing	Egg retrieval with surrogate

conditions with absent vagina and no genital ambiguity. (See also the article in this issue by Allen on intersex disorders.)

Case 16: (Utero) Vaginal Agenesis: Mayer-Rokitansky-Kuster-Hauser Syndrome (Figs. 29–31)

A 16-year-old presented with primary amenorrhea. She was a figure skater, and she, her family, and her health care provider always had thought she had an element of hypothalamic delay. On the other hand, she had full pubertal development but no first menses. She did describe a monthly 1- to 2-day episode of mild to moderate pelvic pain, usually but not always left-sided. Upon examination, no vagina could be identified. The introital skin appeared relatively normal, and there was an element of distensibility to that area, although she had never attempted intercourse (**Figs. 29, 30**). Neither a rectal examination nor an ultrasound revealed a uterus, but an MRI identified bilateral small masses along each pelvic sidewall just below the pelvic brim, consistent with "rudimentary" uterine horns. Ovaries also were identified in the same vicinity.

Although mittleschmertz ovulatory pain was considered a possible cause for her pain, a 3-month course of cyclic oral contraceptives precipitated the pain reproducibly during the pill-free interval. Therefore, despite the rudimentary appearance of the horns on MRI, the patient underwent laparoscopic bilateral uterine horn removal, under the assumption that one or both might harbor endometrium and that the monthly pain was a consequence of cryptomenorrhea (**Fig. 31**). A small nidus of endometrium was identified on histopathology of the left horn but not the right. She did experience minimal premenstrual syndrome molimina and occasional ovulatory pain but had no further episodes of the presumed cryptomenorrhea. The ovarian cyst seen in these pictures was not identified during the earlier imaging; therefore it was assumed to be functional and was expected to involute. It was left in situ.

The patient was diagnosed as having Mayer-Rokitansky-Kuster-Hauser syndrome. She was educated, counseled, and her renal/vertebral systems were imaged. She was instructed on the use of vaginal dilators and ultimately became coital. A very normal-appearing and functional vagina was the end result. Unfortunately, a couple years later she experienced torsion of the right ovary, and the diagnosis was missed. The ovary became completely infarcted and since has been removed laparoscopically. Ovarian

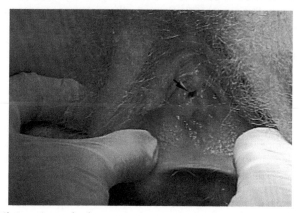

Fig. 29. (Case 16) A patient who has vaginal agenesis. Arrow indicates urethral meatus.

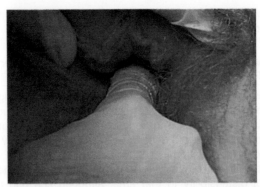

Fig. 30. (Case 16) Distensible "introitus" in a patient who has vaginal agenesis. Dilator therapy would involve a similar maneuver.

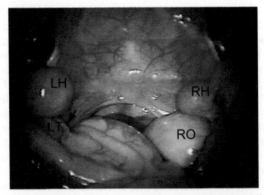

Fig. 31. (Case 16) Pelvis in a patient who has vaginal agenesis showing bilateral non-communicating horns (and right ovarian cyst). The normal left ovary (*arrow*) is only partially visible. LH, left horn; LT, left fallopian tube; RH, right horn; RO, right ovary with cyst; RT, right fallopian tube.

torsion has been reported in patients who have vaginal agenesis (see the article by Breech elsewhere in this issue).[79–82] Several other references on anomalies of the reproductive tract are listed in the discussion of dysmenorrhea early in this article, and **Table 1** presents a very basic comparison of complete androgen insensitivity and Mayer-Rokitansky-Kuster-Hauser syndrome as two conditions with absent vagina.

SUMMARY

Although dysmenorrhea, pelvic mass/pain, genital irritation, and amenorrhea are relatively common complaints, the astute clinician needs a broad differential diagnosis to avoid missing uncommon underlying etiologies such as: Müllerian anomalies and cryptomenorrhea, ovarian teratomas and torsion, labial hypertrophy, vaginal foreign bodies, dermopathies, genital ulcers, imperforate hymen, and the absent vagina. The author hopes that these images will assist health care providers, their students, and their patients.

REFERENCES

1. Carpenter SEK, Rock JA. Pediatric and Adolescent Gynecology. 2nd edition. Philadelphia: Lippincott Williams & Wilkins; 2000.
2. Emans SJH, Laufer MR, Goldstein DP. Pediatric and Adolescent Gynecology. 5th edition. Philadelphia: Lippincott Williams and Wilkins; 2005.
3. Sanfilippo JS, Lara-Torre E, Edmonds K, et al. Clinical Pediatric and Adolescent Gynecology. 1st edition. New York: Informa Healthcare; 2009.
4. Harel Z. Dysmenorrhea in adolescents and young adults: etiology and management. J Pediatr Adolesc Gynecol 2006;19:363–71.
5. Song AH, Advincula AP. Adolescent chronic pelvic pain. J Pediatr Adolesc Gynecol 2005;18:371–7.
6. Spence JE. Vaginal and uterine anomalies in the pediatric and adolescent patient. J Pediatr Adolesc Gynecol 1998;11:3–11.
7. Shulman LP. Müllerian anomalies. Clin Obstet Gynecol 2008;51:214–22.
8. Scarsbrook AF, Moore NR. MRI appearances of Müllerian duct abnormalities. Clin Radiol 2003;58:747–54.
9. Burgis J. Obstructive Müllerian anomalies: case report, diagnosis, and management. Am J Obstet Gynecol 2001;185:338–44 [see comment].
10. Gell JS. Müllerian anomalies. Semin Reprod Med 2003;21:375–88.
11. Steinkampf MP, Manning MT, Dharia S, et al. An accessory uterine cavity as a cause of pelvic pain. Obstet Gynecol 2004;103:1058–61.
12. Laufer MR, Goitein L, Bush M, et al. Prevalence of endometriosis in adolescent girls with chronic pelvic pain not responding to conventional therapy. J Pediatr Adolesc Gynecol 1997;10:199–202.
13. Smith NA, Laufer MR. Obstructed hemivagina and ipsilateral renal anomaly (OHVIRA) syndrome: management and follow-up. Fertil Steril 2007;87:918–22.
14. Breech LL, Laufer MR. Developmental abnormalities of the female reproductive tract. Curr Opin Obstet Gynecol 1999;11:441–50.
15. Breech LL, Laufer MR. Obstructive anomalies of the female reproductive tract. J Reprod Med 1999;44:233–40.
16. Troiano RN. Magnetic resonance imaging of Müllerian duct anomalies of the uterus. Top Magn Reson Imaging 2003;14:269–79 [see comment].
17. Troiano RN, McCarthy SM. Mullerian duct anomalies: imaging and clinical issues. Radiology 2004;233:19–34.
18. Jayasinghe Y, Rane A, Stalewski H, et al. The presentation and early diagnosis of the rudimentary uterine horn. Obstet Gynecol 2005;105:1456–67.
19. Hurst BS, Matthews ML, Marshburn PB. Laparoscopic myomectomy for symptomatic uterine myomas. Fertil Steril 2005;83:1–23 [see comment].
20. Kelly BA, Bright P, Mackenzie IZ. Does the surgical approach used for myomectomy influence the morbidity in subsequent pregnancy? J Obstet Gynaecol 2008;28:77–81.
21. Paul PG, Koshy AK, Thomas T. Pregnancy outcomes following laparoscopic myomectomy and single-layer myometrial closure. Humanit Rep 2006;21:3278–81.
22. Saridogan E, Cutner A. Endoscopic management of uterine fibroids. Hum Fertil (Camb) 2006;9:201–8.
23. Seracchioli R, Manuzzi L, Vianello F, et al. Obstetric and delivery outcome of pregnancies achieved after laparoscopic myomectomy. Fertil Steril 2006;86:159–65.
24. Sizzi O, Rossetti A, Malzoni M, et al. Italian multicenter study on complications of laparoscopic myomectomy. J Minim Invasive Gynecol 2007;14:453–62.
25. Altgassen C, Kuss S, Berger U, et al. Complications in laparoscopic myomectomy. Surg Endosc 2006;20:614–8.

26. Diesen DL, Price TM, Skinner MA. Uterine leiomyoma in a 14-year-old girl. Eur J Pediatr Surg 2008;18:53–5.
27. Grapsa D, Smymiotis V, Hasiakos D, et al. A giant uterine leiomyoma simulating an ovarian mass in a 16-year-old girl: a case report and review of the literature. Eur J Gynaecol Oncol 2006;27:294–6.
28. Leidi L, Brusati M, Vespa MG. A treacherous scar. Am J Obstet Gynecol 2007; 197:553.e1–2.
29. Lieng M, Istre O, Langebrekke A. Uterine rupture after laparoscopic myomectomy. J Am Assoc Gynecol Laparosc 2004;11:92–3.
30. Brandt ML, Helmrath MA. Ovarian cysts in infants and children. Semin Pediatr Surg 2005;14:78–85.
31. de Silva KS, Kanumakala S, Grover SR, et al. Ovarian lesions in children and adolescents—an 11-year review. J Pediatr Endocrinol 2004;17:951–7.
32. Stepanian M, Cohn DE. Gynecologic malignancies in adolescents. Adolesc Med Clin 2004;15:549–68.
33. Templeman CL, Fallat ME. Benign ovarian masses. Semin Pediatr Surg 2005;14: 93–9.
34. Stankovic ZB, Djukic MK, Sedlecki K, et al. Rapidly growing bilateral ovarian cystadenoma in a 6-year-old girl: case report and literature review. J Pediatr Adolesc Gynecol 2006;19:35–8.
35. Reddy J, Laufer MR. Advantage of conservative surgical management of large ovarian neoplasms in adolescents. Fertil Steril 2008.
36. Bildirici K, Kabukcuoglu S, Ozalp SS, et al. Massive ovarian edema: a case report. Eur J Gynaecol Oncol 2004;25:512–4.
37. Chaturvedi R, Lal N. Massive ovarian edema—a diagnostic dilemma: a case report. Indian J Pathol Microbiol 2007;50:578–80.
38. Friedrich M, Ertan AK, Axt-Fliedner R, et al. Unilateral massive ovarian edema (MOE): a case report. Clin Exp Obstet Gynecol 2002;29:65–6.
39. Geist RR, Rabinowitz R, Zuckerman B, et al. Massive edema of the ovary: a case report and review of the pertinent literature. J Pediatr Adolesc Gynecol 2005;18: 281–4.
40. Heiss KF, Zwiren GT, Winn K. Massive ovarian edema in the pediatric patient: a rare solid tumor. J Pediatr Surg 1994;29:1392–4.
41. Kallipolitis G, Sklia E, Milingos S, et al. Laparoscopic treatment of massive ovarian edema. J Am Assoc Gynecol Laparosc 1999;6:513–6.
42. Roberts CL, Weston MJ. Bilateral massive ovarian edema: a case report. Ultrasound Obstet Gynecol 1998;11:65–7.
43. Umesaki N, Tanaka T, Miyama M, et al. Sonographic characteristics of massive ovarian edema. Ultrasound Obstet Gynecol 2000;16:479–81.
44. Umesaki N, Tanaka T, Miyama M, et al. Successful preoperative diagnosis of massive ovarian edema aided by comparative imaging study using magnetic resonance and ultrasound. Eur J Obstet Gynecol Reprod Biol 2000;89:97–9.
45. Casey AS, Pothiawala G, Gehris RP. Basic dermatology in children and adolescents. In: Sanfilippo JS, Lara-Torre E, Edmonds K, et al, editors. Clinical pediatric and adolescent gynecology. New York: Informa Healthcare; 2009. p. 154–76.
46. Jamieson MA. Vaginal discharge and genital bleeding in childhood. In: Sanfilippo JS, Lara-Torre E, Edmonds K, et al, editors. Clinical pediatric and adolescent gynecology. New York: Informa Healthcare; 2009. p. 140–53.
47. Laufer MR, Galvin WJ. Labial hypertrophy: a new surgical approach. Adolesc Pediatr Gynecol 1995;8:39–41.

48. Werlinger KD, Cockerell CJ. Vulvar disease update. Adv Dermatol 2006;22:91–100.

49. Bills G, Kaufman RH, Bornstein J, et al. Clinical question: ask the experts. Recurring painful vulvar ulcers. J Low Genit Tract Dis 2005;9:55–8.

50. Bohl TG. Vulvar ulcers and erosions—a dermatologist's viewpoint. Dermatol Ther 2004;17:55–67.

51. Cheng SX, Chapman MS, Margesson LJ, et al. Genital ulcers caused by Epstein-Barr virus. J Am Acad Dermatol 2004;51:824–6.

52. Juel-Jensen BE. Herpes simplex and zoster. Br Med J 1973;1:406–10.

53. Lautenschlager S. [Herpes simplex and varicella zoster virus infections]. Ther Umsch 2003;60:605–14 [In German].

54. Trager JD. Recurrent oral and vulvar ulcers in a fifteen-year-old girl. J Pediatr Adolesc Gynecol 2004;17:397–401.

55. Wetter DA, Bruce AJ, MacLaughlin KL, et al. Ulcus vulvae acutum in a 13-year-old girl after influenza A infection. Skinmed 2008;7:95–8.

56. Hernandez-Nunez A, Cordoba S, Romero-Mate A, et al. Lipchutz ulcers—four cases. Pediatr Dermatol 2008;25:364–7.

57. Huppert JS, Gerber MA, Deitch HR, et al. Vulvar ulcers in young females: a manifestation of aphthosis. J Pediatr Adolesc Gynecol 2006;19:195–204.

58. Brown D. Herpes zoster of the vulva. Clin Obstet Gynecol 1972;15:1010–4.

59. Moomaw MD, Cornea P, Rathbun RC, et al. Review of antiviral therapy for herpes labialis, genital herpes and herpes zoster. Expert Rev Anti Infect Ther 2003;1:283–95.

60. Wu JJ, Brentjens MH, Torres G, et al. Valacyclovir in the treatment of herpes simplex, herpes zoster, and other viral infections. J Cutan Med Surg 2003;7:372–81.

61. Nicolaou N, Varma S, Blackford S, et al. Case 3: vulval Crohn's disease (VCD). Clin Exp Dermatol 2002;27:535–6.

62. Vettraino IM, Merritt DF. Crohn's disease of the vulva. Am J Dermatopathol 1995;17:410–3.

63. Andreani SM, Dang HH, Grondona P, et al. Rectovaginal fistula in Crohn's disease. Dis Colon Rectum 2007;50:2215–22.

64. Strong SA. Perianal Crohn's disease. Semin Pediatr Surg 2007;16:185–93.

65. Ford CV. Deception syndromes: factitious disorders and malingering. In: Levenson JL, editor. The American Psychiatric Publishing textbook of psychosomatic medicine. Arlington, VA: American Psychiatric Publishing, Inc; 2005. p. 297–309.

66. Jaghab K, Skodnek KB, Padder TA. Munchausen's syndrome and other factitious disorders in children—case series and literature review. Psychiatry 2006;3:46–55.

67. Spiryda LB, Laufer MR, Soiffer RJ, et al. Graft-versus-host disease of the vulva and/or vagina: diagnosis and treatment. Biol Blood Marrow Transplant 2003;9:760–5.

68. Mazur T. Gender dysphoria and gender change in androgen insensitivity or micropenis. Arch Sex Behav 2005;34:411–21.

69. Quint EH, Strickland JL. Management quandary. testicular feminization. J Pediatr Adolesc Gynecol 2001;14:99–100.

70. Conn J, Gillam L, Conway GS. Revealing the diagnosis of androgen insensitivity syndrome in adulthood. BMJ 2005;331:628–30.

71. Fallat ME, Donahoe PK. Intersex genetic anomalies with malignant potential. Curr Opin Pediatr 2006;18:305–11.

72. Galani A, Kitsiou-Tzeli S, Sofokleous C, et al. Androgen insensitivity syndrome: clinical features and molecular defects. Hormones 2008;7:217–29.
73. Hughes IA, Deeb A. Androgen resistance. Baillieres Best Pract Res Clin Endocrinol Metab 2006;20:577–98.
74. Kallipolitis GK, Milingos SD, Creatsas GK, et al. Laparoscopic gonadectomy in a patient with testicular feminization syndrome. J Pediatr Adolesc Gynecol 2000;13:23–6.
75. Levin HS. Tumors of the testis in intersex syndromes. Urol Clin North Am 2000;27: 543–51.
76. Kolon TF. Disorders of sexual development. Curr Urol Rep 2008;9:172–7.
77. Walden U, Rauch R, Hiort O, et al. Diagnosis of 5-alpha-reductase deficiency in a teenage Turkish girl. J Pediatr Adolesc Gynecol 1998;11:39–42.
78. Oakes MB, Eyvazzadeh AD, Quint EH, et al. Complete androgen insensitivity syndrome—a review. J Pediatr Adolesc Gynecol 2008;21:305–10.
79. Folch M, Pigem I, Konje JC. Müllerian agenesis: etiology, diagnosis, and management. Obstet Gynecol Surv 2000;55:644–9.
80. Sonmezer M, Atabekoglu C, Dokmeci F. Laparoscopic excision of symmetric uterine remnants in a patient with Mayer-Rokitansky-Kuster-Hauser syndrome. J Am Assoc Gynecol Laparosc 2003;10:409–11.
81. Laufer MR. Congenital absence of the vagina: in search of the perfect solution. When, and by what technique, should a vagina be created? Curr Opin Obstet Gynecol 2002;14:441–4.
82. Economy KE, Barnewolt C, Laufer MR. A comparison of MRI and laparoscopy in detecting pelvic structures in cases of vaginal agenesis. J Pediatr Adolesc Gynecol 2002;15:101–4.

Disorders of Sexual Development

Lisa Allen, MD, FRCSC

KEYWORDS

- Disorders of sexual development • Gender assignment
- Feminizing genitoplasty and surgical outcomes
- Gender identity • Quality of life • Disclosure

Disorders of sex development (DSDs) are medical conditions in which the development of chromosomal, gonadal, or anatomic sex varies from normal and may be incongruent with each other.[1] The term DSD arose from a conference sponsored by the Lawson Wilkins Pediatric Endocrine Society and the European Society for Pediatric Endocrinology and replaces previous terminology such as intersex disorders or hermaphroditism, terms which in the past were part of cumbersome and/or confusing classification systems and often not well accepted by patients and families.[1] Disorders of sexual development is a more inclusive concept, incorporating medical diagnoses which would not traditionally have been included with intersex conditions, ie, Mullerian agenesis.

This article primarily addresses the medical conditions where infants may be born with ambiguous genitalia leading to decisions with regard to gender assignment. The approach to investigations and diagnosis in the newborn period will be stressed within an interprofessional team. Policies with regard to surgery have developed, with techniques evolving and data emerging from long-term outcome studies. Current medical and surgical management are reviewed. Finally, a developmental approach to disclosure is presented.

The management of patients with DSD diagnoses requires a thoughtful contemplative health care provider. The development of gender identity may not be consistent with the gender assigned in the newborn period and gender dysphoria may manifest. This awareness must be incorporated into any strategy of care. Ideally, treatment, especially surgery (if appropriate), should be undertaken by individuals with specific experience and training. Given the relative rarity of these conditions, an overall incidence of intersex conditions is 1:5500[2] (the incidence of DSD diagnoses will be slightly higher than 1:5500, as it includes conditions not previously classified with intersex terminology), referral of newborns, children, and adolescents for care to multidisciplinary gender teams in large centers can assist in addressing medical, surgical, and psychosocial challenges.

Section of Pediatric Gynecology, Division of Endocrinology, The Hospital for Sick Children, 555 University Avenue, Toronto, ON Canada, M5G 1X8
E-mail address: lallen@mtsinai.on.ca

doi:10.1016/j.ogc.2009.02.001
0889-8545/09/$ – see front matter © 2009 Elsevier Inc. All rights reserved.

DISORDERS OF SEX DEVELOPMENT CLASSIFICATION AND ETIOLOGIES

Disorders of sex development may result from a heterogeneous group of etiologies. The DSD nomenclature divides these etiologies into categories of 46XX DSD, 46XY DSD, Sex Chromosome DSD, Ovotesticular DSD, and 46XX Testicular DSD. Within each category specific diagnoses are made when possible (**Table 1**).

APPROACH TO DIAGNOSIS

In the newborn period, in particular, when an infant is born with ambiguous genitalia reflecting a possible diagnosis of a DSD, there is felt a sense of urgency to provide the family with not only the specific diagnosis but in conjunction a gender assignment. This urgency arises from the cultural pressures that necessitate the usual announcement of "It's a boy" or "It's a girl" to friends, family, and colleagues. However, the complexities of diagnosis and gender assignment require time; it is extremely important to avoid unfounded early judgments that may not be consistent with final diagnoses. The first contacts families have with health care providers are extremely important and are remembered. Within those first meetings the principal issue is to reassure the family upfront about their child's overall health and well-being. It is acceptable to acknowledge the uncertainty that exists in assigning the gender of their child. The genital examination should be reviewed with the parents, along with providing an education with regard to the basic embryology pertaining to sexual development. Educational tools can be invaluable to complement verbal explanations such as developmental Web sites (http://www.sickkids.ca/childphysiology, http://dsdguidelines. org/). Health care providers should explain the process that will be involved to investigate their child. As information becomes available, the results should be shared with families in a timely fashion, actively involving them in the decision-making process. Families may wish to record information sessions with the health care providers to assist them in recall. It is important to find out who the family would like to have to meet with the team. In some family cultures, the grandparents or aunts and uncles may be important to include. Recommendations on the optimal management of newborns and individuals with DSDs suggest a multidisciplinary team involvement.[1,3] These interprofessional teams consist of care providers from pediatric endocrinology, urology, gynecology, genetics, psychology, psychiatry, social work, and nursing. Each team may function differently in consultation processes, but it is advisable to have one individual function as a coordinator, assisting families to move through the process with the team, providing consistency of care and information. In our center, social work and endocrinology are often the first contacts for the family. If all team members are not able to consult together, social work may be able to be present at most consults, helping families to clarify information, particularly if conflicting. It is crucial to give parents the support at this time, to decide with whom they should share information about their baby's health, outside of the parental dyad and what information to share. Ideally, all members of the team will consult before diagnoses are made and gender assignment suggested.

The diagnosis of DSDs involves the usual process of history, physical examination, and investigations.

The history begins with a perinatal history inquiring to determine if there were symptoms of maternal virilization or maternal medication use in pregnancy suggesting an exogenous (maternal) source of androgen. Antenatal karyotyping may be available if amniocentesis or chorionic villus sampling was performed. Occasionally the diagnosis of a DSD may occur antenatally with the discovery of a discrepancy between the prenatal karyotype and genital anatomy on routine ultrasonography or from suspicion

Table 1
Classification and etiologies of disorders of sexual development

Category	Etiology	Diagnosis
46XX DSD	Increased fetal adrenal androgen production	Congenital adrenal hyperplasia (21 hydroxylase deficiency, 11 B Hydroxylase deficiency, 3B-Hydroxysteroid dehydrogenase deficiency, P450 Oxidoreductase) Androgen-secreting tumor
	Fetal gonadal androgen production	Ovotesticular DSD (both ovarian and testicular tissue) 46XX SRY+ testicular DSD (SRY translocation)
	Fetoplacental source	Placental aromatase deficiency Oxidoreductase deficiency
	Transplacental passage of maternal androgens	Maternal androgen secreting tumor or Luteoma of pregnancy Exogeneous androgens (eg, danazol)
	Other	Dysmorphic syndromes Mullerian agenesis Cloacal exstrophy
46XY DSD	Testicular dysgenesis/malfunction	Pure gonadal dysgenesis (XY) Mixed gonadal dysgenesis (often 45X/46XY) Testicular regression Ovotesticular DSD
	Biosynthetic defect—decreased androgen synthesis	5 alpha reductase deficiency Leydig cell hypoplasia or aplasia Nonvirilizing CAH (StAR, 3 beta-Hydroxysteroid dehydrogenase, 17OHD/17-20 lyase, Smith-Lemli-Opitz Syndrome)
	Deficient synthesis or action of AMH	Persistent Mullerian duct syndrome
	End organ unresponsiveness	Androgen receptor defects (complete or partial AIS)
	Other	Dysmorphic syndromes Hypospadius Micropenis Cloacal exstrophy Persistent Mullerian duct syndrome
Sex-Chromosome DSD	—	45XO Turner Syndrome 47XXY Kleinfelter syndrome
Ovotesticular DSD	—	46XX/46XY 45X/46 XY (mixed gonadal dysgenesis)

Abbreviations: AIS, androgen insensitivity syndrome; AMH, antimullerian hormone; CAH, congenital adrenal hyperplasia; DSD, disorders of sexual development; SRY, sex-determining region Y.

of genital ambiguity such as a reduction in penile size, absence of a phallus, scrotal phallic malposition, labial fusion, or indeterminate sex on second trimester ultrasound.[4] A family history of other individuals affected with DSDs may allow more detailed directed imaging or specific testing for prenatal diagnosis, ie, DNA analysis for CYP21 (21-hydroxylase) gene in congenital adrenal hyperplasia (CAH).

The family history, as alluded to in the preceding paragraph, can assist with diagnosis. Questioning should cover not only family members such as siblings or relatives with ambiguous genitalia (ie, X-linked conditions such as androgen insensitivity syndrome [AIS] but also early neonatal death, or relatives with amenorrhea or infertility). Early neonatal death in a male sibling may reflect an undiagnosed CAH condition with salt wasting crisis. Families may not share the diagnosis of DSD with relatives but may disclose issues of infertility. Consanguinity in the parents increases the risk of disorders associated with an autosomal recessive pattern of inheritance such as CAH, testosterone biosynthetic defects, Leydig cell hypoplasia, and 5 alpha reductase deficiency.

On physical examination it is important to assess for features that may suggest a dysmorphic syndrome as opposed to an isolated variation in genital anatomy. A general assessment of health should include an assessment for dehydration, although salt-wasting crises with CAH generally occur between the 4th and 15th day of life.

Examination of the external genitalia cannot provide a diagnosis, nor determine gender assignment; however, it can provide evidence to exclude some diagnosis (ie, with a palpable labioscrotal gonad, CAH in a female infant is unlikely) and is one factor that will be considered in gender assignment.

One of the important features to assess on examination is the presence or absence of unilateral or bilateral palpable gonads. Gonads may need to be milked down into the labioscrotal folds, and a careful examination sweeping from the internal ring along the inguinal canal is necessary (**Fig. 1**).[5] Gonads that are bilaterally palpable are generally testes, albeit they may be dysgenetic.[6] In the algorithm for diagnosis (**Fig. 2**), the presence or absence of palpable gonads along with knowledge of karyotype will help determine further aspects of investigation.

The further examination of the external genitalia can assist with determining the Prader staging of the individual. The Prader scale is a determination of the degree of virilization of the external genitalia on a scale from 1 to 5 reflecting progressive virilization of the external genitalia and the urogenital sinus. By accurately assessing the genitalia and using descriptive terminology such as a Prader scale, health care providers have a consistent vocabulary when making management decisions (**Fig. 3**).

Features to be assessed on the physical examination include phallus size, fusion of labioscrotal folds, rugosity of labioscrotal folds, presence of a persistent urogenital sinus, presence of a vaginal opening, and position of the urethral meatus. The phallus should be measured for both length and width of the corporal bodies, from the base to the tip of the glans. The full-term newborn penis should measure at least 2 cm and is usually 3.5 ± 0.4 cm, a phallus less than 2.3 to 3.6 cm is consistent with

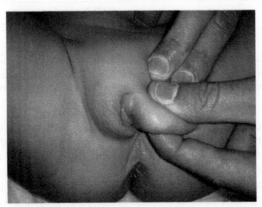

Fig. 1. Palpation for gonads, milking down from inguinal canal into labioscrotal folds.

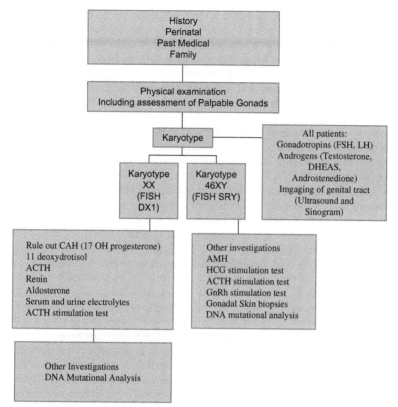

Fig. 2. Algorithm of investigations for disorders of sexual development.

a micropenis.[7,8] Clitoral size in term newborns ranges from 2.0 to 8.5 mm in length, with width from 2.0 to 6.0 mm.[9] A single opening on the perineum may suggest a persistent urogenital sinus; imaging such as a genitogram is required to determine the level of the confluence relative to the perineum. Fusion of the labioscrotal folds

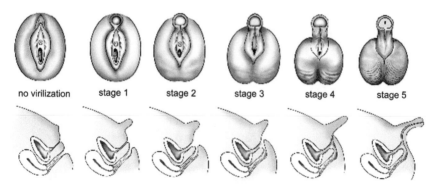

no virilization   stage 1   stage 2   stage 3   stage 4   stage 5

Fig. 3. Prader scale reflecting the degree of virilization of the external genitalia. The internal genitalia reflect the changes in the urogenital sinus that may be seen with a 46XX DSD such as congenital adrenal hyperplasia.

is evident if the distance measured from the anus to the posterior fourchette is more than 50% of the distance measured from the anus to the phallus (clitoris). Labioscrotal fusion and a urogenital sinus is a reflection of earlier in utero exposure to androgens, as these events occur before 14 weeks of gestational age. In hypospadius patients, it is important to assess the location of the urethral meatus along the ventral aspect of the penile shaft and the degree of chordee. Hyperpigmentation of the genital skin and nipples may reflect the excess ACTH (adrenocorticotropic hormone) and proopiomelanocortin in infants with CAH.

In preterm infants, caution must be applied in the interpretation of the findings on external genital examination to avoid overdiagnosis of DSD, as the clitoris may appear prominent in female infants, and descended testes do not occur before 34 weeks of gestational age (**Fig. 4**).[10,11]

Some investigations will be applied to all individuals with DSD to assist with diagnosis, others are more specifically ordered based on results of earlier testing and physical examination. All individuals require karyotyping on peripheral blood, initial rapid testing is available using fluorescence in situ hybridization for X and Y chromosomes (DX1 for X, sex determining region Y [SRY] for Y) but careful assessment of the full karyotype must be performed for definitive assessment especially to rule out mosaicism. Imaging of the internal genital tract usually involves both ultrasound to assess for the presence of a uterus and intra-abdominal or inguinal gonads and also a genitogram of the urogenital sinus, to determine presence of vagina, impression of cervix, and length of confluence (high or low urogenital sinus). Gonadotropins, testosterone, and dihydrotestosterone are part of initial investigations.

CAH is both the most common cause of ambiguous genitalia in the newborn, with a worldwide incidence of 1:14,500[12] and is potentially life threatening, therefore biochemical screening should be performed in any suspected 46XX DSD newborn. Basal 17 hydroxyprogesterone will be elevated in the most common form of CAH, 21 Hydroxylase deficiency, but may not be elevated until 48 hours following birth. Salt-wasting crises will have hyponatremia, hyperkalemia, and dehydration; therefore, serum and urine electrolytes, renin, and aldosterone are important additional testing. Less common forms of CAH account for only 5% of CAH and will require more definitive testing, ie, 11 deoxycortisol for 11 beta hydroxylase deficiency or elevated 17 hydroxypregnenolone and dehydroepiandrosterone for 3 beta hydroxysteroid dehydrogenase deficiency. Borderline results may require ACTH stimulation testing.

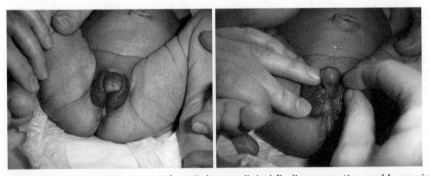

Fig. 4. Ambiguous genitalia in an infant. Relevant clinical findings: rugation and hyperpigmentation of fused labioscrotal folds. Enlarged phallus and solitary perineal opening consistent with urogenital sinus.

More specific testing will generally be guided by the DSD teams caring for these newborns such as gonadal or skin biopsies to determine gonadal mosaicism, androgen receptor binding assays, and analysis of 5 alpha reductase activity. Human chorionic gonadotropin (HcG) stimulation testing will assist with detecting defects in testosterone biosynthesis. Antimullerian hormone measurement can indicate presence of testicular tissue and specifically presence of Sertoli cells. Stimulation with exogeneous testosterone may determine the capacity of the phallus to respond to androgens. Molecular genetic testing for mutations in genes involved in sex development can be performed: CYP21A2 for CAH, androgen receptor gene for AIS, SRY gene for XY gonadal dysgenesis, and mutations in SOX 9 and WT1 gene, which are associated with dysgenetic gonadal development and syndromes such as campomelic dysplasia and Denys-Drash syndrome, respectively.[3,10] Specific genetic testing is not routinely available except in specialized centers. Despite completion of these investigations, a definitive diagnosis may not be able to be reached in the newborn period. In one study, just under half of DSD cases (48.7%) had no definitive diagnosis provided to newborns.[13]

MANAGEMENT: GENDER ASSIGNMENT

Before discussing assignment of gender, one must understand the three components of psychosexual development. Gender identity refers to the intrinsic sense of oneself as female or male. Gender role refers to the set of behaviors typical of one gender or another, these will vary with context such as the surrounding culture. Sexual orientation refers to an individual's erotic responsiveness, that is the gender or genders to whom one is attracted (homosexual, heterosexual, bisexual). Gender identity, gender role and sexual orientation are each components and yet may be distinct.[14]

When assigning gender to a newborn or child, the hope is that the assigned gender will be consistent with the developed internal sense of gender, ie, gender identity. It should be emphasized that a variation in gender role or differences in sexual orientation does not reflect an incorrect gender assignment. For example, in young women with CAH, gender role behaviors have been found to differ from control girls in a more masculinized fashion, however gender identity does not differ substantially from non-CAH control girls.[15–17]

There are many aspects of the child that must be taken into account when assigning gender: karyotype, gonadal function, phenotype (body habitus, Prader staging of external genitalia), internal genitalia (ie, presence of uterus), potential for fertility and sexuality, risk of future malignancy, and prenatal androgen influences on target tissue (including the brain).[18] In addition, information on known quality of life from long-term outcome studies should be discussed and accounted for when assigning gender as a newborn.

Although gender assignment should be solely based on the expected gender identity that an individual will develop over his or her lifetime, international studies indicate that the influence of the society that the individual will be raised in plays a role. Families living in societies that are matrilineal will be more accepting of female gender assignment than those raised in patriarchal societies. The reasons may be cultural, traditional, or economic (ie, lines of inheritance) as to why one gender may be more acceptable to a family than the other and may reflect how men and women are treated within that society. Even within a country, different ethnic groups may have different views on gender assignment.[19,20] These cultural, religious, and family values are additional considerations for the team before gender assignment.

Gender assignment has evolved over time. The concept of gender neutrality was advocated in the 1950s by John Money[21] who believed that an infant remained gender neutral until the age of 2, and that gender assignment along with feminizing genito-plasty surgery and an unequivocable commitment from family and health care providers would result in formation of an internal sense of gender consistent with that assigned. Recent awareness and knowledge indicates that whereas most individuals will be content with the gender assigned, gender dysphoria in individuals with DSD does exist. Gender dysphoria may be sufficiently intense to result in self reassignment of gender, especially as adolescence and adulthood approach. The challenge remains that gender assignment and accompanying medical and surgical treatments that are applied in infancy and childhood are often disconnected from the care of individuals in adolescence and adulthood. Pediatric health care providers must manage infants and children with DSDs with the awareness of the emerging long-term data related to quality of life, sexuality, and psychosocial outcomes. Factors predicting gender dysphoria have not yet been elucidated, gender identity has not consistently been associated with genital appearance, predictors of prenatal androgen exposure (Prader staging), nor age at surgical procedures.[15,22]

The prenatal androgen environment of the fetus and the acceptance of the brain as a gendered organ have started to be taken into account in gender assignment. As an example, in the past, individuals with a diagnosis of 46XY cloacal exstrophy were previously assigned to a female gender because of the absence of functional male genitalia despite normally functioning testes and androgen response in target tissues. Current knowledge that gender identity evolves in these individuals and that 35% to 55% experience either gender dysphoria and/or have self-declared as a male identity, has altered the practice of gender assignment.[23,24] A survey of urologists indicated that 70% would choose a male gender assignment, mostly guided by the belief of the likelihood of brain imprinting by prenatal androgen exposure.[25] However, animal studies suggest that differences between male and female brains are not solely a result of the prenatal androgen exposure during critical periods of brain development but may also be influenced by sex-determining genes even before gonadal function.[26] Differentiation of the human brain cells may be under sex-specific transcriptional control mechanisms.[27] Hence, the gender identity that develops in 46XY cloacal exstrophy can differ from the gender identity that develops in 46XX CAH despite prenatal androgen exposure in both conditions.

The traditional gender assignment for some medical conditions leading to DSDs is listed in **Table 2**.[28]

Once a diagnosis is rendered and a gender assigned, a developmental approach to care should ensue continuing with the multidisciplinary team. An interprofessional

Table 2
Gender assignment in DSD conditions

Diagnosis	Typical Gender Assignment
46XX CAH	Female (advanced Prader stages, late diagnosis consideration to male gender assignment)
Complete AIS	Female
XY cloacal exstrophy	Male
PAIS	Male or female
MGD	Male or female
Ovotesticular DSD	Male or female

Abbreviations: AIS, androgen insensitivity syndrome; CAH, congenital adrenal hyperplasia; DSD, disorders of sexual development; MGD, mixed gonadal dysgenesis; PAIS, partial androgen insensitivity syndrome.

comprehensive approach will ensure that all aspects of care are addressed: medical and surgical management, gender issues, conveyance of information, disclosure, and, importantly, psychosocial issues. Before the introduction of an interprofessional clinic, one center found that these issues were not addressed with consistency. Patients previously involved with individual services had errors in diagnosis in 21% of cases, and had gaps in care: 10% in medical/surgical management, 13% in gender issues, 33% in information and disclosure, and 38% in psychosocial issues (unpublished data).[29]

SURGERY

When undertaken, feminizing genital surgery includes some or all of the following: clitoral surgery for clitoral hypertrophy, urogenital sinus mobilization if present, labioplasty, neovaginal construction, and possible gonadectomy in XY containing karyotypes.

Clitoral surgery has evolved considerably. Originally surgery to reduce the size of the clitoris involved clitoral resection, owing to its obvious severe impact on sexuality, clitoral recession replaced resection in the 1980s.[29,30] Clitoral recession was technically easy, preserved full clitoral sensation but could be associated with painful erectile tissue and the presence of visible bulging corpora upon arousal. The most commonly performed surgery presently is clitoroplasty, removing the enlarged corpora cavernosum of the clitoris while sparing the neurovascular bundle to the glans. Recent reports of further possible enhancement such as the corporal sparing dismembered clitoroplasty are appearing. The latter technique splits the corpora in the midline after detaching them from the glans, and rather than removing this erectile tissue, buries the bodies within the labia bilaterally.[31]

The management of the urogenital sinus varies depending on the level of confluence. For the low urogenital sinus, where the separation of the urethra and vagina occurs within millimeters from the introitus, a simple Y-V flap vaginoplasty can be performed (Fortunoff flap) (**Fig. 5**).[32] Mobilization of the entire urogenital sinus is performed if the urogenital sinus confluence is within 3 cm from the perineum.[33] The excess mucosa of the mobilized urogenital sinus is used to partially construct the posterior and lateral walls of the vagina.[34] Those extremely high urogenital sinuses, higher than 3 cm from the perineum, where the vagina may enter the urogenital sinus proximal to the external urethral sphincter may require neovaginal reconstruction.[33] The trend with feminizing genitoplasty procedures is to perform single-stage surgical procedures, where both clitoral surgery and urogenital sinus surgery is completed at the same point in care. Genitoplasty also involves refashioning the tissues to create labia minora and labia majora.

Although the goals of feminizing genitoplasty are to restore anatomy achieving a more feminine appearance with a patent vagina for menstruation and sexual function, to preserve sensation and promote sexuality, to preserve reproductive capacity, and to prevent urologic sequelae, it is also anticipated that one of the aims is to develop a more stable gender identity, and to promote better psychosocial and psychosexual outcomes.[13,35]

It is clear that the newborn infant may not consent to decisions related to surgery in infancy or childhood. Surgery in infancy and childhood is generally irreversible and may impact on sexual functioning later in life.[36,37] Most health care professionals will advise deferring surgery with Prader 1 and 2 stages, as well as for neovaginal creation. It is recognized that some variations of the genitalia may never require corrective surgery, and as a vagina is nonessential to health during the childhood ages, deferring

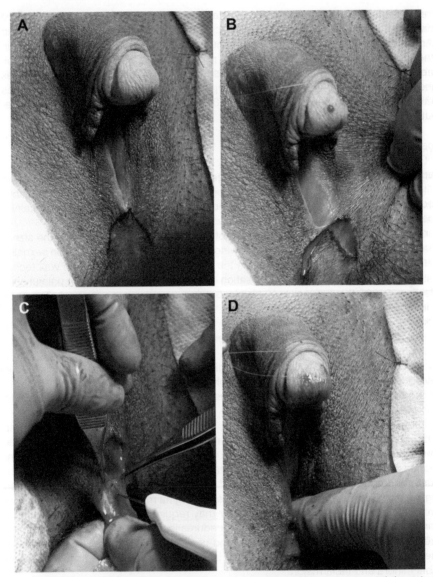

Fig. 5. (*A*) Flap location for Y-V vaginoplasty in low urogenital sinus surgery. Adult patient with 5 alpha reductase deficiency. (*B*) Initial incision for flap. (*C*) Further dissection of flap. (*D*) Flap will then be advanced into apex of a vertical incision made in the posterior wall of the vagina. Postoperative dilating of the blind-ended vagina will create further length and width of the vagina.

treatment to adolescence or adulthood is logical when decisions may be made by the individual rather than for that individual. Assessments of trends in genital surgery over time indicate that parents are choosing to defer surgery in childhood, which in the past was not common.[28]

The dilemma with regard to surgery lies with the more advanced Prader stages (III, IV, and V) and in conditions with potential ongoing androgen action on the external genitalia (Partial androgen insensitivity syndrome or PAIS) where female gender assignment is made (yet gender identity may not develop congruently with assigned gender). Arguments have been made to defer surgery until an age where individuals may provide their own informed consent (full consent policy). However, little information is yet available on the long-term outcomes of individuals where surgery is not undertaken with respect to the influence of discordant genitalia on psychosexual and quality-of-life measures. Most surgery in DSD children still occurs within the first year of life; in one study, 63% of the population had surgery before the age of 6 months.[38]

Consent for surgery from families must include a discussion of the risks of feminizing genitoplasty on genital function later in life (ie, adverse clitoral sensory function), risks of gender self-reassignment, and the high likely need for further revision surgery in adolescence or adulthood, which will be reviewed later in this article.

Most centers caring for newborns and children with DSDs practice on a spectrum of policy between the optimal gender policy and the full consent policy with regard to decisions for surgery, applying an individualized, family-centered, culturally sensitive, and open-minded approach. Although surgery may be performed, a supportive environment allows families to choose to defer surgery. Several guidelines on surgery have been published: the Consensus Statement on Management of Intersex Disorders reflects recommendations from the Lawson Wilkins Pediatric Endocrine Society and the European Society for Pediatric Endocrinology, the statement of the British Association of Pediatric Surgeons Working Party on the Surgical Management of Children Born with Ambiguous Genitalia can be found at www.baps.org.uk.[1]

GONADECTOMY

Gonadectomy is required in some 46XY DSD conditions for two main reasons: risk of malignancy and risk of ongoing virilization with continued androgen exposure (with female gender assignment).

Dysgenetic gonads or intra-abdominal testes carry a varying risk of malignancy. DSD patients are at increased risk of developing seminomas of the testes and dysgerminomas in dysgenetic gonads.[39] Gonadoblastomas may occur in the dysgenetic gonads of children.[40] Less frequent gonadal malignancies include Sertoli cell tumor, yolk sac tumor, teratoma, embryonal carcinoma, choriocarcinoma, and unclassified sex cord stromal tumor.[41–45] Tumor risk can be considered as high, intermediate, or low. The highest risk of malignancy is associated with the dysgenetic intra-abdominal gonad, or in PAIS with nonscrotal gonads where tumor risk may range from 15% to 50%. The lowest risk is in the patient diagnoses of complete androgen insensitivity syndrome (CAIS) and ovotesticular DSD at 2% to 3%. An example of an intermediate risk would be a dysgenetic or PAIS intrascrotal gonad.[39] The general recommendation is to remove streak gonads where any Y-containing chromosomal material is present in childhood including in Turners mosaicism. Turners mosaicism with a Y-containing karyotype carries a malignancy risk of 12%.[39]

In women with CAIS, deferring removal of testes until after the natural process of pubertal development avoids the need for estrogen induction of secondary sexual characteristics for most women and allows the patient to decide about removal after a full consent process. Malignancy risk is not only influenced by the dysgenetic nature of the gonads and by gonad location, but also by age. The tumor risk in DSD patients with Y chromatin material in their genetic makeup increases with age. This is particularly relevant in women with CAIS where the possibility of deferral of gonadectomy to postpuberty is considered. In CAIS the risk of tumor formation is initially low (3.6% at age 25) and rises to 33% at age 50.[40] Rare tumors are reported young, there is a case report of a 17-month-old girl with CAIS, diagnosed with a yolk sac tumor;[44] however, rare tumors can occur in gonads of non-DSD children. Tumor risk is sufficiently low in the first 2 decades of life for CAIS to allow postpubertal timing of gonadectomy.

The other concern with regard to retained gonads is the potential for ongoing virilization of children/adolescents assigned a female gender, ie, with PAIS and 5 alpha reductase deficiency. In these scenarios, gonadectomy during the early neonatal period, before the peak of gonadal function with PAIS or before puberty with 5 alpha reductase deficiency will prevent further masculinizing genital anatomic change.

In some individuals with DSDs the gonad is contained within a hernial sac, if the hernia requires surgical repair, gonadectomy may occur concurrently.

Gonadectomy for intra-abdominal gonads may be approached laparoscopically, whereas for inguinal gonads, the approach is typically via an inguinal incision (Table 3).[46]

MEDICAL

The discussion of the steroid management of the most common cause of ambiguous genitalia, congenital adrenal hyperplasia, is beyond the scope of this article. Principles of hormone replacement therapy will be presented for DSD diagnoses with female gender. The goals of hormone replacement therapy are not only to initiate and maintain secondary sexual characteristic development (including uterine growth) but also to allow for psychosexual development. Bone health will benefit from sex steroid initiation and prevention of osteopenia/osteoporosis is an additional important consideration.[47]

The group of DSD patients who require hormone therapy are those who are hypogonadal, ie, patients postgonadectomy, or in those with Turners syndrome and/or premature ovarian failure. In women with CAIS who did not undergo early gonadectomy, spontaneous pubertal development will usually occur through peripheral aromatization of androgens to estradiol, although no pubic or axillary hair will develop owing to the androgen resistance. The presence or absence of a Mullerian structure (ie, uterus) will determine if estrogen therapy alone is required or a combination of

Table 3 Recommendations for timing of gonadectomy in DSD conditions	
DSD	**Timing of Gonadectomy**
PAIS (with female gender assignment)	At diagnosis, often in first 6 months of life (concern of virilization/malignancy)
Gonadal dysgenesis with Y containing chromosomal material, includes mixed gonadal dysgenesis with streak gonad (intra-abdominal)	Childhood (concern of risk of malignancy)
Androgen biosynthetic defects, ie, 5 alpha reductase deficiency (female gender assignment)	Prepuberty (concern of virilization at puberty)
CAIS	At diagnosis, at time of hernia repair or defer to postpuberty for spontaneous pubertal development (low risk of malignancy)
Gonadal dysgenesis (scrotal testis) (male gender assignment)	Consider biopsy at puberty, may consider sperm banking if feasible

Abbreviations: CAIS, complete androgen insensitivity syndrome; DSD, disorders of sexual development; PAIS, partial androgen insensitivity syndrome.

estrogen-progestin replacement. As hormone replacement therapy will be prescribed consistent with previous gender assignment, its introduction to an individual should serve as a developmental milestone where the contentedness of that individual with their sex of rearing should be assessed. A reluctance by the adolescent to begin hormone replacement therapy may indicate gender dysphoria with the assigned sex and warrants a thorough, sensitive discussion.[48]

The timing of prescribing sex steroids will depend on the natural age of spontaneous puberty and the influence of the surrounding peer group. Many young women will wish to begin thelarche at a similar age to their classmates.

Final predicted adult heights should be followed. For individuals with impaired height potential, ie, those with advanced bone ages (ie, poorly controlled CAH) or with restricted genetic potential (Turners syndrome), benefit may result from a slight delay in introduction of estrogen therapy. Hence, not only chronologic age but bone age should be considered. Endocrinologists in North America most frequently base introduction of hormone replacement therapy (HRT) on a bone age of older than 12, and would consider a chronologic age range of 12 to 14 as appropriate.[49] Newer information on final heights obtained for young women with Turners syndrome indicate no adverse effect on final heights with low-dose transdermal estrogen regimens started at early ages (12 to 13), and better psychoscocial outcomes than the traditional delayed regimens (older than age 15).[50,51] Estrogen replacement may be oral (estradiol or conjugated equine estrogen) or transdermal (patch or gel). The general process is to begin at a low dose, gradually increasing over a period of several years toward the final adult replacement regimen. The optimal young adult dose of estrogen is not clear; our institution uses the doses of HRT in **Table 4**, a higher amount than for bone protection derived from studies in postmenopausal women. These doses are generally accepted as appropriate for young adults in the premature ovarian insufficiency literature.[52] The timing of incremental increase in estrogen is guided by tissue response, ie, Tanner staging of breasts and side effects/tolerance to therapy but is generally every 6 months. An example of a regimen of HRT is to begin with oral estradiol at 0.5 mg/day increasing by 0.5 mg/day every 6 months to a maximum dose of 2 mg/day. Progestin therapy, if required, is introduced at 2 years of unopposed estrogen therapy or with any spontaneous uterine bleeding. Recent concerns with regard to HRT in postmenopausal women have resulted in increased flexibility in dosing regimens, with newer lower dose formulations available. This marketing change has been advantageous for pubertal induction regimens. Transdermal estradiol patches for example are now available in strengths of 25.0, 37.5, 50.0, 75.0, and 100.0 μg.

Table 4	
Hormone replacement therapy in DSD conditions	
Type	**Final Maintenance Dose**
Estrogens	
Oral conjugated equine estrogen	1.25 mg/d
Oral estradiol	2.0 mg/d
Transdermal patch estradiol	100 μg/24 h (100-μg patch applied twice weekly)
Progestins (if Mullerian structure—specifically uterus present)	
Medroxyprogesterone acetate	10 mg/d cyclically 10–14 d/mo
Micronized progesterone	200 mg cyclically 10–14 d/mo

With adolescents and young adults, switching to a combined hormonal contraceptive method may be preferable. This allows an aspect of privacy and anonymity especially if in college/university or other shared accommodation situations where a contraceptive method may not require explanation to peers but hormone replacements may (**Table 4**).

OUTCOMES

The ideal information to guide policies on the management of individuals with DSD is long-term outcome data covering all aspects of quality of life, sexuality, fertility, and psychosocial functioning. There are challenges with regard to interpreting the information that is beginning to become available. The most marked is that management has evolved; surgical techniques have changed; and interprofessional teams recognizing the importance of psychological support, family-centered care, education, and disclosure have now become the standard of care. It will be a while before we see if improved outcomes related to these altered care plans will be evident in adult populations. It is important however not to disregard the evidence that is currently available, recognizing that in some areas research remains sparse. These long-term outcomes must be reflected back to the pediatric health care professionals caring for infants and children where most management decisions are made. Many aspects may influence long-term outcomes, including the family and culture in which the child lives, as well as the specific diagnosis. Information on long-term outcomes has suggested that different diagnoses may carry different prognoses in quality-of-life measures.

GENDER IDENTITY

Gender dysphoria is present in 46XY DSD conditions with normal gonadal function and less commonly in 46XX DSD medical conditions including CAH and in other DSD conditions. Gender dysphoria is more common with female gender assignment than male gender assignment, although dissatisfaction with male sex of rearing can be seen.[20–22]

Several studies have assessed the degree of gender dysphoria and gender change in adolescent and adult women with CAH.[20,22,53] This group of individuals would have experienced prenatal androgen exposure but not the possible gene-related sexual dimorphism of the brain. Zucker and colleagues[53] reported 5.7% (3/53) of 46XX CAH women living in a male social role; only one of the three had self-declared male identity, the remaining 2 individuals were assigned male gender at birth. Dessens and colleagues[20] reviewed multiple studies, comprising 250 46XX CAH individuals assigned female gender at birth, of which 5.2% experienced gender dsyphoria and 1.6% changed gender. Gender dysphoria and gender change were not found to be related to Prader staging. Although the rates of gender dysphoria are lower than that seen in some 46XY DSD conditions with normal gonadal function, the reported rates are higher than in non-DSD populations. Another study (not included in Dessens and colleagues,[20] review) included a population of patients studied in a psychosexual development clinic, that may overestimate the incidence of gender identity issues. It reported five of nine individuals assigned female gender at birth had self-declared male identities for a rate of 55%.[22] Information on gender dysphoria for mixed/partial gonadal dysgenesis (22% to 55%)[22,54] similarly reinforces that all individuals diagnosed with a DSD should have access to psychological counseling and follow-up, asking questions related to gender identity, and assisting those individuals whose self-declared gender identity is different from the assigned gender identity with their dsyphoria especially as adulthood approaches. This may include assisting with gender transition. A trend to more gender dysphoria as an individual ages exists.[21]

Although gender dysphoria may develop with the gender assigned as a newborn to varying degrees with different diagnoses, most individuals overall do not exhibit gender dsyphoria; hence, in addition to genetic factors and prenatal hormone exposure, other factors such as the social environment may influence gender outcome. When discussing generally irreversible surgical procedures with families, part of the counseling must include awareness of the potential for gender dysphoria, with its inherent risk of self reassignment later in life.

SURGICAL OUTCOMES

In the past several years, an increasing number of international clinics and DSD teams have published on the outcomes of childhood surgery for the women they care for. Recognition exists that the cosmesis of external genitalia may not reflect the function of the genitalia. Studies that look at interim results, with only short-term follow-up into childhood may not reflect or correlate with longer term results but at the present time are the only measures available for assessing newer surgical techniques.[29,55] Caution must be advised on interpreting these early results. The best studies will take into account objective measures of sexual functioning at an age where the vagina and clitoris are part of a woman's sexuality as well as quality-of-life measures. The lack of rigorous definitions of complications or outcomes along with differing medical and surgical techniques may be responsible for sometimes conflicting results.

Different surgical groups report disparate cosmetic outcomes of feminizing genitoplasty surgeries. Dissatisfaction with cosmesis from a patient perspective or objective assessments of poor cosmetic results by health care providers ranges from 30% to 100%.[56,57] Alizai and colleagues[58] reported on 14 girls with CAH who were formally assessed by an examination under anesthesia with a urologist, plastic surgeon, and gynecologist and found in 46% the clitoral appearance was deemed to be unsatisfactory because of atrophy or absence. This value is similar to the 41% poor cosmetic results reported by Creighton and colleagues[59] in the United Kingdom after assessment of genital proportion and objective aspects of clitoris, labia, vagina, pubic hair, and skin. The Australian experience reported by Lean and colleagues[60] was more favorable, cosmesis was reported (consistent with the Creighton and colleagues' study) as good if appearance was normal and unlikely to be judged abnormal by non-medically trained individuals, satisfactory if there were up to two minor abnormalities but still unlikely to be judged abnormal by nonmedically trained individuals, and poor if they appeared abnormal or had three or more abnormal features. Using this assessment scheme, 72% had good genital appearance; however, in the detailed description of abnormality, 25% of clitori were small, absent, or large and 38% had a small vaginal introitus.

Repeat surgical procedures, often more minor than initial genitoplasty or vaginal dilation, are commonly required at puberty, even with planned single-stage feminizing genitoplasties. The results from the previous study by Creighton and colleagues[59] found that 98% of their adult population required treatment, of which 77% would be major surgical revisions. Other groups report lesser operative intervention at puberty; major revision surgery was required in only 2 of the 32 patients assessed in an Australian DSD population; however, an additional 49% required minor introital surgery or vaginal dilation. The most frequent reason for further therapy is vaginal stenosis, and while not always defined in studies, stenosis implies a vagina not acceptable for vaginal intercourse. Stenosis occurred in 11%, 36%, and 100% of the following studies assessing outcomes of childhood feminizing genitoplasty: Eroglu and colleagues,[57] Krege and colleagues,[61] and Alizai and colleagues.[58]

The most important message in the evolving surgical literature regarding feminizing vaginoplasty surgery is that the outcomes are not related to the age at which surgery is performed but are influenced by the experience of the surgeon; therefore, referrals to centers with DSD teams and subspecialty surgeons should be mandatory before considering feminizing surgery.[60]

Recent clitoral surgery has evolved to spare the neurovascular bundle when performing clitoroplasty. The clitoris is an intensely innervated structure, with capacity to perceive light pressure, vibration, temperature, and pain.[35] Unfortunately, there is little data on the sexual function of the clitoris following surgery. There is preliminary evidence that clitoral surgery may result in sexual dysfunction, even with newer clitoroplasty techniques. Sexual dysfunction was evident overall in a group of adult women with DSD; however, when clitoral surgery had been performed compared with no clitoral surgery a significantly higher rate of difficulties in sensuality and orgasm subscales of a standardized questionnaire were evident.[37] Objective assessment of genital sensation following feminizing genitoplasty revealed abnormal results for both cold and warm extremes of temperature when applied to the clitoris in women with CAH compared with nonsurgical controls.[36] Further evaluation of sexual function following surgical procedures is extremely important, especially objective assessments with newer surgery techniques.

Incorporating the current knowledge of outcomes of genital surgery in childhood into counseling of families of newborns and children with DSDs may allow families to feel comfortable with choices to avoid surgery on lesser degrees of genital ambiguity knowing that impairment to function and sensation may occur.

In CAIS and Mullerian agenesis (MRKH syndrome), although feminizing genitoplasty is not required, most patients will desire creation of a neovagina. The technique of active vaginal dilatation of the existing vaginal dimple is preferred over all surgical techniques. Although surgical procedures involving split thickness skin grafting (McIndoe procedure), colonic interposition, and laparoscopic-assisted peritoneal vaginoplasty are available, these should be reserved for the rare circumstance of failed vaginal dilation owing to the potential for both surgical complications and stenosis, which may occur with any surgical procedure.

PSYCHOSEXUAL OUTCOMES/QUALITY OF LIFE MEASURES

Quality of life for women includes aspects of intimacy with partners, arousal and sexual function, as well as self-esteem, social functioning, and mental health. Recently, quality-of-life studies are being reported on women with DSD diagnoses compared with either illness controls or population controls. Women with DSD may report delayed sexual milestones, fewer partnerships and sexual experiences, and a lower level of arousal.[53,54,62] Overall lower quality of life, higher anxiety, higher frequency of suicidal thoughts, and lower self-esteem may be more frequent than in population or illness controls.[48,63] Similar to other outcome information, this cannot be generalized to all women with DSD but may be more common with certain diagnoses, ie, CAH, mixed gonadal dysgenesis (MGD) compared with CAIS.[63] Importantly, patients may not feel comfortable bringing these issues to their health care providers for discussion.[54] Hence, psychosocial care provided by mental health staff comfortable with expertise in DSD should be integrated into the interprofessional care team. This will allow not only recognition of challenges but can provide therapy including addressing interpersonal relationships. Sexual therapy may be a valuable adjunct in adulthood.

DISCLOSURE

Disclosure begins with the family at the time of the diagnosis and assessment of their newborn with a DSD and should be considered a lifelong ongoing process that evolves along a developmental time line. The diagnosis of DSD is both challenging to understand and challenging to explain; however, the health care team should consider themselves as having a role in preparing the family and the child/adolescent to receive this diagnosis when they are cognitively and psychologically prepared. In health care teams who care for many DSD patients, the responsibility for disclosure may be shared among team members in conjunction with the family. Guidance around disclosure may be provided by social work or other team members who have developed the expertise to work with the family from infancy.

Helping families to correctly understand the child's diagnosis is the first step on the road to disclosure; families should be encouraged to gather information that can later be used to help them explain to their child decisions that were made with regard to management. Audio files of initial consultations with physicians may prevent inaccuracies in recollection. These audio recordings can be used with the patient at a later age when they have questions about the decisions that were made around their medical care. Parents can be encouraged to practice telling the "story" of their child's diagnosis out loud to them when they are a newborn. This practice allows for a growing comfort level on behalf of the parents with what they may perceive as difficult information, at a time when a child cannot remember. As children's questions arise, they should be answered truthfully although in a developmentally appropriate way. Some milestones in a child/adolescent's life may be natural points to disclose in a stepwise fashion about their medical history, ie, with peers' onset of puberty, with sex education in primary school, biology classes in high school, or with parenting classes. The family should be encouraged to keep the health care team apprised of what has and has not been disclosed to the patient. Parents may need separate appointments with the health care team to explore and rehearse how to disclose information, as well as to assess their own reaction to the process. It is not uncommon for parents to experience a sense of sadness and guilt at new developmental stages of their child's life. It is important for them to get professional mental health support if these feelings become overwhelming. It is a myth to believe that patients are better off not being aware of their diagnosis. The absence of disclosure can lead to angry, alienated patients who feel betrayed by the health care team and their families.

It is very important throughout this process to offer contact with patient support groups. Parents often feel alone and alienated, as do patients as they learn about their conditions. The connection with a group of patients with conditions the same or similar, is key in decreasing the sense of isolation and difference that is reported from these populations.

SUMMARY AND FUTURE DIRECTION

Patients with DSD are infrequently encountered with an incidence 1:5500.[2] Their complex management must address medical, surgical, and psychosexual needs of the individual patient. Evolving information suggests that thoughtful, flexible, family-centered care by specialized interprofessional teams may provide the optimal environment for care. The awareness that current management cannot eliminate all adverse outcomes (eg, gender dysphoria, surgical complications) should drive ongoing research and continual reflection into the optimal care decisions. Long-term outcome studies of newer surgical techniques, the decisions of families to not proceed with surgery, and quality-of-life measures should continue to be objectively assessed to further our knowledge base regarding appropriate management of DSD patients. Continued listening to and dialoguing and collaborating with DSD patients, families, and support/advocacy groups will also add to our understanding of this complex condition. A developmental approach to disclosure of diagnosis to the affected individual is advocated, with age-appropriate teaching materials and educational Web sites as useful adjuncts. Lifelong care should be offered by knowledgeable care providers, with smooth transitions from pediatric to adult health care facilities. The education that the health care team provides to the patient and family should be supplemented with advocacy in the public arena.

ACKNOWLEDGMENT

I acknowledge the dedicated team of health care professionals who make up the Multidisciplinary Urogenital Clinic at The Hospital for Sick Children from whom I have learned so much: Riyanna Babul-Hirji, MS, Darius Bagli, MD, Susan Bradley, MD, David Chitayat, MD, Walid Farhat, MD, Genevieve Kilman, BA, CCLS, Armando Lorenzo, MD, Barb Neilson, MSW RSW, J.L. Pippi Salle, MD, PhD, Dianne Wherret, MD, and Ken Zukker, PhD. A special thank you to Barb Neilson for her comments on the article.

REFERENCES

1. Lee PA, Houk CP, Ahmed SF, et al. Consensus statement on management of intersex disorders. International Consensus Conference on Intersex. Pediatrics 2006;118:e488–500.
2. Sax L. How common is intersex? A response to Anne Fausto-Sterling. J Sex Res 2002;39:174–8.
3. Parisi MA, Ramsdell LA, Burns MW, et al. A gender assessment team: experience with 250 patients over a period of 25 years. Genet Med 2007;9:348–57.
4. Pajkrt E, Chitty LS. Prenatal gender determination and the diagnosis of genital anomalies. BJU Int 2004;93(Suppl 3):12–9.
5. Evaluation of the newborn with developmental anomalies of the external genitalia. American Academy of Pediatrics. Committee on Genetics. Pediatrics 2000;106: 138–42.
6. Arcari AJ, Bergada I, Rey RA, et al. Predictive value of anatomical findings and karyotype analysis in the diagnosis of patients with disorders of sexual development. Sex Dev 2007;1:222–9.
7. Flatau E, Josefsberg Z, Reisner SH, et al. Penile size in the newborn infant. J Pediatr 1975;87:663–4 [letter].
8. Cheng PK, Chanoine JP. Should the definition of micropenis vary according to ethnicity? Horm Res 2001;55:278–81.
9. Oberfield SE, Mondok A, Shahrivar F, et al. Clitoral size in full-term infants. Am J Perinatol 1989;6:453–4.
10. Ogilvy-Stuart AL, Brain CE. Early assessment of ambiguous genitalia. Arch Dis Child 2004;89:401–7.
11. Riley WJ, Rosenbloom AL. Clitoral size in infancy. J Pediatr 1980;96:918–9.
12. Pang SY, Wallace MA, Hofman L, et al. Worldwide experience in newborn screening for classical congenital adrenal hyperplasia due to 21-hydroxylase deficiency. Pediatrics 1988;81:866–74.

13. Thyen U, Lanz K, Holterhus PM, et al. Epidemiology and initial management of ambiguous genitalia at birth in Germany. Horm Res 2006;66:195–203.
14. Houk CP, Hughes IA, Ahmed SF, et al. Summary of consensus statement on intersex disorders and their management. Pediatr 2006;118:753–7.
15. Berenbaum SA. Effects of early androgens on sex-typed activities and interests in adolescents with congenital adrenal hyperplasia. Horm Behav 1999;35:102–10.
16. Berenbaum SA, Bailey JM. Effects on gender identity of prenatal androgens and genital appearance: evidence from girls with congenital adrenal hyperplasia. J Clin Endocrinol Metab 2003;88:1102–6.
17. Meyer-Bahlburg HF, Dolezal C, Baker SW, et al. Prenatal androgenization affects gender-related behavior but not gender identity in 5-12-year-old girls with congenital adrenal hyperplasia. Arch Sex Behav 2004;33:97–104.
18. Mouriquand PD. Possible determinants of sexual identity: how to make the least bad choice in children with ambiguous genitalia. BJU Int 2004;93(Suppl 3):1–2.
19. Ozbey H, Darendeliler F, Kayserili H, et al. Gender assignment in female congenital adrenal hyperplasia: a difficult experience. BJU Int 2004;94:388–91.
20. Kuhnle U, Krahl W. The impact of culture on sex assignment and gender development in intersex patients. Perspect Biol Med 2002;45:85–103.
21. Money J. Ablatio penis: normal male infant sex-reassigned as a girl. Archives of Sexual Behaviour 1975;4(1):65–71.
22. Dessens AB, Slijper FM, Drop SL. Gender dysphoria and gender change in chromosomal females with congenital adrenal hyperplasia. Arch Sex Behav 2005;34:389–97.
23. Meyer-Bahlburg HF. Gender identity outcome in female-raised 46,XY persons with penile agenesis, cloacal exstrophy of the bladder, or penile ablation. Arch Sex Behav 2005;34:423–38.
24. Reiner WG. Gender identity and sex-of-rearing in children with disorders of sexual differentiation. J Pediatr Endocrinol Metab 2005;18:549–53.
25. Diamond DA, Burns JP, Mitchell C, et al. Sex assignment for newborns with ambiguous genitalia and exposure to fetal testosterone: attitudes and practices of pediatric urologists. J Pediatr 2006;148:445–9.
26. Dewing P, Shi T, Horvath S, et al. Sexually dimorphic gene expression in mouse brain precedes gonadal differentiation. Brain Res Mol Brain Res 2003;118:82–90.
27. Mayer A, Lahr G, Swaab DF, et al. The Y-chromosomal genes SRY and ZFY are transcribed in adult human brain. Neurogenetics 1998;1:281–8.
28. Thomas DF. Gender assignment: background and current controversies. BJU Int 2004;93(Suppl 3):47–50.
29. Randolph JG, Hung W. Reduction clitoroplasty in females with hypertrophied clitoris. J Pediatr Surg 1970;5:224–31.
30. Lee PA, Witchel SF. Genital surgery among females with congenital adrenal hyperplasia: changes over the past five decades. J Pediatr Endocrinol Metab 2002;15:1473–7.
31. Pippi Salle JL, Braga LP, Macedo N, et al. Corporeal sparing dismembered clitoroplasty: an alternative technique for feminizing genitoplasty. J Urol 2007;178:1796–800 [discussion: 1801].
32. Fortunoff S, Lattimer JK, Edson M. Vaginoplasty technique for female pseudohermaphrodites. Surg Gynecol Obstet 1964;118:545–8.
33. Pena A. Total urogenital mobilization—an easier way to repair cloacas. J Pediatr Surg 1997;32:263–7 [discussion: 267–8].
34. Rink RC, Metcalfe PD, Cain MP, et al. Use of the mobilized sinus with total urogenital mobilization. J Urol 2006;176:2205–11.

35. Crouch NS, Creighton SM. Long-term functional outcomes of female genital reconstruction in childhood. BJU Int 2007;100:403–7.
36. Crouch NS, Minto CL, Laio LM, et al. Genital sensation after feminizing genitoplasty for congenital adrenal hyperplasia: a pilot study. BJU Int 2004;93:135–8.
37. Minto CL, Liao LM, Woodhouse CR, et al. The effect of clitoral surgery on sexual outcome in individuals who have intersex conditions with ambiguous genitalia: a cross-sectional study. Lancet 2003;361:1252–7.
38. Graziano K, Teitelbaum DH, Hirschl RB, et al. Vaginal reconstruction for ambiguous genitalia and congenital absence of the vagina: a 27-year experience. J Pediatr Surg 2002;37:955–60.
39. Looijenga LH, Hersmus R, Oosterhuis JW, et al. Tumor risk in disorders of sex development (DSD). Best Pract Res Clin Endocrinol Metab 2007;21:480–95.
40. Manuel M, Katayama PK, Jones HW Jr. The age of occurrence of gonadal tumors in intersex patients with a Y chromosome. Am J Obstet Gynecol 1976;124: 293–300.
41. Shahidi H, Robia M. Bilateral germ cell tumors and androgen insensitivity syndrome. J Clin Oncol 2007;25:4686–8.
42. Wysocka B, Serkies K, Debniak J, et al. Sertoli cell tumor in androgen insensitivity syndrome—a case report. Gynecol Oncol 1999;75:480–3.
43. Nojima M, Taguchi T, Ando Y, et al. Huge seminoma developed in a patient with testicular feminization. J Obstet Gynaecol Res 2004;30:109–12.
44. Handa N, Nagasaki A, Tsunoda M, et al. Yolk sac tumor in a case of testicular feminization syndrome. J Pediatr Surg 1995;30:1366–7 [discussion: 1367–8].
45. Chan LY, Wong SF, Yu VS. Advanced stage of dysgerminoma in testicular feminisation: is radical surgery necessary? Aust N Z J Obstet Gynaecol 2000;40:224–5.
46. Chertin B, Koulikov D, Alberton J, et al. The use of laparoscopy in intersex patients. Pediatr Surg Int 2006;22:405–8.
47. Mizunuma H, Soda M, Okano H, et al. Changes in bone mineral density after orchidectomy and hormone replacement therapy in individuals with androgen insensitivity syndrome. Hum Reprod 1998;13:2816–8.
48. Warne G, Grover S, Hutson J, et al. A long-term outcome study of intersex conditions. J Pediatr Endocrinol Metab 2005;18:555–67.
49. Drobac S, Rubin K, Rogol AD, et al. A workshop on pubertal hormone replacement options in the United States. J Pediatr Endocrinol Metab 2006;19:55–64.
50. Carel JC, Elie C, Ecosse E, et al. Self-esteem and social adjustment in young women with Turner syndrome—influence of pubertal management and sexuality: population-based cohort study. J Clin Endocrinol Metab 2006;91:2972–9.
51. Davenport ML. Evidence for early initiation of growth hormone and transdermal estradiol therapies in girls with Turner syndrome. Growth Horm IGF Res 2006; 16(Suppl A):S91–7.
52. Bondy CA. Care of girls and women with Turner syndrome: a guideline of the Turner Syndrome Study Group. J Clin Endocrinol Metab 2007;92:10–25.
53. Zucker KJ, Bradley SJ, Oliver G, et al. Psychosexual development of women with congenital adrenal hyperplasia. Horm Behav 1996;30:300–18.
54. Szarras-Czapnik M, Lew-Starowicz Z, Zucker KJ. A psychosexual follow-up study of patients with mixed or partial gonadal dysgenesis. J Pediatr Adolesc Gynecol 2007;20:333–8.
55. Braga LH, Lorenzo AJ, Tatsuo ES, et al. Prospective evaluation of feminizing genitoplasty using partial urogenital sinus mobilization for congenital adrenal hyperplasia. J Urol 2006;176:2199–204.

56. Gollu G, Yildiz RV, Bingol-Kologlu M, et al. Ambiguous genitalia: an overview of 17 years' experience. J Pediatr Surg 2007;42:840–4.

57. Eroglu E, Tekant G, Gundogdu G, et al. Feminizing surgical management of intersex patients. Pediatr Surg Int 2004;20:543–7.

58. Alizai NK, Thomas DF, Lilford RJ, et al. Feminizing genitoplasty for congenital adrenal hyperplasia: what happens at puberty? J Urol 1999;161:1588–91.

59. Creighton SM, Minto CL, Steele SJ. Objective cosmetic and anatomical outcomes at adolescence of feminising surgery for ambiguous genitalia done in childhood. Lancet 2001;358:124–5.

60. Lean WL, Deshpande A, Hutson J, et al. Cosmetic and anatomic outcomes after feminizing surgery for ambiguous genitalia. J Pediatr Surg 2005;40:1856–60.

61. Krege S, Walz KH, Hauffa BP, et al. Long-term follow-up of female patients with congenital adrenal hyperplasia from 21-hydroxylase deficiency, with special emphasis on the results of vaginoplasty. BJU Int 2000;86:253–8 [discussion: 258–9].

62. Zucker KJ, Bradley SJ, Oliver G, et al. Self-reported sexual arousability in women with congenital adrenal hyperplasia. J Sex Marital Ther 2004;30:343–55.

63. Johannsen TH, Ripa CP, Mortensen EL, et al. Quality of life in 70 women with disorders of sex development. Eur J Endocrinol 2006;155:877–85.

Müllerian Anomalies

Lesley L. Breech, MD[a],*, Marc R. Laufer, MD[b]

KEYWORDS

- Müllerian anomalies • Utero-vaginal anomalies
- Vaginoplasty • Vaginal reconstruction
- Vaginal anomalies

The diagnosis and management of girls and young women with Müllerian anomalies requires not only knowledge of embryologic development, but an awareness of the known associations of structural anomalies of the female reproductive tract with other congenital anomalies, including renal anomalies and anorectal malformations. Recognition of such associations appropriately guides the diagnostic evaluation and allows potential simultaneous operative treatment. Because reproductive anomalies are not rare, most clinicians will encounter these abnormalities within routine gynecologic practice and an organized discussion is advantageous for appropriate diagnosis, management, and possible referral. Familiarity with the anomalies, associations and optimal treatment allows providers to offer the recommended clinical care in a timely way, avoiding unnecessary delays and potential compromise to reproductive success.

EMBRYOLOGY

The reproductive organs in the female consist of external genitalia, gonads, and an internal duct system, the Müllerian ducts. These three components originate embryologically from different primordia and in close association with the urinary system and hindgut. Thus, the developmental history is quite complex. The Müllerian (paramesonephric) duct system is stimulated to develop preferentially over the Wolffian (mesonephric) duct system, which regresses in early female fetal life. The cranial parts of the Wolffian ducts can persist as the epoöphoron of the ovarian hilum; the caudal parts can persist as Gartner's ducts. The Müllerian ducts persist and, with complete development, form the fallopian tubes, the uterine corpus and cervix, and a portion of the vagina.

About 37 days after fertilization, the Müllerian ducts first appear lateral to each Wolffian duct as invaginations of the dorsal coelomic epithelium. The site of origin of the invaginations remains open and ultimately forms the fimbriated ends of the fallopian

[a] Department of Pediatrics, University of Cincinnati College of Medicine, Cincinnati Children's Hospital Medical Center, 3333 Burnet Avenue, ML 4000, Cincinnati, OH 45229, USA
[b] Children's Hospital Boston, 300 Longwood Avenue, Boston, MA 02115, USA
* Corresponding author.
E-mail address: lesley.breech@cchmc.org (L.L. Breech).

Obstet Gynecol Clin N Am 36 (2009) 47–68
doi:10.1016/j.ogc.2009.02.002
0889-8545/09/$ – see front matter © 2009 Elsevier Inc. All rights reserved.

obgyn.theclinics.com

tubes. At their point of origin, each of the Müllerian ducts forms a solid bud. As the solid buds elongate, a lumen appears in the cranial part, beginning at each coelomic opening. The lumina extend gradually to the caudal growing tips of the ducts.

The paired Müllerian ducts continue to grow in a medial and caudal direction until they eventually meet in the midline and become fused together in the urogenital septum. A septum between the two Müllerian ducts gradually disappears, leaving a single uterovaginal canal lined with cuboidal epithelium. Failure of reabsorption of this septum can result in a septate uterus. The most cranial parts of the Müllerian ducts remain separate and form the fallopian tubes. The caudal segments of the Müllerian ducts fuse to form the uterus and part of the vagina. The cranial point of fusion is the site of the future fundus of the uterus. Variations in this site of fusion can result in an arcuate or bicornuate uterus. Complete failure of fusion can result in a didelphic uterus. Although isolated case reports continue to challenge established embryologic mechanisms of Müllerian development, additional reports are necessary to fully evaluate potential variations in embryologic development.

The vagina is formed from the lower end of the uterovaginal canal, which developed from the Müllerian ducts and the urogenital sinus. The point of contact between the two is the Müllerian tubercle. A solid vaginal cord results from proliferation of the cells at the caudal tip of the fused Müllerian ducts. The cord gradually elongates to meet the bilateral endodermal evaginations (sinovaginal bulbs) from the posterior aspect of the urogenital sinus below. These sinovaginal bulbs extend cranially to fuse with the caudal end of the vaginal cord, forming the vaginal plate. Subsequent canalization of the vaginal cord occurs, followed by epithelialization with cells derived mostly from endoderm of the urogenital sinus. Most investigators suggest that the vagina develops under the influence of the Müllerian ducts and estrogenic stimulation. There is general agreement that the vagina is a composite formed partly from the Müllerian ducts and partly from the urogenital sinus.

At about the 20th week, the cervix takes form as a result of condensation of stromal cells at a specific site around the fused Müllerian ducts. The mesenchyme surrounding the Müllerian ducts becomes condensed early in embryonic development and eventually forms the musculature of the female genital tract. The hymen is the embryologic septum between the sinovaginal bulbs above and the urogenital sinus proper below. It is lined by an internal layer of vaginal epithelium and an external layer of epithelium derived from the urogenital sinus (both of endodermal origin), with mesoderm between the two. It is not derived from the Müllerian ducts.

CONGENITAL HYMENAL ABNORMALITIES

The normal hymen can have multiple configurations including annular, crescentic, and fimbriated/redundant. However, failure of the hymen to perforate completely in the perinatal period can result in varying anomalies including imperforate, microperforate, cribiform (sievelike), navicular (boatlike), or septated (**Fig. 1**). Such anomalies are ideally recognized at birth as part of the newborn examination or seen in childhood as part of well-child genital examinations. An abnormal hymen that results in a small orifice may preclude the use tampons, insertion of vaginal cream or suppositories, or the ability to have vaginal intercourse. Providers should be aware that there have been reports of familial occurrences of hymenal abnormalities, and thus alert young women that their daughters may have a similar abnormality.[1]

Imperforate hymen (**Fig. 2**) has an incidence of 1 in 1000 and may present in the neonatal period as hydrocolpos or mucocolpos, resulting from stimulation of the vaginal epithelium. Significant amounts of mucous can be secreted during the

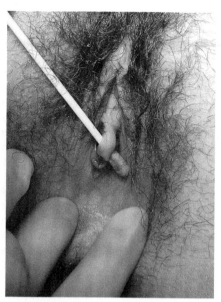

Fig. 1. Septate hymen in menarchal female.

perinatal period secondary to maternal estradiol stimulation.[2] The newborn may have a bulging, translucent yellow-gray mass at the vaginal introitus. Most hydro/mucocolpos is asymptomatic and resolves as the mucous is reabsorbed and estrogen levels decrease. However, large hydro/mucocolpos may obstruct the ureters, resulting in hydronephrosis or even respiratory distress. Neonatal ultrasound

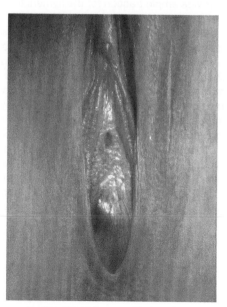

Fig. 2. Imperforate hymen. Notice the thin, transparent hymen stretched over the dark-colored accumulated menstrual blood.

can demonstrate the fluid collection. Resection of the hymen is recommended in the symptomatic infant. Aspiration, without definitive enlargement or a vaginostomy for continued drainage, should be avoided owing to the risks of reaccumulation with recurrence of a mass or ascending infection. Asymptomatic girls with an imperforate hymen can be monitored throughout childhood and avoid the risks of surgery in infancy. The optimal time for surgery is after the onset of puberty (as evidenced by thelarche) but before menarche. The hymen should then be resected to prevent the development of hematocolpos, pain, and possible retrograde menstruation. Pubertal timing allows adequate resection with less risk of scarring and a decrease in the potential need for repeat procedures, given the presence of adequate on-going endogenous estrogen. In the unestrogenized state of childhood it may be difficult to differentiate vaginal agenesis and an imperforate hymen.

Unfortunately, the most common presentation of imperforate hymen is in a pubertal girl with cyclic or persistent pelvic pain and an abdominal mass or perineal bulging with a translucent bluish-tinged hymen secondary to significant hematocolpos, and in severe cases, additional hematometra. Less commonly, mass-effect symptoms including urinary retention or constipation are the patient complaints leading to evaluation. Hematocolpos may become quite large because the vagina is distensible and the obstruction is so distal.

Definitive surgery should take place only after the appropriate evaluation. This should always include an examination of the external genitalia, and a digital rectal examination, if indicated, with radiographic imaging only as necessary to confirm the diagnosis. Pelvic and abdominal ultrasonography will confirm a distal obstruction.

The goal of hymenotomy/hymenectomy is to open the hymenal membrane to allow the egress of menstrual flow, tampon use, and eventually comfortable sexual intercourse. The procedure is usually performed under general anesthesia with the patient in high lithotomy. After the usual sterile preparation and draping, a straight or Foley catheter is used to drain the bladder and properly delineate the urethra. Stay sutures can then be placed to provide ample traction for the hymenotomy and allow stabilization for quick insertion of a suction device to collect the copious amount of thickened, chocolate-colored old blood and menstrual fluid. After evacuation of the hematocolpos, the hymenal orifice can be enlarged with removal of excess tissue to create an orifice of "normal" size. In treatment of the imperforate hymen, puncture without definitive surgical repair should be avoided, because the viscous fluid may not drain adequately and the small perforations will allow ascension of bacteria and the possibility of infection, such as pelvic inflammatory disease or tuboovarian abscess.

Other hymenal anomalies with some degree of perforation are rarely clinically significant in childhood. A navicular configuration may be associated with postvoid dribbling and complaints of incontinence or, in rare circumstances, recurrent urinary tract infections. Most young women present after menarche with complaints of difficulty inserting or removing a tampon or, less commonly, with significant dyspareunia with penetration (**Fig. 3**). These are also usually surgically corrected with a simple outpatient excision.

ANOMALIES OF THE UTERUS, CERVIX, AND VAGINA

Anomalies of the female reproductive tract may result from one of several developmental abnormalities, including agenesis/hypoplasia, vertical fusion (canalization abnormalities resulting from abnormal contact with the urogenital sinus), lateral fusion (duplication), or resorption (septum). Clinicians should be cognizant that patients with each abnormality will present with different symptoms, and will require specific

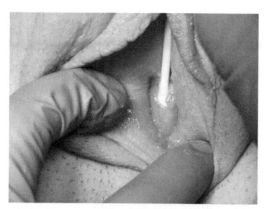

Fig. 3. Redundant posterior hymen causing difficulty with tampon use.

individualized therapy. Common symptoms seen in uterine and vaginal malformations include primary amenorrhea, acute and/or chronic pelvic pain, abnormal vaginal bleeding, or a foul-smelling vaginal discharge (often worse at the time of menses). Non-obstructive anomalies may even be found incidentally on routine examination. Young women with obstructive anomalies are more likely to present with acute symptoms of pain and discomfort.

Genetics

The etiology of anatomic defects of the female genital tract is not fully understood. Most forms of isolated Müllerian duct and urogenital sinus malformations are inherited in a polygenic/multifactorial fashion. Mendelian forms of inheritance with a single gene mutation have been described to explain specific syndromes including the McKusick-Laufman syndrome (MKS), which uncommonly includes vaginal atresia and more commonly includes transverse vaginal septa and the hand-foot-genital syndrome.[1] Hand-foot-genital syndrome includes bilateral great toe and thumb hypoplasia and small hymenal opening with various degrees of incomplete Müllerian fusion with or without two cervices or a longitudinal vaginal septum.

Incidence

The actual incidence of Müllerian anomalies is not definitively known. Reporting issues skew our knowledge of the true incidence. These abnormalities are relatively underreported in infants and are likely overreported in patients being evaluated for reproductive concerns, especially in adult women struggling with infertility.[3–6] In a study of fertile women who were evaluated for Müllerian duct anomalies at the time of tubal ligation, an incidence of 3.2% was identified.[4] Many young women may have an underlying asymptomatic Müllerian duct anomaly; yet, since they have no pain, pelvic mass, or reproductive compromise, they may not come to diagnosis.

Many uterine abnormalities are asymptomatic until attempts at childbearing and thus, are often not diagnosed during adolescence. It is not until adulthood, when patients experience multiple spontaneous pregnancy losses, persistent menstrual abnormalities, or infertility that a definitive diagnosis is made. Patients with segmental agenesis/hypoplasia usually present with primary amenorrhea: however, if a normally functioning endometrium is present, significant cyclic or chronic pelvic pain may develop. It is only if a mucocolpos significant enough to cause symptomatic obstruction occurs as an infant, or hematocolpos at the time of menarche, that children or adolescents with obstructive phenomenon come to diagnosis.

Diagnosis

Identification of recognizable reproductive symptoms is an important key to the diagnosis of a structural defect of the female genital tract. The symptoms include cyclic or constant pain, pain with insertion and removal of a tampon, or the absence of menses. A gynecologic history of amenorrhea, the inability to remove a tampon, or persistent bleeding despite using a tampon is suspicious for a uterovaginal anomaly. Last, the physical examination may reveal an imperforate hymen or only a vaginal dimple with vaginal agenesis. The discovery of a blind vaginal pouch can suggest that the Müllerian contribution to the vagina has been impaired.

Imaging Studies for Reproductive Tract Anomalies

Radiographic imaging provides much needed information to aid in making the correct diagnosis. Delineation of the patient's individual anatomy is essential to develop an appropriate plan for surgical correction. Ultrasound is helpful in identifying the anatomy in all cases of reproductive tract anomalies and can be used as a transabdominal, transvaginal, or transperineal approach.[7–12] MRI can be helpful in determining the anatomy in cases of complicated obstructive anomalies, and is often considered the "gold standard" for imaging of anomalies of the reproductive tract,[13–16] MRI is especially useful in determining the presence or absence of the cervix in complex anomalies or the presence of functioning endometrium in cases of a noncommunicating obstructed rudimentary uterine horn, however, MRI may miss a rudimentary uterine horn if it is located laterally along the psoas muscle and pelvic sidewall.[17] Such a condition may be more likely in prepubertal patients who have very widely spaced uterine horns, as seen in cloacal anomaly or cloacal exstrophy. A hysterosalpingogram (HSG) can be helpful in determining the patency of the Müllerian structures and delineating complex communication with the urologic or colorectal system.[15] An HSG can be uncomfortable unless performed under anesthesia and should be primarily reserved for use in older adolescents and young adults. In cases of complicated Müllerian anomalies, especially in combination with anomalies of the urologic and colorectal systems, additional information regarding anatomy and diagnosis may be obtained during an examination with the patient under anesthesia using cystoscopy, vaginoscopy, laparoscopy, and/or hysteroscopy.[15,18]

Renal and Other Anomalies

Since the development of a normal Müllerian duct occurs in association with the normal development of the mesonephric duct, urinary tract anomalies are the most common abnormality associated with congenital anomalies of the female reproductive tract.[7,19] Urinary tract abnormalities in patients with Müllerian duct anomalies include ipsilateral renal agenesis, duplex collecting systems, renal duplication, and horseshoe-shaped kidneys. In the general population, the incidence of unilateral renal agenesis has been estimated to be between 1 in 600 and 1 in 1200, on the basis of autopsy studies.[20,21] The incidence of associated genital abnormalities in female patients with renal anomalies is estimated to be between 25% and 89%.[20,22]

TRANSVERSE VAGINAL SEPTUM

Transverse vaginal septa are believed to arise from a failure in fusion and/or canalization of the urogenital sinus and Müllerian ducts. Approximately 1 in 80,000 females are born with a transverse vaginal septum. The complete transverse vaginal septum may be located at various levels (low, middle, or high) in the vagina. Approximately 46% of vaginal septa occur in the upper vagina, 40% in the middle vagina, and 14% in the lower vagina.[23] On examination, the vagina may seem foreshortened ending in a blind vaginal pouch. A recto-abdominal bimanual examination may elicit an abdominal/pelvic mass. Transverse vaginal septa are rarely associated with uterine anomalies.[2]

The septa are usually less than 1 cm thick and may completely or incompletely extend from one vaginal sidewall to the other. Transverse vaginal septa commonly have a small central or eccentric perforation.[24] Rarely, pyohematocolpos may be caused by ascending infection through the small perforation. If there is no perforation in the transverse septum, there is a resultant obstruction with hematocolpos from concealed menses; a mass is palpable above the examining finger on rectoabdominal palpation. An obstruction with a transverse septum resulting in hematometra may lead to endometriosis.[25]

Ultrasound or MRI may help define the septum and its thickness preoperatively. A transperineal ultrasound may also confirm the thickness of the distal obstruction or distance from the perineal skin to allow for appropriate preoperative planning. It is also extremely important to identify a cervix, most reliably seen on MRI, to differentiate between a high septum and congenital absence of the cervix. Management varies between a high transverse vaginal septum and cervical agenesis, and attempts of surgical correction of cervical agenesis have been associated with significant complications, including death.[26]

After menarche, patients with an obstructive anomaly present similarly; however, patients with a high septum present more quickly with significant pain because the uterus distends more quickly. Those adolescents with a microperforation in the transverse septum may have egress of some menstrual blood with continued discharge but may present with pyohematocolpos secondary to ascending infection or painful tampon insertion and dyspareunia.

Aspiration of the hematocolpos should always be avoided because of the risks of ascending infection and pyocolpos. Definitive surgical correction is the therapy of choice. Before surgery, some distention of the upper vagina with menstrual blood (hematocolpos) before the development of significant hematometra may be advantageous. This allows the potential to increase the amount of upper vaginal tissue available for reanastomosis. Furthermore, preoperative dilation therapy may decrease the thickness of the septum and increase the amount of lower vaginal tissue available. Thin septa can then be resected followed by primary end-to-end anastomosis of the lower and upper vagina. Thicker septa may require undermining and mobilization of the upper and lower vaginal mucosa before anastomosis, in addition to resection of the fibrotic septal tissue. A common complication of resection of thick septa is scar contracture and vaginal stenosis. A circumferential "Z"-plasty technique allows for scarring along the suture line to contract the incision in a longitudinal fashion rather than a transverse one.[26] Postoperatively, wearing a vaginal mold or initiating early vaginal dilation may further decrease the risk of vaginal stenosis.[27] If there is not enough vaginal mucosa to accomplish a pull-through procedure and reanastomosis of the vaginal mucosa, a graft may be necessary to create a patent vaginal tract.

LONGITUDINAL VAGINAL SEPTUM

Longitudinal vaginal septa may be associated with one of several uterine anomalies including a complete septate uterus, uterine didelphi, and rarely bicornuate uteri. Longitudinal vaginal septa have also been reported to occur in association with anorectal malformations, including imperforate anus with rectovestibular fistula and cloaca.[28] Septa may be partial or extend the complete length of the vagina. As many as 20% of patients will have renal abnormalities.[29] Most reproductive-age patients present with complaints of dyspareunia and/or persistent bleeding despite tampon use, yet many women may be asymptomatic. Prepubertal girls undergoing evaluation and surgical management of anorectal or genitourinary anomalies are most often asymptomatic but, because surgical exposure is best at the definitive repair, most are treated then. The presence of a vaginal septum can usually be visualized on examination of the vaginal introitus. However, if the septum is incomplete and does not occupy the entire vagina, vaginoscopy may be necessary to evaluate the full extent in prepubertal patients (**Fig. 4**). Pelvic examination, with a speculum examination, in reproductive-age young women is usually adequate for visualization.

Treatment is by surgical resection. Resection should be performed in childhood if undergoing other genitourinary procedures or repair of an anorectal malformation; however, when the vaginal septum is an isolated anomaly, it is most often corrected after menarche owing to the later pubertal diagnosis. The septum should be completely removed while taking care to avoid damaging the cervix or cervices, which commonly insert along the septum at a similar level bilaterally (**Fig. 5**). Trauma to the bladder, rectum, and cervical blood supply should be avoided. After resection of the midline septum, closure of the vaginal mucosal defect is performed by suturing the mucosal surfaces together. In reproductive-age women the use of the hand-held harmonic scalpel for excision followed by reapproximation of the vaginal mucosa with interrupted sutures is effective.

OBSTRUCTED HEMI-VAGINA WITH IPSILATERAL RENAL AGENESIS

Longitudinal vaginal septa are often present with uterine didelphis; yet in some cases an obstructing septum is present. The association of the obstructed hemivagina with ipsilateral renal agenesis has been well described in the literature.[30–33] In fact, an acronym has been proposed, OHVIRA (Obstructed Hemivagina and Ipsilateral Renal Anomaly), to describe the syndrome.[34] Patients with an obstructed hemivagina present later than other obstructing vaginal anomalies, presumably because menstrual flow occurs normally from the nonobstructed hemiuterus.[35] However, these patients also complain

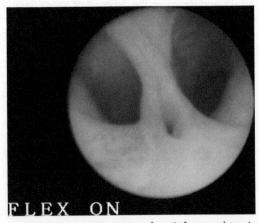

Fig. 4. Vaginal septum viewed on vaginoscopy of an infant undergoing surgical repair of a cloacal anomaly. Notice the rectal communication at the base of the vaginal septum.

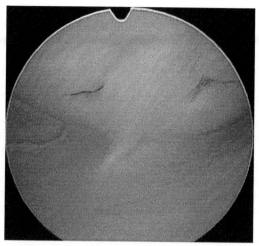

Fig. 5. Vaginoscopy of a prepubertal girl after repair of an anorectal malformation. She had an associated longitudinal vaginal septum that was removed during her definitive repair. Notice the close proximity of the two cervices and the small amount of residual septum remaining posteriorly.

of unilateral cyclic, followed by constant, pain. There may be a microperforation allowing for communication from the obstructed to the nonobstructed side resulting in prolonged or intermenstrual discharge, or very rarely, even pyocolpos.

On physical examination, a mass is felt to bulge from the lateral wall of the vagina toward the midline. After the pelvic examination, radiographic evaluation may also be helpful. Ultrasound is an excellent modality to demonstrate both the uterovaginal anomaly and the urinary anatomy.[36] MRI can provide beautiful images; however, may add significant expense (**Fig. 6**). Diagnostic laparoscopy is rarely necessary.[34] Most

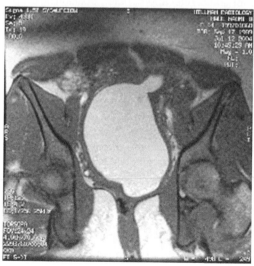

Fig. 6. MRI of the pelvis demonstrating an obstructed right hemivagina in a patient with OHVIRA.

patients with this anomaly can undergo resection of the obstructing septum (the common wall of the hemivaginas) in a fashion much like that described previously for longitudinal vaginal septa. The septal wall is resected to create a single vaginal vault. After resection of the septal wall of the obstructed hemivagina, the patient has normal function with a single vagina, two cervices, and two hemiuteri (uterine didelphis).

VAGINAL ATRESIA / DISTAL VAGINAL AGENESIS / SEGMENTAL VAGINAL AGENESIS

Vaginal atresia, distal vaginal agenesis, or segmental vaginal agenesis occurs when the urogenital sinus fails to contribute to the lower portion of the vagina. The uterus, cervix, and upper vagina develop normally, and the absent mid to lower section of the vagina is replaced by fibrous tissue. The most common presenting symptom is primary amenorrhea. Patients may develop cyclic or chronic pain and a pelvic or abdominal mass as the upper vagina fills with cervical mucus secreted after puberty or obstructed blood after concealed menarche. A physical examination confirms normal secondary development; however, the examination of the external genitalia reveals only a small dimple at the vaginal introitus. A rectoabdominal examination can be helpful to determine the presence of any midline structures (a distended upper vagina, a cervix, and/or uterus). In patients who cannot tolerate a rectoabdominal exam, an ultrasound can provide similar information to assist in differentiating this condition from vaginal agenesis. Ultrasonography, which should be done to assess renal status, also can confirm the presence of an obstructed upper vagina, or the presence of a normal cervix and uterus.[9] Ultrasound with a transperineal approach also will demonstrate the thickness of the segment of agenesis which can be crucial information to guide the surgical approach; MRI is also an excellent modality to determine the presence of a cervix and exclude the diagnosis of cervical agenesis.

In individuals with agenesis or atresia of the distal/lower vagina, an obstruction with a hematocolpos of the upper vagina will result at the time of menarche and requires a surgical procedure to relieve the obstruction at the time of diagnosis. This should ideally be performed when a large hematocolpos has formed but before development of hematometra. The hematocolpos will act as a natural tissue expander hopefully decreasing the need for grafts. After appropriately positioning the patient, a crescentric incision is made where the hymenal ring is or should be located. Careful dissection is performed superiorly through the fibrous area of the absent segment taking precautions to avoid the urethra/bladder and rectum, until the bulging upper vagina is reached. Intraoperative ultrasound guidance can be useful to identify the distended upper vagina in difficult cases.[37] The obstruction is then drained; the vaginal mucosa is identified and a pull-through procedure brings the distended upper vaginal tissue down to the introitus. Foley catheters or urethral sounds, Hegar dilators, or simultaneous rectal examinations are all helpful to determine the limits of the vaginal dissection.

If the distance to the vagina is too great and the vagina will not reach the introitus, an interposition graft has been used to join the introitus and upper vagina. When a bowel graft is necessary, the technique mandates a combined abdominal and perineal approach (**Figs. 7–9**). This surgical technique is more readily performed in childhood, especially if it is performed in the context of more complex reconstruction, such as genitourinary or anorectal surgery.

VAGINAL AGENESIS (MÜLLERIAN APLASIA)

Vaginal agenesis, Müllerian aplasia, or MRKH (Mayer-von Rokitansky-Küster-Hauser) syndrome all include the congenital absence of the vagina and are associated with variable Müllerian duct development. Aplasia of the Müllerian ducts results in not

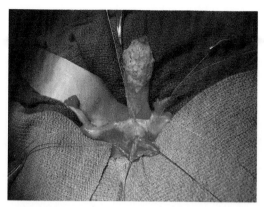

Fig. 7. Intraoperative images of a patient undergoing surgical treatment of distal vaginal agenesis. The native upper vagina would not reach to the introitus.

only absence of the uterine corpus and cervix but also the upper portion of the vagina, which may result in near total or complete vaginal agenesis. Müllerian aplasia is estimated to occur in about 1 in 1000 to 1 in 83,000 female births, but the most widely cited incidence is approximately 1 in 5000 female births.[38] In fact, the most common cause of vaginal agenesis is Müllerian aplasia or MRKH syndrome. Given the close association between the genital and urinary systems throughout fetal development, it is not surprising that approximately one third to one half of patients have associated renal anomalies, including renal agenesis, malrotation, or ectopic kidney.[39–41] Other anomalies associated with vaginal agenesis include anomalies of the skeletal and auditory systems.

Vaginal agenesis is usually accompanied by cervical and uterine agenesis, although approximately 7% to 10% of affected individuals may have a normal but obstructed uterus or a rudimentary uterus with functional endometrium.[42–45] Vaginal agenesis should be differentiated from vaginal atresia/distal vaginal agenesis/segmental vaginal agenesis. Another variant, cervical agenesis or atresia, is the presence of a uterus but agenesis of both the vagina and cervix. Approximately 90% of patients have some degree of Müllerian development, most commonly bilateral fibromuscular uterine

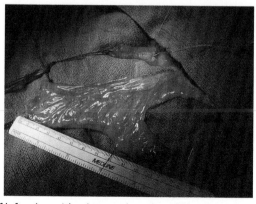

Fig. 8. A segment of left colon with adequate length and blood supply was identified for use as an interposition graft.

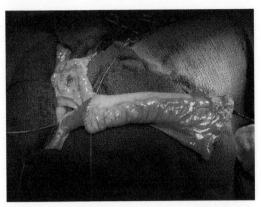

Fig. 9. The colonic interposition graft was then anastomosed to the upper native vagina in an isoperistaltic fashion to reach the introitus comfortably.

remnants located along the pelvic sidewall. However, only 2% to 7% of the uterine remnants will have a functional endometrial lining requiring intervention.[46]

Most patients present with primary amenorrhea around age 15 years, given that they have normal secondary sexual characteristics. Müllerian aplasia is the cause of 10% of cases of primary amenorrhea, second only to gonadal dysgenesis in a tertiary care center.[11] Girls with Müllerian remnants with a functional endometrium may present with cyclic or chronic pain secondary to the accumulation of obstructed menstrual blood.

Evaluation of the patient with near total or complete vaginal agenesis, like other Müllerian anomalies, begins with a genital examination. Most patients will have a vaginal dimple or very foreshortened, blind-ending vagina. The hymenal fringe is usually present along with the small vaginal pouch, as they are both derived embryologically from the urogenital sinus (**Fig. 10**). A pelvic mass will usually be absent and occasionally a peritoneal fold can be palpated on rectoabdominal bimanual examination. Transabdominal pelvic and renal ultrasound will further aid in assessing the reproductive and urologic anatomy and frequently help to determine if a functional

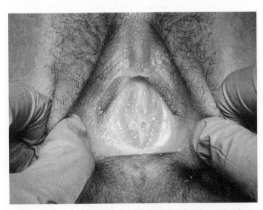

Fig. 10. A view of the introitus of a patient with vaginal agenesis demonstrating the small amount of hymenal fringe that can often be present.

endometrium is present. An MRI may be more accurate in the evaluation of Müllerian structures, but given the expense, it can be reserved for when ultrasound is indeterminate.[36] Laparoscopy may be necessary if noninvasive imaging fails to make an accurate diagnosis and it allows for the removal of obstructed uterine structures. Furthermore, a karyotype will definitively differentiate androgen insensitivity from Müllerian aplasia, if necessary.

Counseling

Of all the Müllerian anomalies, this diagnosis is by far the most upsetting to a girl, young adolescent, or adult woman, and her family. Counseling by an experienced team including nurses, social workers, psychologists and/or psychiatrists is recommended and should be strongly reinforced by the treating health care provider when interacting with patients and families.[47] Although fertility concerns, primarily the inability to carry a pregnancy, are the overriding issue, it is also important to stress to the young woman and her family that she has normal ovarian function with normal production of sex steroids and normal amounts of genetic material. Emphasis on the possibility of fertility options with assisted reproductive technologies and a gestational carrier is crucial,[46,48] in addition to confirming the ability to create a functional vagina.

Treatment

Counseling for the young woman and her family is not only the first step in treatment of Müllerian aplasia, but likely the most important for a long-term successful outcome. Although patients and families may be hesitant to engage in psychotherapy, attention should be given to the psychosocial issues as well as to the correction of the anatomic abnormality. The patient's cooperation and positive attitude are vital to the ultimate success of the creation of a functional vagina.[27] The timing for the nonsurgical or surgical creation of a vagina is purely elective, although many patients feel it is emergent at the time of diagnosis. Because this procedure is not a surgical emergency and it is a decision with lifelong impact, surgical intervention should be delayed until the young woman chooses to proceed with a self-selected specific treatment plan. Because primary nonsurgical creation of a vagina requires continued vaginal dilation, it clearly is inappropriate to consider this approach in children. Surgical procedures to create the vagina which require postoperative dilation should not be performed during childhood. Parents who have been instructed to dilate their daughter's vagina often present distraught and uncomfortable with the procedure. Thus, treatment should wait until the adolescent or young woman is able to determine the treatment and timing of the treatment. Parents may feel anxious and isolated at the time of diagnosis, precipitating interest and inquiry regarding surgical correction. Any technique for creation of a functional vagina should be delayed until the mid to late teens when the young woman can make her own decision, with the support of her family, and is comfortable with and willing to participate in the process. Some women may elect never to create a vagina. It is important to provide patients and their families with resource information presenting all options and support regardless of the treatment selected.

Creation of a Functional Vagina

A vagina may be created by both nonsurgical and surgical approaches.[49,50] A successful outcome, using any method, is a vagina of adequate caliber (diameter and length), with an appropriate amount of secretion or lubrication, positioned as close as possible to an anatomic axis, to accommodate comfortable sexual intercourse. In addition, the vagina should require minimal care for maintenance. None of the current techniques achieves all of these goals, reinforcing the necessity to consider advantages and disadvantages associated with each method.

Nonsurgical Repair

The nonoperative approaches attempt to use progressive invagination of the vaginal dimple to create a vagina of adequate diameter and length. The nonoperative method of creating a functional vagina involves the use of pressure against the vaginal dimple to create a progressive invagination of the mucosa. The Frank approach for creation of a vagina involves the use of graduated hard dilators.[21] The use of vaginal dilators should be offered as first line of therapy to patients with this condition. The rationale for this approach is related to the elimination of surgery, surgical scars, and exposure to anesthesia. Recent studies have shown that the use of dilators is greater than 85% to 90% successful for the creation of a functional vagina.[51,52] It may take months to years to create a functional vagina depending on patient motivation and the frequency of dilation. The Ingram modification of this technique,[43] which involved sitting on a bicycle seat stool, took an average of 11.8 months with a range of 3 to 33 months, but more than 90% were successful in dilation.[44] Although this modification is an interesting adaptation of the Frank method, many young women initially find this technique very awkward. However, as the vagina gains length it can be helpful. The greatest success can be achieved through a combination of education, nursing support, mental health counseling, and a mentor program.

Surgical Repair

Surgical creation of a neovagina is another option for young women who fail nonoperative dilation therapy or who choose surgery after a thorough discussion with the patient (and parents/guardians as indicated) regarding the advantages and disadvantages. Surgical creation of a vagina can be accomplished by one of several techniques.[1,53,54] Discussion should fully describe that many surgical techniques will require postoperative dilation to maintain vaginal adequacy. Generally, surgery should not be used as a first-line option. Many young women are interested in a "quick fix" and think that surgery will achieve this goal. The goals of surgery are to create a neovagina that is of adequate length and width and placed in an anatomically correct axis to provide comfortable, mutually satisfying sexual intercourse. Ideally the neovagina should not require exogenous lubrication, continued postoperative dilation, or have significant surgical complications. Currently, there are multiple operations appropriate for the creation of a neovagina in patients with vaginal agenesis but no consensus on the best approach. The procedure of choice should also be determined by the surgeon's experience and success with the procedure because reoperation increases the risks of injury to surrounding organs.

The modified Abbé-McIndoe is the most commonly performed surgical technique by gynecologists in the United States. It involves harvesting a split-thickness skin graft from the patient's buttocks and placing it over a vaginal mold. An incision is made at the vaginal dimple and adequate space created to the level of the peritoneum for the mold and graft. The labia minora are then temporarily sewn together to prevent the mold from expulsion. The patient is then placed on strict hospital bed rest for 7 days.[55] The mold is then removed and the patient wears a stent continuously for 3 to 6 months, then nightly for an additional 6 months. The patient then must perform regular dilations, continuously wear the surgical mold, or engage in vaginal intercourse to prevent skin-graft contracture and loss of the neovagina. This technique is felt to have a greater than 80% functional success rate.[56] However, it leaves the patient with a potentially disfiguring scar from the donor site. Other complications include graft failure, wound infection, hematoma, and fistula formation.

More recently, investigators have used the modified Abbé-McIndoe technique but substituted other tissues as graft material to avoid unsightly graft site scarring. They include artificial dermis with human recombinant basic fibroblast growth factor spray,[57] autologous buccal mucosa,[58] Interceed absorbable adhesion barrier (Ethicon, Inc, Somerville, NJ),[59] and human amnion.[60,61]

The modified laparoscopic Vecchietti procedure creates a dilationlike neovagina in 7 to 9 days. It involves placement of an acrylic 2-cm olive-shaped bead onto the vaginal dimple that is gradually pulled superiorly by threads laparoscopically placed that are then connected to the traction device placed on the patient's abdomen. The threads are then gradually tightened approximately 1.0 to 1.5 cm per day for a week.[62,63] Postoperatively, the patients must comply with daily vaginal dilation until regularly sexually active.

The laparoscopic Davydov technique uses the patient's own pelvic peritoneum to line the neovagina. It involves dissection of the perineum to create a neovaginal space while laparoscopically mobilizing the peritoneum. The peritoneum is then sutured to the introitus and a purse-string suture closes the cranial end of the neovagina.[62,64] A vaginal mold is left in situ for 6 weeks and the patient then begins daily dilation until regularly sexually active. Complications related to laparoscopic injury and fistula formation have occurred; however, patients report similar sexual function to women with a native vagina.[65]

Patients who fail nonoperative dilation therapy or those seeking little to no postoperative upkeep may be candidates for a bowel vaginoplasty. Bowel vaginoplasty is the preferred method of most pediatric general surgeons, given the immediate and long-term correction of the anomaly. Each bowel segment has advantages and disadvantages. Other than the consideration given to a segment of adequate length and its ability to reach the perineum, the segment chosen should not interfere with fecal continence or the ability to perform necessary simultaneous reconstructive procedures.

Bowel vaginoplasty is performed by selecting an approximately 10-cm segment of bowel that can be mobilized but retain an adequate vascular pedicle to reach the perineum without traction on the pedicle or graft. It may be placed in an isoperistaltic or antiperistaltic fashion in the space dissected from the perineum to the pouch of Douglas between the bladder and rectum.[66,67] Most authors advocate anchoring the proximal bowel neovagina to avoid graft prolapse.[68–71]

Sigmoid vaginoplasty has been the most commonly used bowel segment, given its proximity to the perineum and therefore little difficulty performing a tension-free anastomosis to the introitus. The sigmoid also produces mucous that acts as a natural lubricant. However, some patients have found it excessive and at times malodorous requiring postoperative neovaginal irrigation. Patients do not require routine vaginal dilation given the large lumen, but the anastomosis at the perineum may stenose. As long as the introitus at least retains some patency, this can be addressed after puberty with an outpatient introitoplasty (**Fig. 11**). The disadvantages include the need for a laparotomy (and the resultant scar) unless a skilled laparoscopist is available who can isolate an adequate vascular pedicle.[72] Also included in this procedure are the inherent risks of wound problems at the bowel anastomosis and graft prolapse or even failure.

When an adequate segment of colon is not available for vaginoplasty, small bowel has been used. It is more difficult to mobilize to the perineum, has a smaller lumen, produces excessive mucous, and may be less durable when exposed to the potential trauma of sexual intercourse.[65] Complete stenosis has also been reported.[73]

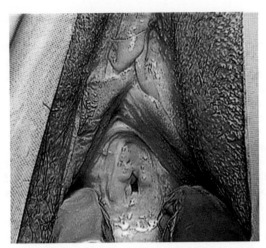

Fig. 11. An introital view after creation of colonic neovagina.

Postoperative sexual satisfaction has been assessed in a validated fashion in only a relatively small number of patients who underwent bowel vaginoplasty. Communal and colleagues[68] administered the standardized Female Sexual Function Index to 16 patients, and Hensle and colleagues[73] administered a validated Female Sexual Dysfunction Questionnaire to 44 patients. Eight of the 11 who responded and who were sexually active reported a 75% "very satisfied" rate, whereas 78% of the 36 who responded endorsed sexual satisfaction, respectively.

The Williams vulvovaginoplasty uses full-thickness skin flaps from the labia majora, creating a neovaginal pouch.[74] Vaginal dilators are then inserted daily postoperatively for a month. Unfortunately, the kangaroolike pouch is positioned at an anatomically odd angle and may have a relatively short length. Furthermore, the labia majora is hair-bearing skin, which will usually result in undesirable cosmesis. Attempts to avoid some of these concerns have included preoperative labia majora tissue expanders, the Creatsas modification, and substituting labia minora.[75–78]

Full-thickness skin grafts also have been performed using the myocutaneous rectus abdominis or gracilis and pudendal thigh fasciocutaneous flaps. Although potentially necessary in patients with more diffuse anomalies, like cloacal exstrophy, these neovaginal grafts are usually one of last resort for a diagnosis of isolated vaginal agenesis given the disfiguring scarring and risks of harvest site wound concerns and graft failure.

RUDIMENTARY UTERINE HORNS

Since approximately 7% to 10% of patients with vaginal agenesis (Müllerian aplasia) may have a rudimentary uterus with some functional endometrium and no outflow tract, it is important to maintain a high index of suspicion for an obstructed rudimentary uterine horn as a cause for recurrent pain in patients with this diagnosis. Ultrasound and/or MRI may be useful in identifying the noncommunicating uterine horn and determining whether functional endometrium is present, as evidenced by a visible endometrial stripe. Not uncommonly, laparoscopy is necessary to diagnose and remove the obstructed rudimentary noncommunicating uterine horn. Patients who have any obstruction to menstrual flow, including an obstructed uterine horn, are at increased risk of endometriosis, but experts believe the endometriosis resolves after relief of the obstruction. Early identification and excision of a blind rudimentary horn will prevent endometriosis by eliminating reflux of menstruation. If a rudimentary is horn is known to be present, patients should be counseled about symptoms of an ectopic pregnancy and the need for immediate evaluation, because spontaneous pregnancies have been reported.[79]

CERVICAL ATRESIA/HYPOGENESIS

Cervical agenesis and dysgenesis are rare[54,80–82] but are extremely important to differentiate from diagnoses like transverse vaginal septum or vaginal atresia/segmental vaginal agenesis. A correct diagnosis allows appropriate counseling before surgical intervention as the classic management recommendation for this condition is hysterectomy. Patients may present with primary amenorrhea, cyclic or chronic abdominal or pelvic pain, and/or a distended uterus. Ultrasonography can aid in defining the anatomy, yet an MRI allows superior identification of the presence and integrity of the cervix.[18] The adequacy of the cervix is the crucial part of the decision to leave the uterine structure in place and anastomose to the native lower vagina or a newly created vagina. The diagnosis and management of this Müllerian anomaly are both challenging and controversial.

DISORDERS OF THE UTERUS
Complete Uterine Septum

The septate uterus has a smooth, normal external surface at the fundus, but the endometrial cavity is split into two by a midline septum. Most uterine fusion/duplication abnormalities do not require surgical intervention; however, the septate uterus is well known for the associated obstetric concerns. If patients experience pain, recurrent miscarriage, infertility, or premature labor, the abnormality should be repaired by hysteroscopic resection.[83–89] The situation is more controversial in young women in whom the diagnosis is made in late adolescence or early adulthood. The decision to surgically intervene before attempts at pregnancy still remains unclear. The presence of a concomitant vaginal septum may influence the timing of intervention. A combined approach may be considered.

Bicornuate Uterus

The uterine fundus is deeply indented, often heart-shaped, in patients with a bicornuate uterus. In most cases, a single cervix is present. The level of the indentation of the fundus can be complete, partial or arcuate. Historically, treatment in the form of a metroplasty, had been recommended. Presently, no surgical intervention is recommended and patients are followed closely for obstetric concerns. In most cases the vagina is normal.

Unicornuate Uterus

A unicornuate uterus is a single uterine horn that has only a single round ligament and fallopian tube, sometimes referred to as a hemiuterus. The opposite uterine horn (hemiuterus), round ligament, and fallopian tube, derived from the opposite Müllerian duct, may be absent or underdeveloped. Variations in the degree of hemiuterine development can occur producing a noncommunicating uterine horn (hemiuterus) on the contralateral side with or without active endometrium. A single unicornuate uterus communicates with a single cervix and a normal vagina. As suspected with unilateral impairment in Müllerian development, associated renal anomalies are common.

Patients with a unicornuate uterus are at increased risk of premature labor and breech presentation.[42,90] As in other obstructive anomalies, endometriosis and subsequent fertility issues may be significant in patients with an associated obstructed uterine horn or hemiuterus.

PREGNANCY OUTCOME IN WOMEN WITH MÜLLERIAN DUCT ANOMALIES

Women with Müllerian duct anomalies seem to have an increased rate of unexplained infertility, endometriosis, spontaneous abortion, breech presentation, and premature delivery.[5,91–94] More long term outcome data are necessary to fully determine the obstetric prognosis of women with Müllerian duct anomalies associated with other urogenital or anorectal malformations. Women who have had vaginal atresia/lower vaginal agenesis/segmental vaginal atresia corrected by the creation of a neovagina are able to become pregnant and to maintain a pregnancy, if a well developed cervix and uterus are present. Patients with vaginal agenesis always should be counseled regarding opportunities for adoption and surrogacy. The wider use of assisted reproductive technologies also will enhance the reproductive capacity of women with congenital abnormalities of the reproductive tract.

ADDITIONAL READING

Laufer MR, Goldstein DP, Hendren WH. Structural abnormalities of the female reproductive tract. In: Emans SJ, Laufer MR, Goldstein DP. Pediatric and Adolescent Gynecology (Fifth Edition), Philadelphia: Lippincott Williams & Wilkins Publishing Company, 2005. p. 334–416.

REFERENCES

1. Usta IM, Awwad JT, Usta JA, et al. Imperforate hymen: report of an unusual familial occurrence. Obstet Gynecol 1993;82:655–6.
2. American Society for Reproductive Medicine Practice Committee. Current evaluation of amenorrhea. Fertil Steril 2006;86:S148–55.
3. Counseller VS. Congenital absence and traumatic obliteration of vagina and its treatment with inlaying Thiersch grafts. Am J Obstet Gynecol 1938;36:632–8.
4. Frank R. The formation of an artificial vagina without operation. Am J Obstet Gynecol 1938;35:1053–5.
5. Rock JA, Zacur HA, Dlugi AM, et al. Pregnancy success following surgical correction of imperforate hymen and complete transverse vaginal septum. Obstet Gynecol 1982;59:448–51.
6. Stray-Pedersen B, Stray-Pedersen S. Etiologic factors and subsequent reproductive performance in 195 couples with a prior history of habitual abortion. Am J Obstet Gynecol 1984;148:140–6.
7. Croak AJ, Gebhart JB, Klingele CJ, et al. Therapeutic strategies for vaginal Mullerian agenesis. J Reprod Med 2003;48:395–401.
8. Duckler L. Squamous cell carcinoma developing in an artificial vagina. Obstet Gynecol 1972;40:35–8.
9. Laufer MR. Congenital absence of the vagina: in search of the perfect solution. When, and by what technique, should a vagina be created? Curr Opin Obstet Gynecol 2002;14:441–4.
10. Murray JM, Gambrell RD Jr. Complete and partial vaginal agenesis. J Reprod Med 1979;22:101–5.

11. Reindollar RH, Byrd JR, McDonough PG. Delayed sexual development: a study of 252 patients. Am J Obstet Gynecol 1981;140:371–80.
12. Singh J, Devi YL. Pregnancy following surgical correction of nonfused mullerian bulbs and absent vagina. Obstet Gynecol 1983;61:267–9.
13. Buttram VC Jr, Gibbons WE. Mullerian anomalies: a proposed classification. (An analysis of 144 cases). Fertil Steril 1979;32:40–6.
14. Soares SR, Barbosa dos Reis MM, Camargos AF. Diagnostic accuracy of sono-hysterography, transvaginal sonography, and hysterosalpingography in patients with uterine cavity diseases. Fertil Steril 2000;73:406–11.
15. Solomons E. Conception and delivery following construction of an artificial vagina; report of a case. Obstet Gynecol 1956;7:329–33.
16. Wierrani F, Bodner K, Spangler B, et al. "Z"-plasty of the transverse vaginal septum using Garcia's procedure and the Grunberger modification. Fertil Steril 2003;79:608–12.
17. Markham SM, Parmley TH, Murphy AA, et al. Cervical agenesis combined with vaginal agenesis diagnosed by magnetic resonance imaging. Fertil Steril 1987; 48:143–5.
18. Mayer CAJ. Ober Verdoppelungen des Uterus and ihre Arten, nebst Bemerkun-gen uber Hasenscharte ind Wolfsrachen. J Chir Auger 1829;13:525.
19. Petrozza JC, Gray MR, Davis AJ, et al. Congenital absence of the uterus and vagina is not commonly transmitted as a dominant genetic trait: outcomes of surrogate pregnancies. Fertil Steril 1997;67:387–9.
20. Martinez-Mora J, Isnard R, Castellvi Λ, et al. Neovagina in vaginal agenesis: surgical methods and long-term results. J Pediatr Surg 1992;27:10–4.
21. Sadler TW. Langman's medical embryology. Philadelphia: Williams & Wilkins; 1990.
22. Bakri YN, al-Sugair A, Hugosson C. Bicornuate nonfused rudimentary uterine horns with functioning endometria and complete cervical-vaginal agenesis: magnetic resonance diagnosis. Fertil Steril 1992;58:620–1.
23. Casey AC, Laufer MR. Cervical agenesis: septic death after surgery. Obstet Gynecol 1997;90:706–7.
24. Strickland JL, Cameron W, Kranz K. Long-term satisfaction of adults under-going McIndoe vaginoplasty as adolescents. Adolesc Pediatr Gynecol 1993; 6:135–7.
25. Batzer FR, Corson SL, Gocial B, et al. Genetic offspring in patients with vaginal agenesis: specific medical and legal issues. Am J Obstet Gynecol 1992;167: 1288–92.
26. Bennett MJ, Berry JV. Preterm labour and congenital malformations of the uterus. Ultrasound Med Biol 1979;5:83–5.
27. Lin PC, Bhatnagar KP, Nettleton GS, et al. Female genital anomalies affecting reproduction. Fertil Steril 2002;78:899–915.
28. Peña A, Levitt MA, Bischoff A, et al. Rectovestibular fistula—rarely recognized associated gynecologic anomalies. J Pediatr Surg 2009; Accepted.
29. Heinonen PK. Complete septate uterus with longitudinal vaginal septum. Fertil Steril 2006;85:700–5.
30. Buss JG, Lee RA. McIndoe procedure for vaginal agenesis: results and compli-cations. Mayo Clin Proc 1989;64:758–61.
31. McIndoe A, Banister J. An operation for the cure of congenital absence of the vagina. Br J Obstet Gynaecol 1938;45:490–4.
32. Shatzkes DR, Haller JO, Velcek FT. Imaging of uterovaginal anomalies in the pedi-atric patient. Urol Radiol 1991;13:58–66.

33. Simon C, Martinez L, Pardo F, et al. Mullerian defects in women with normal reproductive outcome. Fertil Steril 1991;56:1192–3.
34. Smith NA, Laufer MR. Obstructed hemivagina and ipsilateral renal anomaly (OHVIRA) syndrome: management and follow-up. Fertil Steril 2007;87:918–22.
35. Joki-Erkkila MM, Heinonen PK. Presenting and long-term clinical implications and fecundity in females with obstructing vaginal malformations. J Pediatr Adolesc Gynecol 2003;16:307–12.
36. Troiano RN, McCarthy SM. Mullerian duct anomalies: imaging and clinical issues. Radiology 2004;233:19–34.
37. Kresowik J, Ryan GL, Austin JC, et al. Ultrasound-assisted repair of a unique case of distal vaginal agenesis. Fertil Steril 2007;87:976, e979–912.
38. Pellerito JS, McCarthy SM, Doyle MB, et al. Diagnosis of uterine anomalies: relative accuracy of MR imaging, endovaginal sonography, and hysterosalpingography. Radiology 1992;183:795–800.
39. Oppelt P, Renner SP, Kellermann A, et al. Clinical aspects of Mayer-Rokitansky-Kuester-Hauser syndrome: recommendations for clinical diagnosis and staging. Humanit Rep 2006;21:792–7.
40. Pittock ST, Babovic-Vuksanovic D, Lteif A. Mayer-Rokitansky-Kuster-Hauser anomaly and its associated malformations. Am J Med Genet A 2005;135:314–6.
41. Strubbe EH, Willemsen WN, Lemmens JA, et al. Mayer-Rokitansky-Kuster-Hauser syndrome: distinction between two forms based on excretory urographic, sonographic, and laparoscopic findings. AJR Am J Roentgenol 1993;160:331–4.
42. The American Fertility Society classifications of adnexal adhesions, distal tubal occlusion, tubal occlusion secondary to tubal ligation, tubal pregnancies, mullerian anomalies and intrauterine adhesions. Fertil Steril 1988;49:944–55.
43. Ingram JM. The bicycle seat stool in the treatment of vaginal agenesis and stenosis: a preliminary report. Am J Obstet Gynecol 1981;140:867–73.
44. Roberts CP, Haber MJ, Rock JA. Vaginal creation for mullerian agenesis. Am J Obstet Gynecol 2001;185:1349–52.
45. von Rokitansky KE. Ober die sogenannten Verdoppelungen des Uterus. Med Jb Ost Staat 1938;26:39.
46. Evans TN, Poland ML, Boving RL. Vaginal malformations. Am J Obstet Gynecol 1981;141:910–20.
47. Rotmensch J, Rosenshein N, Dillon M, et al. Carcinoma arising in the neovagina: case report and review of the literature. Obstet Gynecol 1983;61:534–6.
48. Simpson JL. Genetics of the female reproductive ducts. Am J Med Genet 1999;89:224–39.
49. Scanlan KA, Pozniak MA, Fagerholm M, et al. Value of transperineal sonography in the assessment of vaginal atresia. AJR Am J Roentgenol 1990;154:545–8.
50. Suidan FG, Azoury RS. The transverse vaginal septum: a clinicopathologic evaluation. Obstet Gynecol 1979;54:278–83.
51. Cramer DW, Ravnikar VA, Craighill M, et al. Mullerian aplasia associated with maternal deficiency of galactose-1-phosphate uridyl transferase. Fertil Steril 1987;47:930–4.
52. Fedele L, Dorta M, Brioschi D, et al. Magnetic resonance imaging in Mayer-Rokitansky-Kuster-Hauser syndrome. Obstet Gynecol 1990;76:593–6.
53. Hauser GA, Schreiner WE. [Mayer-Rokitansky-Kuester syndrome. Rudimentary solid bipartite uterus with solid vagina]. Schweiz Med Wochenschr 1961;91:381–4 [In German].

54. Nussbaum Blask AR, Sanders R, Rock JA. Obstructed uterovaginal anomalies: demonstration with sonography. Part II: teenagers. Pediatr Radiol 1991;179:84–8.
55. McIndoe A. The treatment of congenital absence and obliterative conditions of the vagina. Br J Plast Surg 1950;2:254–67.
56. Klingele CJ, Gebhart JB, Croak AJ, et al. McIndoe procedure for vaginal agenesis: long-term outcome and effect on quality of life. Am J Obstet Gynecol 2003;189:1569–72.
57. Noguchi S, Nakatsuka M, Sugiyama Y, et al. Use of artificial dermis and recombinant basic fibroblast growth factor for creating a neovagina in a patient with Mayer-Rokitansky-Kuster-Hauser syndrome. Humanit Rep 2004;19:1629–32.
58. Lin WC, Chang CY, Shen YY, et al. Use of autologous buccal mucosa for vaginoplasty: a study of eight cases. Humanit Rep 2003;18:604–7.
59. Motoyama S, Laoag-Fernandez JB, Mochizuki S, et al. Vaginoplasty with Interceed absorbable adhesion barrier for complete squamous epithelialization in vaginal agenesis. Am J Obstet Gynecol 2003;188:1260–4.
60. Ashworth MF, Morton KE, Dewhurst J, et al. Vaginoplasty using amnion. Obstet Gynecol 1986;67:443–6.
61. Nisolle M, Donnez J. Vaginoplasty using amniotic membranes in cases of vaginal agenesis or after vaginectomy. J Gynecol Surg 1992;8:25–30.
62. Ismail IS, Cutner AS, Creighton SM. Laparoscopic vaginoplasty: alternative techniques in vaginal reconstruction. BJOG 2006;113:340–3.
63. Veronikis DK, McClure GB, Nichols DH. The Vecchietti operation for constructing a neovagina: indications, instrumentation, and techniques. Obstet Gynecol 1997; 90:301–4.
64. Langebrekke A, Istre O, Busund B, et al. Laparoscopic assisted colpoiesis according to Davydov. Acta Obstet Gynecol Scand 1998;77:1027–8.
65. Giannesi A, Marchiole P, Benchaib M, et al. Sexuality after laparoscopic Davydov in patients affected by congenital complete vaginal agenesis associated with uterine agenesis or hypoplasia. Humanit Rep 2005;20:2954–7.
66. Karateke A, Gurbuz A, Haliloglu B, et al. Intestinal vaginoplasty: is it optimal treatment of vaginal agenesis? A pilot study. Surgical method of sigmoid colon vaginoplasty in vaginal agenesis. Int Urogynecol J Pelvic Floor Dysfunct 2006;17: 40–5.
67. O'Connor JL, DeMarco RT, Pope JCT, et al. Bowel vaginoplasty in children: a retrospective review. J Pediatr Surg 2004;39:1205–8.
68. Communal PH, Chevret-Measson M, Golfier F, et al. Sexuality after sigmoid colpopoiesis in patients with Mayer-Rokitansky-Kuster-Hauser Syndrome. Fertil Steril 2003;80:600–6.
69. Ekinci S, Karnak I, Ciftci AO, et al. Sigmoid colon vaginoplasty in children. Eur J Pediatr Surg 2006;16:182–7.
70. Khen-Dunlop N, Lortat-Jacob S, Thibaud E, et al. Rokitansky syndrome: clinical experience and results of sigmoid vaginoplasty in 23 young girls. J Urol 2007; 177:1107–11.
71. Parsons JK, Gearhart SL, Gearhart JP. Vaginal reconstruction utilizing sigmoid colon: complications and long-term results. J Pediatr Surg 2002;37:629–33.
72. Darai E, Toullalan O, Besse O, et al. Anatomic and functional results of laparoscopic-perineal neovagina construction by sigmoid colpoplasty in women with Rokitansky's syndrome. Humanit Rep 2003;18:2454–9.
73. Hensle TW, Shabsigh A, Shabsigh R, et al. Sexual function following bowel vaginoplasty. J Urol 2006;175:2283–6.

74. Williams EA. Congenital absence of the vagina: a simple operation for its relief. J Obstet Gynaecol Br Commonw 1964;71:511–2.

75. Chudacoff RM, Alexander J, Alvero R, et al. Tissue expansion vaginoplasty for treatment of congenital vaginal agenesis. Obstet Gynecol 1996;87:865–8.

76. Creatsas G, Deligeoroglou E. Expert opinion: vaginal aplasia: creation of a neovagina following the Creatsas vaginoplasty. Eur J Obstet Gynecol Reprod Biol 2007; 131:248–52.

77. Creatsas G, Deligeoroglou E, Makrakis E, et al. Creation of a neovagina following Williams vaginoplasty and the Creatsas modification in 111 patients with Mayer-Rokitansky-Kuster-Hauser syndrome. Fertil Steril 2001;76:1036–40.

78. Purushothaman V. Horse shoe flap vaginoplasty—a new technique of vaginal reconstruction with labia minora flaps for primary vaginal agenesis. Br J Plast Surg 2005;58:934–9.

79. Lodi A. [Clinical and statistical study on vaginal malformations at the Obstetrical and Gynecological Clinic in Milano, 1906–50.] Ann Ostet Ginecol 1951;73: 1246–85 [In Italian].

80. Bates GW, Wiser WL. A technique for uterine conservation in adolescents with vaginal agenesis and a functional uterus. Obstet Gynecol 1985;66:290–4.

81. Economy KE, Barnewolt C, Laufer MR. A comparison of MRI and laparoscopy in detecting pelvic structures in cases of vaginal agenesis. J Pediatr Adolesc Gynecol 2002;15:101–4.

82. Willemsen WN. Combination of the Mayer-Rokitansky-Kuster and Klippel-Feil syndrome—a case report and literature review. Eur J Obstet Gynecol Reprod Biol 1982;13:229–35.

83. Coney PJ. Effects of vaginal agenesis on the adolescent: prognosis for normal sexual and psychological adjustment. Adolesc Pediatr Gynecol 1992;5:8–12.

84. Duncan PA, Shapiro LR, Stangel JJ, et al. The MURCS association: Mullerian duct aplasia, renal aplasia, and cervicothoracic somite dysplasia. J Pediatr 1979;95: 399–402.

85. Fielding C. Obstetric studies in women with congenital solitary kidneys. Acta Obstet Gynecol Scand 1965;44:555–62.

86. Raga F, Bonilla-Musoles F, Blanes J, et al. Congenital Mullerian anomalies: diagnostic accuracy of three-dimensional ultrasound. Fertil Steril 1996;65:523–8.

87. Thompson DP, Lynn HB. Genital anomalies associated with solitary kidney. Mayo Clin Proc 1966;41:538–48.

88. Valdes C, Malini S, Malinak LR. Ultrasound evaluation of female genital tract anomalies: a review of 64 cases. Am J Obstet Gynecol 1984;149:285–92.

89. Weijenborg P, Kuile M. The effect of a group programme on women with the Mayer-Rokitansky-Kuster-Hauser Syndrome. Br J Obstet Gynaecol 2000;107: 365–8.

90. Farber M. Congenital atresia of the uterine cervix. Semin Reprod Endocrinol 1986;4:33–8.

91. Abbe R. New method of creating a vagina in a case of congenital absence. Med Rec 1898;54:836–8.

92. Erdogan E, Okan G, Daragenli O. Uterus didelphys with unilateral obstructed hemivagina and renal agenesis on the same side. Acta Obstet Gynecol Scand 1992;71:76–7.

93. Garcia RF. Z-plasty for correction of congenital transferse vaginal septum. Am J Obstet Gynecol 1967;99:1164–5.

94. Kuster H. Uterus bipartitus solidus rudimentarius cum vagina solida. Z Geburtshilfe Gynakol 1910;67:692.

Urologic Issues in the Pediatric and Adolescent Gynecology Patient

Elizabeth B. Yerkes, MD

KEYWORDS

- Urinary tract infection • Incontinence • Enuresis
- Vulvovaginitis • Constipation • Dysuria
- Interlabial mass • Biofeedback

Based on the close proximity of the organ systems and difficulty in localizing symptoms, there is natural overlap between the fields of pediatric and adolescent urology and gynecology. This article lends the urologist's perspective on perineal pain, repetitive posturing or perineal compression, vulvovaginitis, vaginal discharge, and interlabial masses. The fine points of obtaining an elimination history are shared, and the management of recurrent urinary tract infection (UTI) and UTI-type symptoms is discussed. The spectrum of daytime incontinence and elimination disorders is outlined to guide initial management in these challenging patients. A somewhat surprising role of constipation, or functional fecal retention, in genitourinary complaints recurs throughout the article (**Box 1**). The benefits of learning pelvic floor relaxation, through basic voiding modification or formal biofeedback therapy, for management of genitourinary complaints are addressed. Two review cases are included at the end of the article to put the history and physical examination to work.

The reader should understand that evidence-based management of these complaints continues to evolve, with new terminology and classification systems at every turn.[1,2] The term *dysfunctional elimination syndrome* replaced the term *dysfunctional voiding* as we gained an appreciation of the close relation between urinary symptoms, constipation, recurrent UTIs, and vesicoureteral reflux.[1] New terminology was recently presented by the International Children's Continence Society (ICCS),[2] and further updates are likely forthcoming. This article is intended to provide a practical guide for initial evaluation and management of the common issues. An effort is made to include current (in italics) and some more familiar terminology to avoid confusion.

Regardless of the terminology, it is important to pinpoint the specific issues for any given child so that the program may be tailored to her needs. Successful therapy is

Northwestern University's Feinberg School of Medicine, Division of Urology, Children's Memorial Hospital, 2300 Children's Plaza #24, Chicago, IL 60614, USA
E-mail address: eyerkes@childrensmemorial.org

Obstet Gynecol Clin N Am 36 (2009) 69–84
doi:10.1016/j.ogc.2008.12.006
0889-8545/08/$ – see front matter © 2009 Elsevier Inc. All rights reserved.

Box 1
Constipation and the pediatric and adolescent gynecology patient

Recurrent UTI or UTI-type symptoms

Daytime incontinence

Repetitive posturing or perineal compression

Perineal pain

Vulvovaginitis, recurrent or persistent

Lichen sclerosus

time-intensive, in the office and by telephone, but clinical progress yields great dividends in terms of the self-esteem and social adjustment of the child or teen with urinary issues.

NEUROPHYSIOLOGY OF THE GENITOURINARY TRACT

A limited review of pelvic neurophysiology and reflex mechanisms is a relevant prelude to any discussion of genitourinary issues. Voluntary control of micturition requires modulation of sacral reflex pathways by the brain stem. Storage and elimination involve the sacral parasympathetic and somatic nerves. Urine is stored at low pressures, based on the viscoelastic properties of the bladder. During filling, there is a normal increase in sphincter tone. The first step of voluntary micturition is relaxation of the striated urinary sphincter. Without relaxation of the external sphincter, coordinated or synergic micturition cannot occur.[3] This highlights the importance of pelvic floor relaxation in the pediatric and adolescent gynecology (PAG) patient who has urinary complaints. Nonrelaxation or overactivity of the pelvic floor can be learned in response to a painful stimulus, stressful social circumstances, or psychologic disturbance.[4] Active sphincter contraction during a bladder contraction (detrusor external sphincter dyssynergia) is, however, highly suspicious for a neurologic process and should be thoroughly evaluated.[5]

Sensory information from the external genitalia and rectum also travels along the sacral nerve roots. This relation accounts for the common association of genitourinary and fecal issues and explains some of the difficulties in localizing genitourinary symptoms. Sensation and function are impaired to varying degrees in children with abnormalities of the conus medullaris, distal spinal canal, or sacral nerve roots (ie, tethered cord syndrome, sacral agenesis).

EVALUATION OF GENITOURINARY COMPLAINTS

A comprehensive elimination history should be obtained to establish a diagnosis and direct management. Unfortunately, the child or teen is often embarrassed and affected by comments from peers or family members. The emotionally charged situation is further complicated by difficulty in localizing and articulating associated symptoms. A supportive rapport is important, but straight talk for the child and parent is also necessary to maintain a working relationship.

The history should include daytime voiding habits, nighttime continence, fluid intake and diet, frequency and quality of bowel movements, and any posturing or holding behaviors noted. The child's altered perception of time, combined with the parents' lack of specific knowledge of the child's independent toilet habits, also makes the accuracy of the initial information suspect.

Completion of an intake and elimination diary is a useful tool for all parties to understand the situation. From a practical standpoint, this is best accomplished on weekends, but elimination habits may differ at home and at school. The patient and parent should be provided with a sample diary (**Table 1**) and a urine hat or other measuring device. Timing and quality of bowel movements should be recorded. Fluid intake is an important element, because bladder sensation is impaired by slow bladder filling.

It is also useful to learn how incontinence episodes are being handled by the parent and child. Is the child hiding underwear? Are absorptive pads or garments used? Have others noticed an odor or made unhelpful comments? Have there been punishments?

Eliciting a history of developmental or behavioral conditions and diagnoses is important, because these conditions may affect the child's ability to achieve continence and may limit the provider's ability to obtain a clear history. It may have an impact on her recognition of or response to bladder activity, as in attention-deficit/hyperactivity disorder, sensory integration disorders, developmental delay, spastic quadriplegia, and spinal dysraphism. Spastic quadriplegia may affect her ability to get to the bathroom in time. A history of sexual abuse, another major traumatic life event, or an underlying behavioral or psychiatric diagnosis would indicate a need for early involvement of child psychology in the treatment program.[6–8]

Any concerns regarding the child's development or any changes in her coordination or stamina may suggest a neurologic influence. Significantly delayed ambulation in an otherwise developmentally normal incontinent child could suggest occult spinal dysraphism or tethered cord. Back, buttock, or posterior leg pain or changes in gait could suggest a tethered cord. Acute vision changes or changes in sensation or coordination could also suggest a neurologic condition.

After eliciting a full history and gaining the confidence of the child and parent, a comprehensive examination is completed. Special attention is given to the abdomen, genitalia, spine, and lower extremities. The abdominal examination may reveal a distended or painful bladder or palpable stool in the lower abdomen. Examination of the genitalia would detect any congenital anomaly, inflammation, mass, evidence of trauma or abuse, or urine pooled within the vaginal vault. The anus is inspected for lesions and for general tone and anal wink, but a formal digital examination is not typically warranted. The entire spine is screened for neurocutaneous abnormalities, such as a dimple, hairy tuft, vascular malformation, lipoma, skin appendage, or short or asymmetric gluteal cleft **Fig. 1**. Assessment of the lower extremities includes general coordination and sensation, symmetric tone, deep tendon reflexes, development of the calf muscles, and contour of the pedal arch, again looking for suggestion of a neurologic process.

A clean-catch urine specimen should be obtained on all voiding patients. A urinalysis with microscopy screens for glucose and protein, and it allows quantification of hematuria, pyuria, and epithelial cells. A culture is obtained if infection is suspected based on symptoms or history. Consider repeating the specimen before treatment if

Table 1					
Elimination diary					
Date	Time	Food intake (eg, 1 slice of pizza, 1 apple)	Fluid intake (eg, 8 oz of milk, 12 oz of cola)	Amount of urine voided (oz)	Bowel movement (Large and hard, small hard pebbles, "hot dog")	Other (Dry, damp, wet, soaked; urgency; pain; bowel accident; "potty dance" or other posturing)

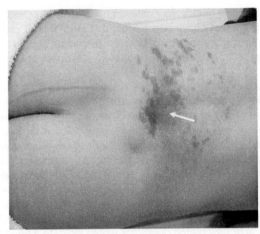

Fig. 1. Neurocutaneous abnormality of the lumbosacral spine. Arrow demonstrates hairy tuft overlying vascular patch.

the urinalysis and culture results are inconsistent, particularly if the urinalysis seems benign but the culture is positive.

Although not necessarily warranted during initial management of genitourinary complaints, there are several radiologic studies that may be elected. Adequacy of bladder emptying can be assessed by ultrasound (**Fig. 2**). Imaging of the kidneys by ultrasound or a voiding cystourethrogram would be indicated only in the setting of febrile or recurrent urinary infection or high suspicion for an anatomic or neurologic abnormality.

A plain film of the abdomen is useful in assessing the fecal load and its role in the patient's complaints, although there is no universally accepted classification and there is some variability in correlation with symptoms.[9,10] Attention to the rectal impaction and the amount of formed stool throughout the colon is important (**Fig. 3**). The abdominal radiograph may also reveal a gross bony abnormality in occult spinal dysraphism or sacral agenesis (**Fig. 4**). Use of a visual aid, such as the Bristol Stool Scale, to help the child describe the stool,[11] in combination with a thorough elimination diary, is usually adequate. The parent, however, may require firm radiographic proof of constipation to comply with medical therapy.

Transabdominal ultrasound for measurement of the rectal diameter is gaining attention as a tool for diagnosing constipation and monitoring therapeutic progress.[12,13]

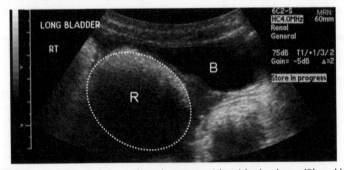

Fig. 2. Longitudinal ultrasound view of modest postvoid residual volume (B) and large rectal fecal load (R).

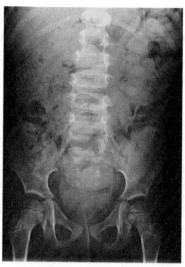

Fig. 3. Abdominal radiograph to assess fecal load. Note extensive stool in the rectum and throughout the colon.

The diameter is measured in the transverse view when at least 3 hours have passed since the last bowel movement and if there is no acute urge to defecate. A mean diameter of 4.9 cm in constipated children versus 2.1 cm in controls has been demonstrated, although there is some crossover in diameter between clinically constipated children and normal children.[12] Office ultrasound and digital rectal examination are equally efficacious in diagnosing fecal impaction, limiting the indication for digital examination. Ultrasound could eliminate further radiographs or unpleasant examinations as the child's progress is monitored, and it could provide visual proof of constipation for the skeptical parent.[13]

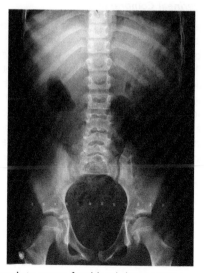

Fig. 4. Abdominal radiograph to assess fecal load demonstrates sacral agenesis.

COMMON ISSUES IN THE PEDIATRIC AND ADOLESCENT GYNECOLOGY PATIENT: THE UROLOGIST'S PERSPECTIVE

The following complaints are seen in the urology office and the PAG office. Note that constipation figures prominently for each complaint. Suggestions for management of constipation are discussed elsewhere in this article.

Perineal Pain

Evaluation of perineal pain should begin by determining if the pain is related to urination (*dysuria*) or if it is seemingly random. If dysuria is present, attempt to determine whether there is primarily pain as the urine hits the perineum (*external dysuria*) or whether there is suprapubic discomfort or urethral burning (*internal dysuria*). This distinction is difficult for younger patients to understand. Once infection is ruled out, application of a bland ointment, such as vitamin A and D containing petrolatum-based ointment, provides a barrier to moisture and protects the tissues. Hydration to reduce irritation from concentrated urine may also be helpful.

It is important to determine whether some element of constipation is present. Habitual withholding of defecation with increased pelvic floor tone can result in perineal discomfort and dysuria. Constipation can lead to an overactive bladder or a large-capacity bladder with poor sensation and poor emptying.[14] Bladder spasms associated with the overactive bladder may be experienced as pain at the urethral meatus. Provide a visual aid, such as the Bristol Stool Scale, to help the patient describe her stools.[11] If no such aid is readily available, food analogies, such as "grapes," "Baby Ruth," or "hot dog," are easily understood. Large soft stools daily or large soft stools more than once daily could also indicate a significant fecal load.

Query regarding potential injury, including prior severe dermatitis or vaginitis, traumatic radiologic testing, anal fissure, and sexual abuse. Examination for vaginal discharge and for evidence of trauma or abuse is performed. While examining the perineum, ask the child to put one finger on the painful area. Intense pain or hypersensitivity with otherwise normal-appearing tissue may suggest a pain syndrome or neuropathy.

Repetitive Posturing or Perineal Compression

Posturing is typically a response to uninhibited bladder contractions associated with an overactive bladder or with postponement of urination. The parent may have observed the posturing or repetitive behavior for years but never connected it to postponement of urination. Vincent's curtsy is the classic maneuver in which the child suddenly squats, pressing a heel into the perineum. The child may fidget, dance, hold the genitalia, or "freeze" with the legs pressed together or crossed. The posturing may occur in a standing, seated, or squatting position. Each of these maneuvers directly compresses the perineum or contracts the pelvic floor to abort the bladder contraction reflexively and prevent loss of urine. Although aware that an urgent event has occurred, the child may subsequently deny the need to visit the toilet.

Vulvovaginitis and Vaginal Discharge

Evaluation and management of constipation should be part of the management of vulvovaginitis as well. Constipation is commonly present in children who have bacterial and nonspecific vulvovaginitis and anogenital dermatologic conditions.[15,16] If the vaginitis is chronic and painful, the child may learn to withhold bowel movements for fear of pain, further aggravating the constipation and perineal colonization with coliform bacteria.

If the constipation is not addressed, the child may be refractory to conventional treatments. Adherence to a consistent bowel program results in remission of bacterial vaginitis.[16]

Lichen sclerosus of the anogenital region most commonly presents with pruritus, but constipation is present in more than 60% of these cases.[15] Failure to recognize and treat the constipation may further aggravate this chronic dermatologic condition.

An ectopic ureter to the distal urethra, perineum, or vagina should be included in the differential diagnosis for an infant with episodic thick vaginal discharge. The typical presentation of constant dampness from an ectopic ureter is not discernable in children before toilet training.

Interlabial Masses of Urethral Origin

A variety of interlabial masses present during early childhood, most of which are benign lesions. Attention to presenting features and local landmarks typically allows the diagnosis without radiographic evaluation. Several of these lesions are related to the vagina, but several are urethral in origin. These lesions are briefly discussed in this section.

Paraurethral cysts or Skene's cysts typically present in infancy as a smooth whitish painless paraurethral mass with fine overlying vessels. The lesions result from obstruction of the paraurethral gland ducts. The eccentric position of the cyst may cause deviation or splaying of the urinary stream or may deform the anterior vaginal wall. Most lesions rupture spontaneously or resolve within the first several months. If the cyst persists or is symptomatic, simple incision or needle aspiration results in full resolution as well.[17]

A rather large purplish congested mass fills much of the vestibule in cases of prolapsed ureterocele. The ureterocele has an eccentric position that may make it difficult to visualize the urethral meatus, but labial retraction reveals a normal hymen. The prolapse can result in bladder outlet obstruction or urosepsis if bacteriuria is present. Ectopic ureteroceles are typically associated with the upper pole of a duplicated system and naturally distort the bladder outlet. If the diagnosis is in question, renal and bladder ultrasound can guide initial management.[17] Before onset of congestion, the acute prolapse can reduce spontaneously. Urgent urologic consultation is indicated for any prolapsed ureterocele.

Urethral prolapse most commonly presents with bloody spotting in the underwear, although dysuria, urinary retention, and perineal discomfort occur in some girls. The prolapse may be circumferential or partial; in circumferential prolapse, the tissue resembles a congested donut surrounding the urethral meatus. Focal ischemia may be present **Fig. 5**. Four- to 5-year-old African-American girls are the most commonly affected. The shearing of mucosa is not well understood but may be attributable to the prepubertal hypoestrogenic state or straining. A recent history of coughing or constipation is often elicited. Conservative therapy consists of sitz baths, management of constipation, and application of a short course of conjugated estrogen cream or emollients to help the tissue recess. Surgical excision is indicated in the event of necrosis, refractory inflammation, or persistent symptoms after conservative therapy.[17]

URINARY TRACT INFECTION AND URINARY TRACT INFECTION TYPE SYMPTOMS

UTIs are one of the most common medical issues addressed by pediatric urologists. The first step in management is to ascertain whether there is truly infection or whether there are only UTI-type symptoms, such as external dysuria, urinary frequency, urinary urgency, and urge incontinence. The behavioral modifications used to treat UTIs and

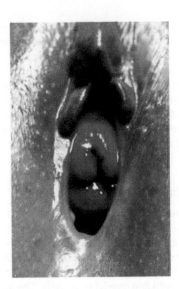

Fig. 5. Urethral prolapse.

UTI-type symptoms are essentially the same, but antibiotic therapy (treatment or prophylactic) or radiographic evaluation would be reserved for true infections.

As previously discussed, abnormal voiding habits, constipation, and UTIs are closely related.[1,9,10,18] Infections and abnormal elimination occur in a vicious cycle. As a result of painful urination during an infection, the child may learn to postpone urination. Postponement may increase the risk for recurrent infection, but the pelvic floor contraction used to postpone urination may result in incomplete and high-pressure voiding and inefficient defecation (**Fig. 6**). Constipation further impairs the efficiency of urination[14] and may increase perineal colonization, thereby increasing the risk for infection and so on. Constipation could be the entry point for this cycle as well. Constipation can result in unstable bladder contractions (*overactive bladder*), involuntary loss of urine, poor coordination of micturition, and a large-capacity bladder

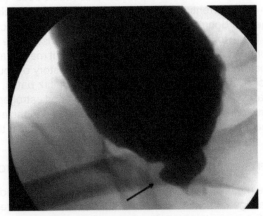

Fig. 6. "Spinning top" urethra on voiding cystourethrogram suggests incomplete relaxation of pelvic floor during urination.

with inefficient emptying (*underactive bladder*). Invagination of the posterior bladder wall, mechanical obstruction of the bladder outlet, irritation of the trigone, and impaired bladder contractility by shared neural pathways are potential means by which rectal distention from constipation can affect bladder function (**Fig. 7**).[14,19]

Vesicoureteral reflux is also commonly present in children who have a UTI. In most cases, the reflux is identified during radiographic evaluation of a first UTI. In general, infection does not cause vesicoureteral reflux, and reflux does not cause a UTI. The presence of reflux, however, complicates UTIs by allowing the bacteria access to the upper urinary tract. In cases of high-grade (high volume) reflux, urinary stasis occurs as refluxed urine returns to the bladder again after voiding. Bacteriuria may be more difficult to clear when urinary stasis is present. Abnormal elimination habits decrease the likelihood of spontaneous resolution of vesicoureteral reflux and also increase the likelihood of UTIs.[1,14]

Common causes of UTIs in girls include poor fluid intake, infrequent or inefficient urination, and constipation. Close proximity of the urethra to the vagina and rectum, the short female urethra, and inherited bacterial adherence factors increase the risk for infection. These factors cannot be changed, making efficient elimination of urine and stool more important in girls.

Fluid intake is important for several reasons. Intake drives urine production, which, in turn, results in more timely urination and clearance of bacteria from the lower urinary tract. Water intake is one cornerstone of the management of constipation.

Infrequent urination may not be easily remedied in the child who has progressed from postponement of urination to a large underactive bladder, but the more rapid bladder filling with increased fluid intake helps to restore the sensation of bladder filling necessary to initiate urination. Timed trips to the restroom (*timed voiding*) at least every 2 hours during the day is one early intervention for children and teens with UTIs and other urinary complaints.

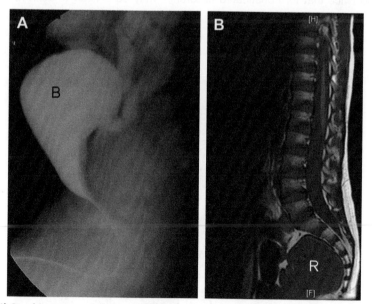

Fig. 7. (*A*) Stool in rectum deforms the bladder base and bladder outlet on voiding cystourethrogram. (*B*) Profound rectal distention (R) noted on MRI to rule out tethered cord. Rectal distention can impair bladder contractility by shared neural pathways.

Inefficient urination may be attributable to incomplete sphincter relaxation or poor bladder contractility. Repositioning on the toilet to optimize relaxation of the external sphincter and pelvic floor is taught at the first visit and reinforced at return visits (**Fig. 8**). One must appreciate that this position may be difficult or embarrassing to assume at school, given the lack of foot support and the need to remove undergarments completely. It is important to sit on the toilet at school and to continue voiding at timed intervals, however. A Valsalva maneuver to release urine is discouraged because it tightens the pelvic floor.[14] Other relaxation techniques, such as yoga breathing, blowing bubbles, and counting slowly, may be helpful.

Biofeedback for pelvic floor retraining is effective for children whose elimination habits are refractory to the previously discussed measures. This noninvasive therapy involves electromyographic (EMG) monitoring of the external sphincter complex by means of perineal patch electrodes. Uroflowmetry is used to assess the quality of the urinary stream, and ultrasound is used to check postvoid residual volumes. Multiple sessions are used to help the child identify the appropriate muscles and practice relaxation of the complex. The afferent EMG output can be linked to interactive computer games, with the game controlled by contraction and relaxation of the appropriate muscle groups. Progress is measured by the game score.[20]

Anecdotally, children who have been particularly affected emotionally by their elimination issues seem to thrive during the one-on-one sessions with the provider and take pride in their progress. Biofeedback therapy has been shown to improve daytime incontinence, abnormal voiding patterns, constipation, and other urinary complaints. Resolution or improvement of vesicoureteral reflux is also enhanced with this therapy.[21]

Management of constipation is much more art than science. Each child has a unique constitution and response to medical intervention. Basic principles of adequate water intake, increased dietary fiber, and timed toileting with support of the feet apply to all children. Specific recommendations for dietary fiber intake (age + 5 g for normal children and twice that for constipated children)[14] may be difficult to achieve in picky

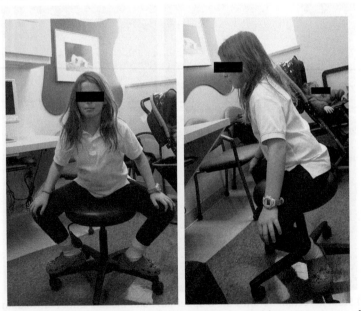

Fig. 8. Repositioning on the toilet for pelvic floor relaxation and for management of vaginal reflux.

eaters or younger children, but tasteless fiber supplements are available over the counter. Time should be set aside for toileting 30 minutes after a large meal to take advantage of the gastrocolic reflex. This quiet time may help the child to become more aware of descent of stool within the rectum. The feet should be positioned so that the angle between the upper and lower leg is 90° to allow pelvic floor relaxation. Valsalva maneuvers or straining to push the stool out is discouraged, because the anal sphincter closes with this maneuver.[14]

There are several other options for bowel management, and the program should be tailored to the child's needs and progress. Experience and preferences of the provider and willingness of the family to accept elements of the program play a role in the regimen as well. Adjustments in the program should be made every 2 to 3 weeks as needed rather than on a daily reactive basis. Polyethylene glycol powder is used by many pediatric urologists and is well tolerated by the patient. Cramping and diarrhea are the most common side effects that complicate treatment in some children.[22] A gradual upward titration of the daily dose to achieve the optimal result may minimize these side effects. In more severe cases, impacted stool in the rectosigmoid colon may be addressed with enemas for 1 to 2 days before starting an oral bowel program. Rectal suppositories, mineral oil, magnesium hydroxide solution (Milk of Magnesia), and senna laxatives are also commonly used.[14] Each child needs a unique program and requires follow-up to keep the family on track. Referral to a pediatric gastroenterologist for troublesome cases is appropriate.

SORTING OUT DAYTIME INCONTINENCE

As with any condition, an accurate history is extremely important in the management of daytime incontinence. Various nontechnical terms, such as *wetness*, *accidents*, *dampness*, *leakage*, or *dripping*, may be better understood than "incontinence." Beyond establishing the interval of urination and adequacy of fluid intake from the elimination diary, it is important to characterize the timing and severity of incontinence. Children who have never achieved daytime continence may have an anatomic abnormality, such as an ectopic ureter or female epispadias with bladder neck incompetence **Fig. 9**. Neurologic impairment or developmental issues may also result in primary incontinence. Secondary onset of incontinence after toilet learning should also raise concern for a neurologic process, but behavioral issues or poor elimination habits are a far more common cause of secondary incontinence.

It is useful to distinguish damp panties from accidents that soak through the undergarment and outer layer. Although many children are reluctant to give specific details, it is important to know whether the child is bothered enough to change clothes or wear a pad during the day or whether the child barely seems to notice wet clothing. A desire to become dry is essential as the treatment program gets underway.

Timing of involuntary urine loss and potential associated activities should also be noted. The following terminology is consistent with the most recent ICCS guidelines.[2] Wetness that occurs while the child is "busy" playing or that occurs only at home or only at school suggests *voiding postponement*, a behavioral issue that can result in true bladder dysfunction. *Stress incontinence* is uncommon in children in the absence of a neurologic or anatomic abnormality. Incontinence associated with laughing, crying, coughing, or while playing sports may, however, be attributable to *overflow* of urine after voiding postponement. *Giggle incontinence* describes centrally mediated complete bladder emptying associated with laughing or another strong emotion. The condition is believed to be related to cataplexy and may be attributable to an imbalance between cholinergic and monoaminergic input. Methylphenidate has been used successfully to

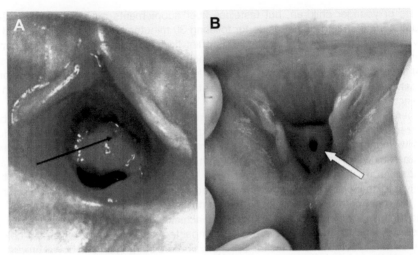

Fig. 9. (*A*) Ectopic ureteral meatus on thicked anterior rim of hymen. (*B*) Female epispadias. Arrow indicates anteriorly-placed vagina. Note bifid clitoris and patulous urethra.

manage this challenging condition,[23] but many families are not willing to consider this medication. Others believe that strong bladder contractions can be precipitated by laughter and that most giggle incontinence occurs in girls with other daytime symptoms. These researchers support use of anticholinergic medication for management of giggle incontinence.[24] Incontinence that occurs only within 10 minutes of finishing on the toilet is mostly likely attributable to *vaginal reflux* of urine during urination.

Getting a true idea of the child's sensation and awareness of impending or recent incontinence can be difficult because the child often seems uncertain how to answer or may experience incontinence in more than one setting. The child may also fear repercussions based on her answer. It is important to establish a supportive rapport and make the child aware that her answers are important in correcting the situation. The parent often perceives that the child does not feel anything, particularly if the child failed to interrupt her activities or if she continued to wear wet garments. If the parent witnesses posturing or holding behaviors, a strong urgency or a bladder contraction has likely occurred.

If the child indicates that she is aware of the need to urinate at the last minute but cannot make it to the restroom in time, the condition may be *overactive bladder* (bladder instability) or *voiding postponement*. If she first feels something as the urine is coming out, *stress incontinence* or *overflow incontinence with an underactive bladder* is the more likely situation. If she reports that she feels nothing until the underwear is soiled, she may be experiencing *vaginal reflux* or *overflow incontinence with an underactive bladder*. If she does not seem to feel anything or notice that she is wet, there may be a neurologic basis for the impaired sensation. Developmental or behavioral concerns should be strongly considered as well. A differential diagnosis for daytime incontinence is listed in **Box 2**.

Because of the close relation between elimination habits, UTIs, and daytime incontinence, the management of daytime incontinence is rather similar to the management of UTIs. In addition to hydration and treatment of constipation, timed voiding is a reasonable early recommendation for all patients with daytime incontinence.[25] Repositioning on the toilet is important to improve pelvic floor relaxation and to minimize vaginal reflux of urine. Biofeedback is used for more difficult cases.

Box 2
Differential diagnosis of daytime incontinence
UTI
Overactive bladder
Voiding postponement
Vaginal reflux
Giggle incontinence
Sphincteric incompetence (anatomic or neurogenic)
Ectopic ureter
Behavioral or developmental

The use of anticholinergic medications to reduce bladder overactivity or alpha-blockade to improve outlet relaxation should be reserved as second-line therapy after modification of elimination habits. Medications are now infrequently recommended as empiric management of daytime incontinence.[2,25] Radiographic evidence of adequate bladder emptying is desirable before a trial of anticholinergic medication, and the child must continue to adhere to the timed voiding program. Alpha-blocker therapy should be considered as an alternative to biofeedback in the management of urinary retention and voiding dysfunction.[26] The medication is well tolerated, and the therapy is far less time-consuming for the family. Combination therapy of alpha-blockade and biofeedback is useful in refractory cases.[27]

SPECIAL TESTING

Specialized testing is not required in most children with the complaints addressed in this article. Children who fail to improve with behavioral management or in whom the diagnosis is not clear may benefit from further testing.

An MRI scan may be ordered when there is a high suspicion for occult spinal cord pathologic findings. Because of its ability to image fluid-filled structures without the use of contrast, MRI is effective for detection of an ectopic ureter associated with a poorly functioning renal unit.

Formal urodynamic testing is indicated for refractory daytime incontinence or in complicated cases without an obvious etiology.[28] This specialized test provides information regarding sensation, capacity, storage pressure, contractility, leak or voiding pressure, residual volume, and sphincter activity. Several of these data points are available with much less invasive testing, including the elimination diary, postvoid ultrasound, and noninvasive uroflow. Formal urodynamic testing is located near the end of the algorithm for patients with elimination concerns. Similarly, cystoscopy has limited indications in children who have infections, incontinence, or other dysfunction of elimination.[29]

SUMMARY

There is significant overlap between urology and pediatric and adolescent gynecology. A detailed history is essential to establish a diagnosis and formulate an appropriate treatment plan. The emotional subtitles accompanying many of these complaints are important to recognize. Tremendous support and compassion are required for many of the girls and their parents. With more scientific data available each day, management of voiding issues and recurrent UTIs is becoming less "art" and more "science," but individualization of therapy is likely to remain important in the management of this diverse group of girls.

REVIEW CASES
Review Case 1

An 8-year-old girl is brought to the office by her parents with the concern that she "grabs her vagina" often in public. She has done this since she toilet trained with some difficulty at the age of 2 years. When confronted by her parents, she says her bottom hurts. She has daytime accidents at least twice per week, and she always runs to the restroom at the last minute, especially when busy playing. The parents have also noted that the child suddenly stops and stares or squats down when playing. After a few minutes, she resumes normal activities. She has had at least two UTIs and often complains of pain with urination. The parents report that the bowel movements are normal.

Examination reveals normal prepubertal genitalia with the exception of deep erythema of the vestibule without discharge. The anus is normal. Examination of the spine and extremities is normal.

After your assessment is complete, which medication would most likely address the child's situation?

A. Oxybutynin (anticholinergic)
B. 1% hydrocortisone to the vulva
C. Methylphenidate
D. Trimethoprim-sulfamethoxazole prophylaxis
E. Polyethylene glycol

Review Case 2

A 6-year-old girl presents with intermittent thick vaginal discharge without pruritus. As a thorough elimination history is elicited, the mother notes that the child is toilet trained but has always been a little damp during the day and is wet every night. She voids five to six times daily. The girl is not certain why she is wet, because there is no warning. The mother has not witnessed any posturing to suggest voiding postponement. There is no loss of urine with coughing, laughing, or gymnastics. The bowel movements are type 4 and 5.[11]

On examination, there is mild erythema consistent with nonspecific vulvovaginitis but no frank discharge. The clitoris is normal. With outward retraction of the labia, a small amount of fluid is noted in the vagina. There is no foreign body. There are no abnormalities of the lumbosacral spine or lower extremities.

Which of the following pairs of diagnoses remain in your differential?

A. Giggle incontinence and constipation
B. Occult spinal dysraphism and stress incontinence
C. Voiding postponement and epispadias
D. Vaginal reflux and ectopic ureter
E. Constipation and stress incontinence

ANSWERS TO REVIEW CASES
Review Case 1

The answer is E. Several of the reported behaviors suggest that the child is having uninhibited bladder contractions or spasms. She aborts the bladder contraction by squatting or freezing in position and squeezing the pelvic floor. The parents describe a form of Vincent's curtsy, one of several postures used by these girls to postpone urination. Empiric treatment with anticholinergic medication covers up the underlying problems and is not indicated at this point. Although the parents report normal bowel function, only the child is in a position to describe the stools and can do so when provided with a visual aid[11] or other familiar terms. This child most likely has constipation or functional fecal retention contributing to the bladder contractions, UTIs, and vaginitis. If an adequate history cannot be obtained, a plain film of the abdomen should identify constipation. Polyethylene glycol is one option for initial management of constipation, but fluid and fiber are essential as well. Although topical agents soothe and treat the vaginitis, bland ointment is likely a better choice than topical corticosteroids in this case.

In addition to management of constipation and timed voiding, biofeedback is likely to be beneficial for this child to learn appropriate pelvic floor relaxation.

Review Case 2

The answer is D. The history and examination largely ruled out at least one of the diagnoses in each pair. This child most likely has vaginal reflux or ectopic ureter, although occult dysraphism remains possible, even with a normal examination.

Vaginal reflux typically manifests with dampness shortly after a trip to the restroom. The next step would be instruction in repositioning on the toilet (see **Fig. 6**).

An ectopic ureter that inserts into the distal urethra, perineum, or vagina results in "constant" dampness despite otherwise normal voiding habits. The degree of wetness depends on the function remaining in the renal unit. Intermittent discharge (from a dilated ureter with stasis) is also a common complaint. The next step would be evaluation with renal and bladder ultrasound, looking for a dilated distal ureter or evidence of a suspicious renal anomaly. MRI of the abdomen and pelvis with delayed contrast views is useful if suspicion remains high after a normal ultrasound.

REFERENCES

1. Koff SA, Wagner TT, Jayanthi VR. The relationship among dysfunctional elimination syndromes, primary vesicoureteral reflux and urinary tract infections in children. J Urol 1998;160:1019–22.
2. Neveus T, von Gontard A, Hoebeke P, et al. The standardization of terminology of lower urinary tract function in children and adolescents: report from the Standardization Committee of the International Children's Continence Society. J Urol 2006; 176:314–24.
3. Normal micturition. In: Blaivas J, Chancellor M, Weiss J, et al, editors. Atlas of urodynamics. 2nd edition. Malden (MA): Blackwell Publishing Inc.; 2007. p. 11.
4. Hinman F, Baumann FW. Vesical and ureteral damage from voiding dysfunction in boys without neurologic or obstructive disease. J Urol 2002;167:1069–73 (reprinted from 1973).
5. Videourodynamics. In: Blaivas J, Chancellor M, Weiss J, et al, editors. Atlas of urodynamics. 2nd edition. Malden (MA): Blackwell Publishing Inc.; 2007. p. 64.
6. Ellsworth PI, Merguerian PA, Copening ME. Sexual abuse: another causative factor in dysfunctional voiding. J Urol 1995;153:773–6.
7. Davila GW, Bernier F, Franco J, et al. Bladder dysfunction in sexual abuse survivors. J Urol 2003;170:476–9.
8. Von Gontard A, Hollmann E. Comorbidity of functional urinary incontinence and encopresis: somatic and behavioral associations. J Urol 2004;171:2644–7.

9. Blethyn AJ, Jenkins HR, Roberts R, et al. Radiological evidence of constipation in urinary tract infection. Arch Dis Child 1995;73:534–5.
10. Giramonti KM, Kogan BA, Agboola OO, et al. The association of constipation with childhood urinary tract infections. J Pediatr Urol 2005;1:273–8.
11. Lewis SJ, Heaton KW. Stool form scale as a useful guide to intestinal transit time. Scand J Gastroenterol 1997;32(9):920–4.
12. Klijn AJ, Asselman M, Vijverberg MAW, et al. The diameter of the rectum on ultra-sonography as a diagnostic tool for constipation in children with dysfunctional voiding. J Urol 2004;172:1986–8.
13. Joensson IM, Siggaard C, Rittig S, et al. Transabdominal ultrasound of rectum as a diagnostic tool in childhood constipation. J Urol 2008;179:1997–2002.
14. Chase JW, Homsy Y, Siggaard C, et al. Functional constipation in children. J Urol 2004;171:2641–3.
15. Maronn ML, Esterly NB. Constipation as a feature of anogenital lichen sclerosus in children. Pediatrics 2005;115(2):e230–2.
16. Van Neer PAFA, Korver CRW. Constipation presenting as recurrent vulvovaginitis in prepubertal children. J Am Acad Dermatol 2000;43(4):718–9.
17. Rink RC, Yerkes EB. Surgical management of female genital anomalies, intersex (urogenital sinus) disorders and cloacal anomalies. In: Gearhart JP, Rink RC, Mouriquand PDE, editors. Pediatric urology. Philadelphia: W.B. Saunders; 2001.
18. Loening-Baucke V. Urinary incontinence and urinary tract infection and their reso-lution with treatment of chronic constipation of childhood. Pediatrics 1997;100: 228–32.
19. Miyazato M, Sugaya K, Nishijima S, et al. Rectal distention inhibits bladder activity via glycinergic and GABAergic mechanisms in rats. J Urol 2004;171: 1353–6.
20. Herndon CDA, Decambre M, McKenna PH. Interactive computer games for treat-ment of pelvic floor dysfunction. J Urol 2001;166:1893–8.
21. Kibar Y, Ors O, Demir E, et al. Results of biofeedback treatment on reflux resolu-tion rates in children with dysfunctional voiding and vesicoureteral reflux. Urology 2007;70:563–6.
22. Erickson BA, Austin JC, Cooper CS, et al. Polyethylene glycol 3350 for constipa-tion in children with dysfunctional elimination. J Urol 2003;170:1818–20.
23. Sher PK, Reinberg Y. Successful treatment of giggle incontinence with methyl-phenidate. J Urol 1996;156:656–8.
24. Chandra M, Saharia R, Shi Q, et al. Giggle incontinence in children: a manifesta-tion of detrusor instability. J Urol 2002;168:2184–7.
25. Allen HA, Austin JC, Boyt MA, et al. Initial trial of timed voiding is warranted for all children with daytime incontinence. Urology 2007;69:962–5.
26. Austin PF, Homsy YL, Masel JL, et al. α-Adrenergic blockade in children with neuropathic and nonneuropathic voiding dysfunction. J Urol 1999;162:1064–7.
27. Yucel S, Akkaya E, Guntekin E, et al. Can alpha-blocker therapy be an alternative to biofeedback for dysfunctional voiding and urinary retention? A prospective study. J Urol 2005;174:1612–5.
28. Kaufman MR, DeMarco RT, Pope JC IV, et al. High yield of urodynamics performed for refractory nonneurogenic dysfunctional voiding in the pediatric population. J Urol 2006;176:1835–7.
29. Parekh DJ, Pope JC IV, Adams MC, et al. The use of radiography, urodynamics studies and cystoscopy in the evaluation of voiding dysfunction. J Urol 2001; 165:215–8.

Genital Trauma in the Pediatric and Adolescent Female

Diane F. Merritt, MD[a,b,c,d],*

KEYWORDS

• Genital trauma • Accidental genital injuries
• Straddle injuries • Female genital cutting or mutilation
• Sexual abuse • Sexual assault

Genital injuries in female children and adolescents may occur in the context of multiple injuries (as in a motor vehicle accident) or as an isolated injury to the genitals (as in a straddle injury). Some children are victims of an isolated assault or repeated abuses, and some incidents are accidents that are unlikely to ever occur again. A thoughtful approach is necessary to be supportive to the child or teen, who may be bleeding, in pain, and frightened, and to the patient's parents or guardians who have concerns about the assessment and repair of an acute injury and the long-term significance for future reproduction. The clinician has an obligation to assess whether the history provided is compatible with the injuries found on genital examination. Inconsistencies between the history and physical examination should arouse suspicion of sexual assault or abuse.

The approach to the injured child follows the traditional assessment of vital signs, airway, breathing, circulation, and evaluation of the sites and sources of trauma. In the case of genital trauma, the severity of the injury and the amount of bleeding determine where and how the examination should take place. If the injury is not severe, the child may be examined in a doctor's office or emergency department without sedation. Force or restraint should not be used for a genital examination. When the child or adolescent is unable or unwilling to allow an adequate examination to be accomplished, light conscious sedation for the assessment of genital injuries has been suggested but may be of limited use. General anesthesia may allow a better examination, assessment, and repair.[1]

[a] Department of Obstetrics and Gynecology, Pediatric and Adolescent Gynecology, Washington University School of Medicine, 660 S. Euclid Avenue, Saint Louis, MO 63110, USA
[b] Barnes Jewish Hospital, One Barnes-Jewish Hospital Plaza, Saint Louis, MO 63110, USA
[c] Saint Louis Children's Hospital, One Children's Place, Saint Louis, MO 63110, USA
[d] Missouri Baptist Medical Center, 3015 North Ballas Road, Saint Louis, MO 63131, USA
* Department of Obstetrics and Gynecology, Campus Box 8064, 660 S. Euclid, Saint Louis, MO 63110.
E-mail address: merrittd@wustl.edu

Obstet Gynecol Clin N Am 36 (2009) 85–98
doi:10.1016/j.ogc.2009.01.003
0889-8545/09/$ – see front matter © 2009 Elsevier Inc. All rights reserved.
obgyn.theclinics.com

HOW TO PERFORM AN EXAMINATION IN A CHILD OR ADOLESCENT

Evaluation of the external genitalia in the pediatric and adolescent population requires a different technique and approach than used in the examination of an adult. An understanding of variations in normal anogenital anatomy is essential, as is an understanding of the physical findings that can mimic signs of trauma or sexual abuse.

There are several techniques to facilitate the examination of a young patient. After the clinician obtains parental permission to perform the genital examination, the child can be held in the parent's lap, or the child can lie supine on the examination table. By placing the child in either a frogleg or knee–chest position, the examiner will be able to assess for normal genital anatomy.[2] Use of labial separation frequently fails to provide the examiner with a complete view of the girl's vestibule. The application of lateral traction to the labia majora does provide a much better view of the girl's vestibule and the vaginal canal. If the posterior hymen is redundant, the folds may obscure an injury. The prone knee–chest position allows the hymen to unfold and drop down, and the vaginal canal also may drop open, resulting in a better view of both the hymen and the contents of vaginal canal.[3,4] Concerns have been raised regarding an examination method that places a girl or child in a face-down position.[5]

A study comparing the effectiveness of examination methods in helping the clinician detect acute and nonacute injuries in pubertal and prepubertal girls assessed the three different examination methods: supine labial separation, supine labial traction, and the prone knee–chest position. Each method had advantages, but the examiner had a greater chance of identifying additional signs of trauma by combining the methods than by using any single technique alone.[6]

If an injury such as a vulvar hematoma, a laceration, or vaginal bleeding is present, the full extent of injury may be difficult to determine, especially if the child is unwilling or unable to cooperate for an adequate examination. In such situations, examination with sedation or under general anesthesia may be necessary. Standard vaginal speculums should not be used to examine a prepubertal child, because they are designed for adults. Vaginoscopy is an important tool used by the pediatric gynecologist; depending on the age and level of cooperation of the child, this procedure may be done with or without anesthesia. Placement of a pediatric cystoscope into the vagina with gentle opposition of the labia provides fluid distension to allow adequate visualization of the vaginal vault in children. In this manner, injuries to the vagina can be assessed, and foreign objects may be found (**Fig. 1**). When the vagina of an adolescent is examined, the speculum selected for use should be the proper size for the patient. A Graves speculum can be used to evaluate an adult, but a narrower Pederson speculum is easier to place in a young woman or virginal teen (**Fig. 2**).

ETIOLOGY AND MANAGEMENT OF ACCIDENTAL GENITAL INJURIES
Straddle Injury

Straddle injuries occur when the soft tissues of the vulva are compressed between an object and the underlying bones of the pelvis. This trauma may result in ecchymoses (bruises), abrasions, and lacerations. Extravasation of blood into the loose areolar tissue in the labia, along the vagina, the mons, or clitoral area may cause a hematoma to form. Examples of commonplace accidental straddle injuries include falling onto the frame of a bicycle, playground equipment, or piece of furniture. Nonpenetrating injuries usually involve the mons, clitoris, and labia and result in linear lacerations, ecchymoses, and abrasions. Lacerations may require repair under local or general anesthesia.

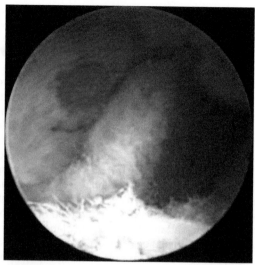

Fig. 1. Image of vaginoscopy in a 4-year-old child with a 3-week history of vaginal spotting and bleeding. A foreign body is seen next to the cervix in the left vaginal fornix. The object was removed, and the bleeding stopped. The foreign body grossly contained cotton fibers, and the culture was positive for *beta-hemolytic Streptococcus* and *Bacteroides* species. (*Courtesy of* Diane F. Merritt, MD, Saint Louis, Missouri.)

Vulvar Hematomas

Vulvar hematomas (often sustained as a result of a straddle injury) can be very painful and may prevent a child or adolescent from urinating because of pain and swelling. If the hematoma is not large, and the perineal anatomy is not distorted, and if the patient

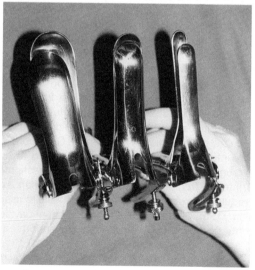

Fig. 2. The vaginal speculum comes is a standard length of 4 inches. The Graves speculum (*left*) is 1.5 inches wide, and the Pederson speculum (*middle*) is 1.0 inches wide. The narrow Pederson speculum (*right*) is 0.75 in wide and is ideal for placement in a young adolescent to view the vagina and cervix. (*Courtesy of* Diane F. Merritt, MD, Saint Louis, Missouri.)

has no difficulty emptying her bladder, she can be managed conservatively with immediate application of ice packs and bed rest. As the hematoma resolves, the blood will track along the fascial planes. The ecchymotic discoloration may take weeks to resolve. If the patient has a larger vulvar hematoma and is unable to void, one should place an indwelling urinary catheter and continue bladder drainage until the swelling resolves. Very large vulvar hematomas may dissect into the loose areolar tissue along the vaginal wall and along the fascial planes overlying the symphysis pubis and lower abdominal wall. Pressure from an expanding hematoma may cause necrosis of the skin overlying the hematoma. Evacuating the hematoma will reduce pain, hasten recovery, and prevent necrosis, tissue loss, and secondary infection. When incising large vulvar hematomas, one should incise along the medial mucosal surface near the vaginal orifice. Because the periclitoral area has a rich blood supply, hematomas in this area require careful isolation of the bleeding vessels. If adequate hemostasis is not attained, the patient will be at risk for bleeding and reaccumulation of the hematoma. When the bed of the hematoma has been debrided of clot and devascularized tissue, and hemostasis has been attained, one should place a closed system drain (ie, Jackson-Pratt) to prevent reaccumulation of blood, to reduce pain, and to reduce the risk of bacterial growth. The drain should exit the skin in a dependent position, and the skin should be closed primarily. The drain can be removed in 24 hours in most cases.[1]

Accidental Penetrating Injuries

Penetrating injuries occur if the victim falls on a sharp or pointed object, and impales herself. Many common household objects are the agent of impalement, including in-lawn sprinkling systems, pipes, fence posts, trailer hitches, and furniture (chair tops, bedposts, legs of stools). The vagina, urethra and bladder, anus, rectum, and peritoneal cavity can be pierced by sharp or pointed objects. The physical findings may appear to be quite minimal, but the patient may have a more serious underlying injury. In a report of 34 perineal impalements, several patterns emerged. Most injuries occurred in the home. Many children either slipped or fell in the bathroom on bathtub toys, soap dispensers, or the shower diverter valves or fell onto objects when climbing out of the tub or when running out of the bathroom after bathing. Slippery surfaces and the lack of protective clothing were stated to be the common contributing factors. Bedroom accidents occurred when children were jumping from one bed to another, a common play activity with obvious risk. Infants and children should be supervised in the bathtub, because they may be at risk for drowning and scalding injuries if the bath water is too hot. They are also at risk for trauma from falls onto objects, but even the presence of supervising adults did not completely prevent these accidents.[7]

Accidental penetrating injuries may closely mimic the injuries associated with sexual assault. For this reason the medical history is essential. Corroboration of the events by an eyewitness is very informative. The family can be asked to bring the object for assessment by the trauma team, or the authorities may investigate the scene of the injury. Because the internal trauma may be more severe than externally apparent, these patients may require an examination under anesthesia to assess fully the extent of the penetrating injury (**Fig. 3**). If the rectum or peritoneal cavities are entered, an exploratory laparotomy or laparoscopy are should be preformed to determine the full extent of injuries and to initiate repairs.[1]

There is some controversy in the trauma literature regarding the role of routine fecal diversion in the management of anorectal injuries, and there are reports on primary repair of anorectal injuries without proximal colostomy. The financial, psychologic, and social disadvantages of a colostomy should be considered also. Onen and colleagues[8] recommend a colostomy to improve the outcome for unstable patients

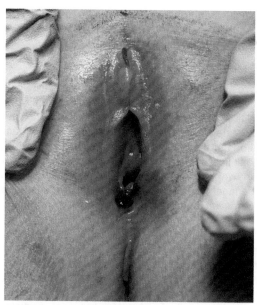

Fig. 3. This girl jumped over a metal pole and landed on it. The injury noted in the four-chette appears minor, but under general anesthesia the anal sphincter was found to be completely transected and required repair. (*Courtesy of* Diane F. Merritt, MD, Saint Louis, Missouri.)

who have a genital injury score of V, severe contamination, and prolonged delay before medical attention is received (**Table 1**).[1]

Accidental vaginal insufflation injuries

Vaginal insufflation injuries occur when females fall off jet skis and water skis, slide down water chutes, or come in direct contact with pool or spa jets. As pressurized water enters the vagina, the walls may overdistend and tear. Significant blood loss can occur. Such injuries may produce no sign of external genital trauma, and only careful vaginal examination (often under anesthesia) will reveal the source of bleeding and true extent of injury. Children and women who participate in water sports can decrease their risk for vaginal insufflation injuries by using protective clothing such as neoprene wetsuits or cut-off jeans while water or jet skiing. On waterslides,

Table 1	
Classification for genital injuries in female children	
Genital Injury Score	**Extent of Injury**
I	Isolated genital injury distal to hymen
II	Isolated genital injury including hymen
III	Isolated genital injury including vagina
IV	Hymeneal or vaginal injury plus partial tear of anorectum
V	Vaginal injury plus complete tear of anorectum

Data from Onen A, Ozturk H, Yayla M, et al. Genital trauma in children: classification and management. Urology 2005;65(5):987.

head-first entries usually are forbidden to prevent head and neck injury, but also it is wise for girls to cross their ankles or to keep their feet together when entering water from a waterslide to prevent genital trauma.[9–11]

Crush or Shear Injuries

Crush injuries may result from motor vehicle accidents, falls, or during collapse of a building caused by structural problems, natural catastrophes (earthquakes), bombings, or warfare. Any time a pelvic fracture occurs, genital injuries may arise when fragments of a pelvic bone penetrate the vagina and lower urinary tract. This penetration may lead to lacerations of the bladder, urethra, or vagina. Shear forces can lead to lacerations when a fall is associated with rapid abduction of the lower extremities or when a patient is run over by a motor vehicle. As reported by Boos and colleagues,[12] two children had perianal lacerations and two had hymenal lacerations when the wheel of the vehicle passed longitudinally over the child's torso.

Animal and Human Bites

Animal bites are rare but may be a cause of genital trauma. Animal bites usually are caused by dogs that are family pets or are known to the victim. Most canine bites involve the extremities, but in children may involve the face, neck, and buttocks. Human bites tend to occur in children as a result of playing or fighting, whereas in adults they usually are the result of aggressive behavior, participation in sports, or sexual activity. Mammalian bites may cause significant damage to delicate tissue of the genitalia. Microorganisms contained in saliva may cause infections resulting in local cellulitis or facilitate inoculation and transmission of communicable diseases. Both syphilis and HIV may be transmissible via a bite wound.[13,14] Human bites should be treated promptly by immediate irrigation with a bactericidal and virucidal solution (1% povidine-iodine) using an 18- to 19-gauge needle and debridement of the wound. The prophylactic use of antibiotics is controversial because of the lack of adequate clinical studies. Simple scrapes and abrasions are unlikely to benefit from antibiotic treatment. Antibiotics may be given if there is deep puncture or crushing, if the victim has underlying diabetes mellitus or an immunodeficiency, or if the wound is obviously infected. Genital bites are at high risk for infection because the loose subcutaneous tissue may facilitate bacterial spread.[15] Management of the bite wound involves irrigation, debridement, and antibiotic prophylaxis. Tetanus vaccination should be administered as part of wound care of mammalian bites, but no studies have assessed the benefit of this strategy. Vaccination need not be performed if there is a record of a tetanus shot being given in the previous 5 years. The need for rabies immunization should be assessed on an individual basis, as should primary versus secondary wound closure.[16,17]

Accidental and Inflicted Burns

Scalds are the leading cause of burn-related hospitalizations and emergency department visits for young children. Most of the older pediatric burn literature focused on tap-water scalding as a preventable cause of pediatric burns, but several recent publications point out that the bulk of scald injuries are not tap water–related and instead are associated with mealtime preparation of food. The most common behaviors include children pulling a hot substance from the stove, microwave, or countertop or having liquid spilled on them while the caregiver is cooking or is carrying the child and a hot liquid.[18] Prevention of scald injuries requires raised awareness of these common household events in addition to reducing the temperature in domestic hot-water tanks and testing the water temperature before placing an infant or child in the bath.[19,20] Accidental immersion burns, in which a child falls into a container of hot liquid, typically have irregular borders and non-uniform depth as the victim struggles to escape the hot liquid. This thrashing also causes splash marks, which, although they sometimes may be found in forced immersion, are more characteristic of accidental immersion. Accidental burns are rarely full-thickness burns, because they typically involve shorter contact time. In accidental splash and spill burns, the head, neck, and trunk are commonly involved when the hot liquid is pulled or knocked over from a higher surface and spilled over by the child. Accidental contact burns often are patchy and superficial, because the child quickly withdraws from the hot object or the falling object brushes across the skin. They may or may not show a clear imprint.

The child abuse literature recognizes that inflicted burns may occur. Scalds are the most frequent form of burn abuse.[21] "Tide marks" (ie, clear lines of demarcation) characterize nonaccidental bath scalds. These scalds also tend to have uniform burn depth and commonly involve the buttocks, perineum, and lower extremities. Stocking and glove burns occur when a child's hands and/or feet are immersed forcibly in hot water, resulting in symmetric, circumferential, and well-demarcated burns. Zebra stripes result from sparing of the flexural creases secondary to the body's flexed position in the hot liquid. Donut-hole sparing occurs when the child's buttocks are pressed against the bathtub, which is relatively cooler than the water in it. Simultaneous scald burns to buttocks, feet, and perineum are highly suspicious for physical abuse and warrant a thorough investigation, as do well-demarcated burns around the buttocks or bilateral symmetric glove and stocking burns.

Inflicted contact burns are deeper, may be multiple, and have well-demarcated margins. They commonly are caused by hot irons, radiators, hair dryers, curling irons, and stoves. Contact burns with uniform depth and well-demarcated margins located on typically protected areas of the body suggest abuse. Cigarette burns are a common form of burn abuse. Inflicted cigarette burns appear as 7- to 10-mm round, well-demarcated burns that have a deep central crater. They heal with scarring because they extend well into the dermis. Cigarette burns commonly appear grouped on the face, hands, and feet. When accidental, they tend to be oval or eccentric and more superficial, because the child usually brushes against the cigarette. The location of a burn, although not pathognomonic, can be helpful when ruling out abuse. Face, hands, legs, feet, perineum, and buttocks tend to be predominant sites in abuse. The perineum and buttocks, in particular, are infrequently involved in accidental burns, and burns in this area often are inflicted as punishment for toilet training accidents.[21] Batteries placed in the vagina may result in chemical burns and have been described in the literature.[22] Genital burns can occur from the use of medications intended to treat genital warts (eg, imiquimod, podophyllin, or trichloroacetic acid). Such chemical burns should be treated immediately by irrigation to neutralize the chemicals and prevent further damage. The management of genital and perineal burns includes cooling the burn for 20 minutes with cold tap water within 3 hours of the injury to reduce pain and wound edema. It is unknown how effective topical application of antimicrobials and dressings are for the treatment of minor burns. A mixture of a topical antibiotic ointment and estrogen cream has been helpful for minimizing scarring from mucosal burns of the female genital tract. Silver sulphadiazine cream has been used historically in the management of burn wounds to minimize the risk wound infection, but no randomized trials or controlled clinical trials have evaluated its clinical effectiveness. There is no current consensus about the optimal dressing for burns in the genital area.

Coitally Related Vaginal Injuries

Whenever an adolescent presents with vaginal trauma, consensual intercourse or sexual assault should be considered in the differential diagnosis. The patient may be too embarrassed or distressed to explain her injuries, and she may not give an accurate account of how the injury occurred. The diagnosis may be incorrectly attributed to a hymenal tear or menstrual bleeding, and the diagnosis of a more serious injury may be overlooked or delayed unless a proper pelvic examination is done to evaluate vaginal bleeding. Minor lacerations of the introitus and lower vagina can occur with initial coitus. Adolescents who sustain deep vaginal lacerations from coitus may present with intense vaginal pain, profuse or prolonged vaginal bleeding, and shock. Predisposing factors for coital injury include initial or hurried intercourse; incompatibility of sexual organ sizes (especially during a first sexual experience); intoxication or substance use by either or both partners; extreme and vigorous sexual penetration with coital positioning of the female in dorsal decubitus with hyperflexion of the thighs or in sitting positions; clumsiness; pregnancy; vaginal spasm; retroversion of the uterus; insertion of foreign bodies; and sexual assault. Vaginal lacerations and perforation may arise because of lack of physiologic preparation of the genitalia from sexual arousal, as may happen when sexual intercourse occurs when the participants' fear discovery. Patients who have vaginal agenesis may sustain deep lacerations from failed attempts at penetration. Urethral intercourse may occur in patients who have vaginal agenesis.[1,23–25]

GUIDELINES FOR THE MEDICAL CARE OF SEXUALLY ABUSED CHILDREN AND ADOLESCENTS

Guidelines for the care of the child or adolescent who has experienced sexual abuse are best found in the literature dedicated to this topic. The American Academy of Pediatrics recently published guidelines, and there are comprehensive reviews that address the current knowledge base in this field.[26–28]

Sexual abuse includes coerced or forced vaginal, anal, intercrural, and oral–genital fondling or penetration. Victims of sexual assault might sustain extragenital physical injury that occurs during resistance or is inflicted deliberately by the assailant. Sexual violence entails a number of negative effects that may the affect victim's health: pregnancy, spread of sexually transmissible diseases, exposure to HIV/AIDS, increased risk for adoption of undesirable sexual behavior (eg, early initiation of sexual activity, multiple sexual partners), and negative effects on mental health.[29] It is unwise for families or professionals to assume that, because there are no symptoms, sexual abuse has not taken place or that, if it has taken place, it has not involved penetration. No child or adolescent alleging sexual abuse should be denied a medical examination purely because they have no symptoms. In a study by Kelly and colleagues,[30] most of the children who had diagnostic findings consistent with sexual assault had no physical symptoms. In a published study of 2384 children referred for possible sexual abuse, 96.3% of all children had a normal examination. In this series, the incidence of abnormal medical findings was only 5.5%, even in children who had a history of anal or vaginal penetration.[31]

Female Genital Mutilation/Female Circumcision

The United Nations World Health Organization defines female genital mutilation (FGM), often referred to as "female circumcision," as the "partial or total removal of the female external genitalia or other injury to the female genital organs for cultural and other non-therapeutic reasons." It is estimated that 100 to 140 million girls and women in the world have undergone some form of FGM, and 3 million girls are at risk from the practice each year (**Box 1**).[32] Type 1 and 2 FGM account for 80% of the cases worldwide. Type 3 is the most extreme and accounts for 15% of the cases but is the practice of choice in several African countries. Girls may undergo this procedure between the age of 4 and 14 years, but it can take place in infancy, late adolescence, before

> **Box 1**
> **Categories of female genital mutilation**
>
> Type 1: Excision of the precipice (the fold of skin surrounding the clitoris), with or without excision of part of the entire clitoris
>
> Type 2: Excision of the clitoris with partial or total removal of the labia minora (the smaller inner folds of the vulva)
>
> Type 3: Excision of part or all of the external genitalia and stitching or narrowing of the vaginal opening
>
> Type 4: Unclassified, which includes pricking, piercing, or incising of the clitoris and/or labia; stretching of the clitoris and/or labia; cauterization by burning of the clitoris and surrounding tissue; scraping of tissue surrounding the opening of the vagina (angurya cuts) or cutting of the vagina (gishiri cuts); introduction of corrosive substances or herbs into the vagina to cause bleeding or to tighten or narrow the vagina; and any other procedure that can be included in the definition of female genital mutilation
>
> *Data from* UNAIDS, UNDP, UNECA, UNESCO, UNFPA, UNHCHR, UNHCR, UNICEF, UNIFEM, WHO. Eliminating female genital mutilation: an interagency statement. Geneva (Switzerland): World Health Organization Press; 2008.

marriage, or at the time of the first pregnancy. Because of the immigration of women from areas where FGM is practiced to other countries, medical care providers all over the world now are caring for these women. The World Health Organization, the International Council of Nurses, the International Confederation of Midwives, and the International Federation of Gynecologists and Obstetricians have openly condemned this practice of willful damage to healthy organs for nontherapeutic reasons. FGM is considered a form of violence against girls and women. The immediate health consequences of FGM include severe pain, shock, hemorrhage, and sepsis. Victims may suffer from urinary retention, menstrual retention, ulceration of the genital region, and injury to adjacent tissue. Long-term complications include cysts and abscesses, keloid scar formation, damage to the urethra resulting in urinary incontinence, dyspareunia, sexual dysfunction, and difficulties with childbirth. During vaginal deliveries, the infibulated woman must be opened to allow passage of the baby. If this opening is not done, she is at risk for formation of vesicovaginal and rectovaginal fistulas, as well as undue suffering, including increased risk of stillbirth and maternal death. The practice of FGM poses a serious challenge for the medical community. Obstetricians confronted by circumcised women must determine the safest way of monitoring pregnancy, given the constraints. Another ethical dilemma arises when women request reinfibulation after giving birth. In the past, physicians have resewn the genitals in an attempt to be culturally appropriate. Most recently, various medical communities have issued guidelines stating that no woman should be recircumcised after giving birth. The conflict between patient wishes and medical guidelines can create professional and ethical dilemmas for the health care worker.[33]

SPECIAL CONSIDERATIONS
Effect of Hormones

The influence of estrogen on tissues is well known. Newborns of both genders often have breast buds because of exposure to maternal hormones. The impact of estrogen on the external genital structures of a newborn is labial swelling, prominence of the clitoris, edema of the hymen, a mucous vaginal discharge, and even occasional withdrawal bleeding or spotting from endometrial sloughing. By 6 to 8 months of age, these changes gradually subside, and the infant's breast buds usually are no longer palpable.[34] Lack of endogenous estrogen production in childhood is associated with flattening of the labia, decrease in the size of the clitoris, and thinning of the hymen. The introital mucosa appears shiny and reddened, and trauma or infections may result in bleeding. Vulvar infections in children most commonly are related to poor hygiene, because the introital tissues are vulnerable to exposure to fecal pathogens. Traumatic distention of the prepubertal hymen or vagina may result in tearing, because the tissues do not allow for stretching, but minor injuries may heal rapidly. At puberty, changes related to estrogen include breast development, enlargement of the labia minora, edematous and pink changes in the hymenal tissues, and a watery mucus vaginal discharge (physiologic leukorrhea). Once exposed to estrogen, the postpubertal vagina and hymen are more distensible and less likely to tear with gentle distention (tampon use). Blunt forceful penetrating trauma may result in lacerations, but even an astute clinician cannot tell if a postpubertal woman has had genital penetration based on the physical examination.[35,36]

Healing Times for Injuries

In a multicenter, retrospective study, photographs were used to document the healing process and outcome of hymenal and nonhymenal genital injuries in prepubertal and pubertal girls whose ages ranged from 4 months to 18 years. An interesting difference was found. In prepubertal girls 88% of hymenal lacerations were in the posterior location, whereas in adolescents 60% were posterior and 23% were lateral at either the 3 o'clock or 9 o'clock location. The documented rapid resolution of these injuries (**Table 2**) makes it imperative that a child or an adolescent be examined as soon as possible when there is a suspicion of a possible sexual assault.[37,38]

DIAGNOSES THAT CAN BE CONFUSED WITH SEXUAL ABUSE OR INJURY

Normal variations in genital anatomy often are misinterpreted as evidence of old trauma or past injuries. The pediatric hymen may have bumps associated with intravaginal ridges or septae or polyps. Labial adhesions, lichen sclerosus, and urethral prolapse are common conditions that require a degree of clinical experience to diagnose and manage (**Fig. 4**). Molluscum contagiosum, viral-associated ulcerations, vertically transmitted warts, vaginal foreign bodies, and vulvo-vaginitis (either nonspecific or with identified pathogens) caused by poor genital hygiene may be misleading. It is valuable for families, health professionals, and legal authorities to have early

Table 2 Time required for nonhymenal genital injuries to heal or resolve	
Type of Injury	**Time of Resolution**
Abrasions	2–3 days
Edema	5 days
Ecchymoses (bruising)	2–18 days
Labial hematoma	2 weeks to 4 weeks; may require surgical drainage
Petechia	24 hours
Blood blisters	30 days in prepubertal girl, 24 days in pubertal girl
Superficial lacerations	2 days with new vessel formation in the prepubertal girls, scar tissue formation in pubertal girls
Deeper lacerations	May require surgical repair

Data from McCann J, Miyamoto S, Boyle C, et al. Healing of nonhymenal genital injuries in prepubertal and adolescent girls: a descriptive study. Pediatrics 2007;120(5):1000–11.

access to expert opinion that may prevent an unnecessary investigation for sexual abuse. Any prepubertal child who has physical symptoms and in whom there is a concern about sexual abuse should be seen urgently by a trained examiner, so that the child can receive appropriate diagnosis and treatment. Some of these children will, in fact, have been sexually abused, but when the concern is based largely on their symptoms, many will not.[30] The role of the clinician in these situations is to provide expertise or to refer the patient and her family to someone who has expertise in the normal variants of genital anatomy and abnormal genital findings.[30]

ADVOCACY

Research is ongoing to determine which children and adolescents are at greatest risk for traumatic stress disorders (either immediate or delayed) because of victimization of a sexual or nonsexual nature. It is thought that accidental trauma or an isolated sexual assault at the hands of a stranger may be less provocative of psychopathology because the family exists as an intact supportive unit. Various protective factors for children in adverse circumstances include intelligence, parental attachment, external interests, coping skills, peer relations, and temperament. Unfortunately, there is a powerful relationship between adverse childhood experiences and the risk of substance and illicit drug abuse, depressed affect, and attempted suicide.[39]

"Poly-victimization" refers to children who have experienced a pattern of on-going or multiple victimizations instead of a single traumatizing event.[40] Previously victimized children, especially those who experienced child maltreatment or family violence or bullying, seem to be at greater risk for subsequent victimizations and are at greater risk for anxiety and depression. These children may blame themselves and be less

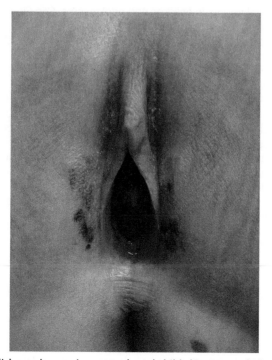

Fig. 4. Untreated lichen sclerosus in a prepubertal child. (*Courtesy of* Diane F. Merritt, MD, Saint Louis, Missouri.)

resilient. Conversely, if the child lives in a cultural setting in which the victim sees other children also being victimized, the child may be able to discount his or her personal culpability and become less vulnerable. More research needs to be done on determining whether cumulative events take a greater toll than isolated events.

Advocacy for children and adolescent victims of violent genital injuries has reached an international level. The United Nations Secretary General's Study on Violence against Children[41] paints a detailed picture of the nature, extent, and causes of violence against children and proposes recommendations on how to prevent and respond to it. The World Health Organization held a global launch of the World Report on Child Injury and Prevention in December 2008. More information on this program can be found at http://www.who.int/violence_injury_prevention/child/injury/world_report/en/.

Individual health care providers play an important role in the identification, support, and referral of children and adolescents who suffer from violence as well as in the management of its consequences.[42,43]

SUMMARY

Genital injuries in children and adolescents may occur accidentally or as the result of an act of violence. This article discusses the etiologies and management of genital trauma. Awareness needs to be heightened among individual providers of medical care, as well as in the international community, to protect young girls from becoming victims of violence and to provide avenues for recovery.

REFERENCES

1. Merritt DF. Genital trauma in children and adolescents. Clin Obstet Gynecol 2008; 51(2):237–48.
2. Huffman JW. Gynecologic examination of the premenarcheal child. Pediatr Ann 1974;3:6–18.
3. Redman JF, Bissada NK. How to make a good examination of the genitalia of young girls. Clin Pediatr 1976;15(10):907–8.
4. Emans SJ, Goldstein DP. The gynecologic examination of the prepubertal child with vulvovaginitis: use of the knee–chest position. Pediatrics 1980;65(4):758–60.
5. Overstolz G, Baker-Gibbs E. The use of the prone knee–chest position: examiner habit or necessity? J Forensic Nurs 2002;1:12–5.
6. Boyle C, McCann J, Miyamoto S, et al. Comparison of examination methods used in the evaluation of prepubertal and pubertal female genitalia: a descriptive study. Child Abuse Negl 2008;32(2):229–43.
7. Sugar NF, Feldman KW. Perineal impalements in children: distinguishing accidents from abuse. Pediatr Emerg Care 2007;23(9):605–16.
8. Onen A, Oztürk H, Yayla M, et al. Genital trauma in children: classification and management. Urology 2005;65(5):986–90.
9. Perlman SE, Hertweck SP, Wolfe WM. Water-ski douche injury in a premenarcheal female. Pediatrics 1995;96(4 Pt 1):782–3.
10. Haefner HK, Anderson F, Johnson MP. Vaginal laceration following a jet-ski accident. Obstet Gynecol 1991;78(5 Pt 2):986–8.
11. Lacy J, Brennand E, Ornstein M, et al. Vaginal injury from a high pressure water jet in a prepubescent girl. Pediatr Emerg Care 2007;23(2):112–4.
12. Boos SC, Rosas AJ, Boyle C, et al. Anogenital injuries in child pedestrians run over by low-speed motor vehicles: four cases with findings that mimic child sexual abuse. Pediatrics 2003;112(1 Pt 1):e77–84.

13. Vidmar L, Poljak M, Tomazic J, et al. Transmission of HIV-1 by human bite. Lancet 1996;347(9017):1762.
14. Fiumara N, Exner J. Primary syphilis following a human bite. Sex Transm Dis 1981;8(1):21–2.
15. Rosen T. Penile ulcer from traumatic orogenital contact. Dermatol Online J 2005; 11(2):18.
16. Gomes CM, Ribeiro-Filho L, Giron AM, et al. Genital trauma due to animal bites. J Urol 2000;165(1):80–3.
17. Ball V, Younggren BN. Emergency management of difficult wounds: part I. Emerg Med Clin North Am 2007;25(1):101–21.
18. Lowell G, Quinlan K, Gottlieb LJ. Preventing unintentional scald burns: moving beyond tap water. Pediatrics 2008;122(4):799–804.
19. Kai-Yang L, Zhao-Fan X, Luo-Man Z, et al. Epidemiology of pediatric burns requiring hospitalization in China: a literature review of retrospective studies. Pediatrics 2008;122(1):132–42.
20. Rimmer RB, Weigand S, Foster KN, et al. Scald burns in young children—a review of Arizona burn center pediatric patients and a proposal for prevention in the Hispanic community. J Burn Care Res 2008;29(4):595–605.
21. Kos L, Shwayder T. Cutaneous manifestations of child abuse. Pediatr Dermatol 2006;23(4):311–20.
22. Yanoh K, Yonemura Y. Severe vaginal ulcerations secondary to insertion of an alkaline battery. J Trauma 2005;58(2):410–2.
23. Bechtel K, Santucci K, Walsh S. Hematoma of the labia majora in an adolescent girl. Pediatr Emerg Care 2007;23(6):407–8.
24. Jeng CJ, Wang LR. Vaginal laceration and hemorrhagic shock during consensual sexual intercourse. J Sex Marital Ther 2007;33(3):249–53.
25. Sloan MM, Karimian M, Ilbeigi P. Nonobstetric lacerations of the vagina. J Am Osteopath Assoc 2006;106(5):271–3.
26. Kellogg N. American Academy of Pediatrics Committee on Child Abuse and Neglect. The evaluation of sexual abuse in children. Pediatrics 2005;116(2): 506–12.
27. Adams JA, Kaplan RA, Starling SP, et al. Guidelines for medical care of children who may have been sexually abused. J Pediatr Adolesc Gynecol 2007;20(3): 163–72.
28. Adams JA. Guidelines for the medical care of children evaluated for suspected sexual abuse: an update for 2008. Curr Opin Obstet Gynecol 2008;20(5):435–41.
29. Alempijevic D, Saiv S, Pavlekic S, et al. Severity of injuries among sexual assault victims. J Forensic Leg Med 2007;14(5):266–9.
30. Kelly P, Koh J, Thompson JM. Diagnostic findings in alleged sexual abuse: symptoms have no predictive value. J Paediatr Child Health 2006;42(3):112–7.
31. Heger A, Ticson L, Velasquez O, et al. Children referred for possible sexual abuse: medical findings in 2384 children. Child Abuse Negl 2002;26(6–7): 645–59.
32. UNAIDS, UNDP, UNECA, UNESCO, UNFPA, UNHCHR, UNHCR, UNICEF, UNIFEM, WHO. Eliminating female genital mutilation: an interagency statement. Geneva (Switzerland): World Health Organization Press; 2008.
33. Baron EM, Denmark FL. An exploration of female genital mutilation. Ann N Y Acad Sci 2006;1087:339–55.
34. Abnormal puberty and growth problems. In: Speroff L, Fritz MA, editors. Clinical endocrinology and infertility. 7th edition. Philadelphia: Lippincott Williams and Wilkins; 2005. p. 362.

35. Underhill RA, Dewhurst J. The doctor cannot always tell. Medical examination of the "intact" hymen. Lancet 1978;1(8060):375–6.
36. Kellogg ND, Menard SW, Santos A. Genital anatomy in pregnant adolescents: "normal" does not mean "nothing happened." Pediatrics 2004;113(1 Pt 1):e67–9.
37. McCann J, Miyamoto S, Boyle C, et al. Healing of nonhymenal genital injuries in prepubertal and adolescent girls: a descriptive study. Pediatrics 2007;120(5):1000–11.
38. McCann J, Miyamoto S, Boyle C, et al. Healing of hymenal injuries in prepubertal and adolescent girls: a descriptive study. Pediatrics 2007;119(5):e1094–106.
39. Dube SR, Anda RF, Felitti VJ, et al. Childhood abuse, household dysfunction, and the risk of attempted suicide throughout the life span: findings from the Adverse Childhood Experiences Study. JAMA 2001;286(24):3089–96.
40. Finkelhor D, Ormrod RK, Turner HA. Poly-victimization: a neglected component in child victimization. Child Abuse Negl 2007;31(1):7–26.
41. The United Nations Secretary General's study on violence against children. Sponsored by OHCHR, UNICEF, WHO. 2005. Available at: http://www.violencestudy.org/r25. Accessed November 2, 2008.
42. Gender and Women's Health, Family and Community Health, Injuries and Violence Prevention, Noncommunicable Diseases and Mental Health. Guidelines for medico-legal care of victims of sexual violence. World Health Organization. Geneva (Switzerland): World Health Organization Press; 2003.
43. WHO Department of Violence and Injury Prevention and Disability. Violence, injuries and disability biennial report, 2006–2007. Geneva (Switzerland): World Health Organization Press; 2008.

The Adolescent Sexual Health Visit

Taraneh Shafii, MD, MPH[a,*], Gale R. Burstein, MD, MPH[b,c]

KEYWORDS

- Adolescent • Sexually transmitted disease
- Sexually transmitted infection • Sexual history • Risk behavior

Adolescents are a challenging population to reach. Yet, despite their stereotypical outward appearance of shunning and ignoring authority figures, when medical providers are able to create a safe, confidential, nonjudgmental, and empowering atmosphere, adolescents are surprisingly open and candid about themselves, their health, and their behavior, including sexuality. The caveat being that providers must ask the sensitive health questions, as adolescents are often reticent to initiate questions about sex or concerns of sexually transmitted infection (STI) symptoms.

Addressing sexual health, screening, and counseling to prevent sequelae of risky sexual behavior are essential components of the adolescent visit to the gynecologist. Discussing sexuality and taking a sexual history may cause feelings of discomfort for the provider and adolescent patient alike. Taking the time to build rapport and trust and the guarantee of confidentiality are key to engaging adolescent patients to discuss their personal health concerns with their provider, thereby permitting him or her to provide optimal care.

This article offers recommendations to facilitate dialog with the adolescent patient, addresses special considerations for the adolescent examination, discusses the use of some of the newly available tests for STIs, and suggests the recommended approach to management of STIs in adolescents.

WHY IS IT IMPORTANT TO DISCUSS SEXUALITY WITH ADOLESCENT PATIENTS?

Adolescence is a period of significant physical, cognitive, and psychosocial growth and development. For most, adolescence is a time of relative good health, requiring few visits to health care providers. Most health morbidity and mortality that plague

[a] Section of Adolescent Medicine, Department of Pediatrics, University of Washington School of Medicine, Harborview Medical Center, 325 9th Avenue, Box #359777, Seattle, WA 98104, USA
[b] Department of Pediatrics, SUNY at Buffalo School of Medicine and Biomedical Sciences, 95 Franklin Street, Room 984, Buffalo, NY 14202, USA
[c] Epidemiology and Surveillance, Erie County Department of Health; 219 Bryant Street, Buffalo, NY 14222, USA
* Corresponding author.
E-mail address: tshafii@u.washington.edu (T. Shafii).

Obstet Gynecol Clin N Am 36 (2009) 99–117
doi:10.1016/j.ogc.2009.01.001
0889-8545/09/$ – see front matter © 2009 Elsevier Inc. All rights reserved.

obgyn.theclinics.com

adolescent health are from consequences of high-risk behaviors, exemplified in adolescent sexual behavior.

ADOLESCENTS AND SEXUALLY TRANSMITTED INFECTIONS

In the United States, 65% of high school 12th grade students have had vaginal intercourse, and more than one third of all high school students have had sex in the past 3 months, with 15% having had four or more lifetime partners.[1] The adverse health consequences of adolescent high-risk sexual behaviors are demonstrated in the astronomic rates of STIs.

Adolescents and young adults have the highest STI rates compared with other age groups, with half of the almost 19 million STI cases in the United States diagnosed annually occurring in 15- to 24-year-olds.[2] Among females, the highest reported gonorrhea and chlamydia rates are among 15- to 19-year-olds followed by 20- to 24-year-olds with the next highest. Among males, the highest reported rates are among young adults age 20 to 24 years, with 15- to 19-year-old males following in close second.[3] In the United States, HIV/AIDS is now the seventh leading cause of mortality in young adults younger than 25 years, and it accounts for 13% of all cases diagnosed annually. HIV Infection diagnosed in those younger than 25 years old is acquired predominantly through heterosexual contact.

WHY ARE ADOLESCENTS AT HIGH RISK FOR ACQUIRING SEXUALLY TRANSMITTED INFECTIONS?

Factors that increase adolescents' risk for STIs can be categorized as (1) biologic susceptibility, (2) psychosocial development, (3) health care use and compliance, and (4) concern for confidentiality, ethical, and legal issues. These four factors contribute to adolescent health risk and influence high-risk behavior in the environment of evolving sexuality and sexual behavior as youth progress through puberty (**Fig. 1**).

Biologic Factors

Because of developing physiologic characteristics, adolescent females are more vulnerable to STIs than adult females. The immature and incompletely estrogenized cervix is characterized by persistence of columnar epithelium extending to the ectocervix, referred to as cervical ectopy (**Fig. 2**). Columnar epithelium is more susceptible to invasion by pathogens, such as *Neisseria gonorrhoeae* and *Chlamydia trachomatis*

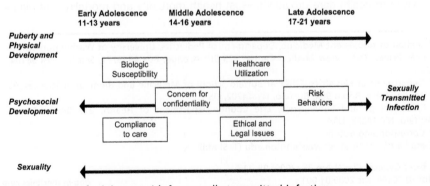

Fig. 1. Schematic of adolescent risk for sexually transmitted infections.

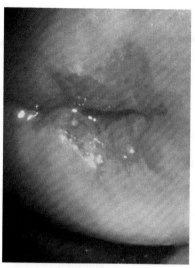

Fig. 2. Cervical ectopy. (*From* Seattle STD/HIV Prevention Training Center at the University of Washington/Claire E. Stevens; with permission.)

than squamous epithelium, which covers the vagina and the mature adult female cervix. Adolescent females tend to have thinner cervical mucus than adult females, thereby presenting a weaker barrier to pathogens infecting the cervix and upper reproductive tract.

Lower estrogen levels present in early adolescence result in thinner genital tissue. In addition, insufficient sexual arousal results in inadequate vaginal lubrication before penetration. This combination places adolescent females at increased risk for trauma or irritation to the female genital tissue, creating potential portals of entry for pathogens.

Psychosocial Development

To guide their approach to the patient, before initiating an interview with an adolescent, it is helpful for providers to be sensitive to adolescent psychosocial development. Adolescence spans approximately a 10-year period consisting of three phases: early adolescence, age 11 to 13 years, or middle school age; middle adolescence, age 14 to 16 years, or high school age; and late adolescence, age 17 to 21 years, or late high school and college (**Table 1**). Many of the developmental issues of older adolescents, however, are also operative in the young adult (eg, early 20s).

EARLY ADOLESCENCE (11 TO 13 YEARS)

Early adolescence is marked by the onset of puberty and physical changes that are often rapid, dramatic, and may occur asynchronously and at different rates from their peers. The underlying question of this age group, 'Am I normal?'[4] continuously is being assessed in the classroom, in the locker room, and at sleepovers. During the physical examination, especially the breast and genital examination, it is of utmost importance that the provider reassures the adolescent that everything looks healthy and normal for her developmental stage.

Early adolescence marks the conscious awakening of sexual feelings and usually manifests as sexual fantasies and masturbation, all of which may be confusing and

Table 1
Physical, psychosocial, and sexual development in adolescents

	Early Adolescence	Middle Adolescence	Late Adolescence
Physical growth	Onset of puberty; rapid changes at different timing and rate from peers	Full physical maturation obtained by females with menarche; more variable in males with continued growth	Full adult physical development obtained by all
Body image	Am I normal? Concern about body and pubertal changes	Start acceptance of body changes; preoccupied with making body more attractive	Accepting and comfortable with pubertal changes and body
Cognition	Concrete, unable to think abstractedly or plan ahead; poor impulse control	Able to conceptualize and think abstractly; may revert to concrete thinking in times of stress; propensity for risk-taking behavior	Abstract thought and ability to anticipate future and plan accordingly; increased self-efficacy
Independence/ peers	Increased interest in friends with a decreased focus on family activities; same-sex friendships predominate	Height of conformity to peer values, appearance and behavior; family conflict; dating in couples or groups common	Establishment of personal values and goals; reacceptance of family; conformity to and influence of peer group fades
Sexuality	Sexual myths, fantasies, masturbation; usually no sexual contact with partner	Sexual contact ranges from hand-holding to intercourse; often exploratory; serial monogamy common	Sexual intercourse achieved by most; focus on intense relationship with one partner; serial monogamy may persist

Data from Radzik M, Sherer S, Neinstein LS. Psychosocial development in normal adolescents. In: Neinstein LS, Gordon CM, Katzman DK, et al, editors. Adolescent health care: a practical guide. 5th edition. Philadelphia: Wolters Kluwer/Lippincott Williams and Wilkins; 2007.

guilt-producing to the youth. Sexual myths are common (eg, you can't get pregnant the first time you have sex), as are dirty jokes amongst peers (eg, think back to the antics of middle school boys). Sexual activity at this stage is usually nonphysical and manifests as phone calls and passing of notes and text messages. Clinicians must recognize that in some populations, however, adolescents are initiating sexual intimacy at this age, including oral sex and anal and vaginal intercourse. In fact, 7% of youth in the United States report first vaginal intercourse before 13 years of age.[1]

Early adolescent cognitive abilities are concrete, and young adolescents are unable to think abstractly, conceptualize, or develop a plan for the future. For example, when asked if she is sexually active, the concrete adolescent may think the provider is asking if she is active during sex, or she may think the provider is asking if she is having sex that day, instead of asking whether she has ever had sex. The cognitive abilities at this developmental stage explain why many young adolescents do not plan ahead or anticipate the need for condoms when sexually active.

Using a condom presents an additional challenge for these youth. In the setting of heightened arousal and emotion, their manual dexterity is limited and they may have difficulty with complex tasks requiring multiple steps like opening a condom package and putting the condom on the penis. These limitations are supported in the findings that younger adolescents are less likely to use condoms or other forms of contraception, and if used, are more likely to have difficulty.[5–8]

MIDDLE ADOLESCENCE (14 TO 16 YEARS)

Full physical maturation is attained by most in middle adolescence, with menarche being the hallmark in females. Sexuality is heightened during this stage, involves more physical contact and is often exploratory and experiential[9] rather than an expression of emotional attachment. Sexual activity at this stage progresses to dating in groups or as couples, hand-holding, touching, kissing, and mutual masturbation. As the average age of sexual debut in the United States is 16.5 years, providers must assume that their middle adolescent patient (1) already may be engaging in oral, anal, or vaginal intercourse; (2) is, therefore, at risk of acquiring STIs; and (3) should be screened by sexual history and laboratory testing. Many adolescents do not seek health care until well after first intercourse.[10–14]

Adolescents in this stage develop capabilities for abstract thinking and conceptualization, yet their ability to carry out such behavior may be limited. In addition, adolescents may revert back to concrete thinking during times of stress, which adds to their susceptibility to high-risk behaviors in intense, hormonally or emotionally driven situations (eg, sexual activity).

This new abstract thinking skill leads to a belief in their own personal fable. They presume that "nothing bad will happen to me... those things only happen to other people." Although most adolescents in this age group understand that driving while intoxicated or engaging in unprotected sex can lead to harmful consequences, their perceived omnipotence and immortality provide them with a false sense of security.[4] Although these assumptions seem reckless to adults, they may point to the adolescents' level of brain and cognitive development and their limited judgment to identify and acknowledge potentially deleterious situations. Also, adolescents' seemingly cavalier attitude in part, may reflect the paucity of life experience. Adolescents may have to validate for themselves the possibility of an adverse outcome to high-risk behavior (eg, becoming infected with chlamydia from unprotected sex). Regardless, the concern for these middle-adolescents is their propensity for engaging in high-risk behaviors that may be fueled further by peer, alcohol, or drug use influences that compromise inhibitions and result in unexpected, yet adverse, health consequences.

LATE ADOLESCENCE (17 TO 21 YEARS)

By the end of late adolescence, full adult physical maturation has been attained. Sexual orientation is established, and intimacy and commitment with a single individual are the basis of sexual relationships.[4] Abstract thought is established more firmly for most. Late adolescents are able to plan for and effectively use condoms. Interestingly, older adolescents' condom use decreases as their use of hormonal contraception increases, providing an opportunity for STI transmission.

SERIAL MONOGAMY

An interesting societal trend contributing to adolescent sexual risk is the adolescent relationships pattern, described as serial monogamy. Adolescents have relationships of relatively short duration (eg, 2 weeks or 2 months) with one partner, but change partners more frequently. So although they may be monogamous, which may be interpreted as a lower risk relationship, as they accrue an increased number of partners over time, they are in fact still at significant risk for STI exposure. Each new partner brings a renewed need for the potential challenge of negotiating safe sex once more. To assess true STI exposure risk and obtain a more valid assessment of sexual risk behaviors, providers should enquire about the number of partners in the past 3, 6, and 12 months.

TREND FOR EARLIER PUBERTY, EARLIER SEXUAL DEBUT, AND DELAYED MARRIAGE

In the United States, the median age of menarche is approximately 12.4 years (12.1 years in black females); the median age of first sexual intercourse is 16.5 years,[4] and the average age of marriage is the late 20s (an increase in approximately 5 to 8 years from the 1950s). Therefore, the average number of years when females are fertile, hormonally primed for sexual activity, and not married has increased significantly over the past 50 years, resulting in the potential for a higher number of sexual partners and increased likelihood for STI contact and acquisition.

SAME-SEX SEXUAL ACTIVITY AND HOMOSEXUALITY

Same-sex sexual activity is not uncommon in adolescence; it is often exploratory and does not necessarily predict future homosexuality. In the 2002 National Survey of Family Growth, 11% of 15- to 19-year-old girls and 14% of 20- to 24-year-old women reported ever having "any same-sex contact."[15]

Adolescence is the period when sexual orientation is discovered and established. Although there have been societal trends in openness and acceptance of homosexuality in the past decade, the recognition of feeling different from one's peers, being attracted to the same sex, experiencing sexuality contrary to the messages of mainstream society, and fearing rejection and abandonment by one's family and friends may be catastrophic for the young person. Gay, lesbian, bisexual, transgender, and questioning youth are at an increased risk for substance abuse, school failure, homelessness, sexual activity, victimization, body image and eating disorders, depression, and suicide.[9]

Sensitivity and awareness of these possible issues are important when interviewing and obtaining a sexual history from an adolescent. Take for example a 15-year-old girl who comes to the office for her first gynecology visit, and the provider asks, "So do you have a boyfriend?" If the young woman in this scenario is struggling with her sexuality, this approach may be detrimental; the health care provider, as a health authority, is modeling that heterosexuality is the only acceptable orientation. As the adolescent may feel embarrassed and ashamed by her doubts, the provider may have alienated the youth, when instead, he or she could have offered a safe venue for discussion of sexual feelings and important sexual health information and resources of support.

Survey data suggest that anywhere from 3% to 10% of adults in the United States report being lesbian or gay. Adolescents are in the process of understanding and accepting their sexuality as evident in the lower proportion (1% to 4%) of adolescents who report being gay, lesbian, or bisexual and the greater proportion (1% to 11%) who report being unsure about their sexual orientation.[4,15]

An alternative example of initiating a conversation about sex would be:

"You are at the age when you start figuring out if you are interested in or attracted to guys, girls or both ... have you thought about that yet? Have you ever had sex with a guy, girl or both?"

Health care providers are in the unique position to normalize sexuality to youth of all orientations by the words and objectivity used to discuss the topic. By acknowledging different sexual orientations, providers send the message that individual attractions are within the range of normal sexual behavior. This allows the struggling gay or transgender youth to begin to accept herself and provides a medical resource for support and information to field questions and concerns. For the heterosexual youth, providers are modeling a position of acceptance and tolerance for sexual minorities.

AGE DIFFERENTIAL IN SEXUAL PARTNERS AND REPORTING LAWS

A significant number of adolescent females engage in sexual relationships with older males, increasing their likelihood of STI exposure and decreasing their power and capacity to negotiate condom use. Adolescent females with partners who are at least 2 years older are at increased risk for STIs.[5,6,8] Reporting laws for statutory rape and sexual misconduct vary by state. Providers need to be aware of the laws in their state.

ESTABLISHING RAPPORT

Building rapport is the most important skill a provider needs in taking care of adolescents. Most adolescent adverse health consequences are the direct results of risk-taking behaviors. To create an environment where the patient feels safe disclosing sexual behaviors and health concerns, providers need to establish a good rapport with their adolescent patients. A few simple techniques may help reassure the adolescent that her provider is trustworthy (**Box 1**).

Box 1
Techniques for establishing rapport with adolescents

Introduce yourself to the adolescent first, look her in the eye, shake her hand and sit down during the interview

Acknowledge the adolescent as your primary patient by directing your questions primarily to her rather than her parents.

Use conversation icebreakers to allow time for the adolescent to become more comfortable and get a sense of who you are.

Allow the adolescent to remain dressed during the interview and sit in a chair rather than on the examination table.

Interview the adolescent without her family present for sensitive questions.

Ensure confidentiality and provide a safe environment for her to be honest.

Practice reflective listening and take time to listen to what the adolescent is saying and not saying.

Facilitate a comfortable experience for the adolescent by providing adolescent-friendly and easy-to-access office and staff.

Acknowledge the Adolescent as the Primary Patient

Although it may be common for mothers to initiate and accompany their daughters on their first visit to the gynecologist, the adolescent is the primary patient; the parents/guardians are secondary. To communicate this at the visit, upon entering the room, look at the adolescent first, make eye contact, address her and shake her hand, before acknowledging the accompanying caregiver. Remember to sit down! Whether in the room for 5 minutes or 20 minutes, sitting down reaffirms to the adolescent that she is important; the provider is not in a hurry, and she has the provider's undivided attention.

Just as in introductions, speak directly to the adolescent when initiating the interview. "What brings you in today?" Younger adolescents may look at the parent/guardian instead of answering the question. That is the cue to first interview the accompanying adult; yet the provider should take every opportunity to return the interview to the adolescent, "Do you agree?" "Is that how it feels?" "You tell me how it feels." For older adolescents, start the interview of nonsensitive questions with the patient and end by asking the parents/guardians if they have anything to add and to state their specific concerns (as this may differ significantly from the adolescents). Parents/guardians are valuable in providing past medical history and family history for any age adolescent who may not know the details of her health history.

Interview the Adolescent without Accompanying Adults Present

Despite mothers accompanying their daughters to the office visit, providers should assume that mothers do not know the extent of their daughters' sexual activity. After the parents/guardians have provided necessary health information and voiced their concerns, ask the parent/guardian to leave the examination room to obtain private time with the adolescent patient. Separating the parents/guardians and the adolescent is imperative and serves several purposes:

Being interviewed alone empowers the adolescent to be responsible for her own health.
The time together helps to create a therapeutic alliance between the provider and patient.
Time alone with the patient allows providers the opportunity to obtain a confidential sexual history and screen for behavioral risks.

Never ask an adolescent about sexual activity in front of a parent/guardian; the answer will most likely be, "no." Most adults honor the request to step out briefly, especially when the practitioner explains that they will be informed of any serious health concerns and are allowed to return to the examination room for the conclusion of the visit.

A useful technique to ensure parents/guardians will be comfortable leaving their adolescent alone with the provider is to normalize the process during the initial interview. "You are at the age where it is time to start taking on some of the responsibility for your health yourself; therefore, I would like to spend some time with you alone without your parents present." "It is my practice with all patients your age to spend some time talking to you without your parents present." "It is our clinic policy regarding adolescents to do a portion of the visit separate from the parents." Inviting parents/guardians back into the room for the end of the visit to hear the assessment and management plan, (that is, with your patient's approval), (1) prevents them from feeling alienated, (2) allows them to continue to be engaged in their adolescent's health at some level, and (3) assists with reinforcement of the care plan, as adolescents often have difficulty following through with medical directions.

Other simple steps providers can take to initiate the rapport and comfort-building process before they even see their patient include providing an adolescent-friendly space in the waiting room, and placing age-appropriate magazines, brochures and posters or even a computerized health education module for teens available in the waiting and examination rooms. Hiring staff members who enjoy adolescents and are skilled in communicating with them on the telephone and in the office helps to alleviate the adolescent's anxiety for the office visit and increases the likelihood that they will return for ongoing care. Allowing the adolescent to remain dressed during the interview and covered as much as possible during the examination contributes to feelings of safety and a sense of being in control of their bodies and their environment.

THE INTERVIEW

Effective communication with adolescents requires a sensitive, flexible, and developmentally oriented approach. Because diagnosis and treatment are the emphasis of medical training, most providers have not received formal training in interviewing techniques or the opportunity to practice these skills with adolescent patients. In a busy gynecologic practice, taking the time necessary to establish rapport and interview the adolescent may not be feasible; alternatives are to have a nurse or midlevel provider (eg, nurse practitioner, physician assistant) dedicated to this purpose, as it must be done to provide optimal care.

Adolescents can be particularly challenging to interview. Their ability to reason lies somewhere between the continuum of concrete operations of childhood and formal operations of adulthood. Asking questions about sexuality also can be a particularly difficult subject to approach. Most adolescents (and adults) prefer to avoid initiating a conversation about sex. Providers must be comfortable with the subject of sexuality to be able to make the adolescent feel comfortable discussing this sensitive and private issue. It is worthwhile for providers to reflect on their own personal experiences of puberty, adolescence, and sexuality to better understand and identify with their patients. Health care providers must set personal views aside and provide patients with comprehensive reproductive health care. If providers feel uncomfortable discussing sexuality and sexual behaviors with their adolescent patients, it is their obligation to refer these patients to colleagues who are able to provide appropriate care. What follows are useful strategies for interviewing adolescent patients, with special emphasis on obtaining information most helpful in assessing sexual risk behaviors and risk for STIs.

OUTLINE THE OFFICE VISIT

Outlining what is going to take place during the office visit helps to decrease the adolescent's anxiety. "First, I am going to talk to you and your mom; then I would like to talk to you by yourself for a bit. Then I will examine you, and if we need to do any tests, I may need to get a blood or urine sample from you." An adolescent will feel much more comfortable if she knows what to expect. Because genital examinations are a source of great anxiety and embarrassment for youth, if a genital examination will take place, the provider should inform the adolescent patient. If a pelvic examination will be performed, a full explanation is imperative, especially if this is the patient's first examination. Showing the adolescent the speculum, and even letting her handle it, usually diminishes rather than escalates anxiety. Diagrams or plastic genitalia models and mirrors during the examination are useful to educate youth, as most young females are unaware of their anatomy and do not know the proper terms. Many young women never have seen their own anatomy.

ENSURE CONFIDENTIALITY

At the opening of the interview, the provider must define his or her confidentiality policy and under what circumstances confidentiality will be breached (eg, suicidal/homicidal thoughts, physical/sexual abuse). "What you and I talk about is confidential from your family, which means I am not going to tell them what we talk about, unless I am worried that you are hurting yourself, hurting someone else, or someone is hurting you." An adolescent must understand that the provider is *her* health care provider, not the parents'. Most adolescents will not admit to engaging in any risk behaviors if she believes parents/guardians will be informed.

Health insurance presents another challenge for providing confidential care to adolescents. Most commercial health plans itemize services so the bill that is sent to the adolescent's family may divulge the type of care provided. So before guaranteeing confidential care to their adolescent patients, providers must be savvy to whether the STI test they ordered will show up on the parent's bill. Providers who care for commercially insured sexually active adolescents can use as ICD-9 codes symptoms (eg, dysmenorrhea, irregular menses) and general clinical findings (ie, vaginal discharge, pyuria, urinary complaints or symptoms of vulvitis) rather than specific STI diagnoses, such as trichomonas or chlamydia. Tools to enhance confidentiality and coding are available on the North American Society for Pediatric and Adolescent Gynecology at: www.naspag.org/Professionals/clinicalResources.cfm.

ASK NONTHREATENING QUESTIONS FIRST

Begin the interview with nonthreatening questions, with subsequent progression to more sensitive questions. Small talk (eg, ask casually about school, upcoming or past vacations, sports) can be quite useful, because:

- It is an icebreaker and gives the patient time to feel out the provider and adjust to her surroundings.
- It gives the provider a sense of how the rest of the interview will flow; is the patient shy or relaxed.
- If the parent/guardian is present, it gives the provider insight into the parent–child dynamic.

Next ask the adolescent about her health concerns. It is important to have and display genuine interest and concern throughout the interview; nothing is more effective in establishing rapport. An adolescent's perception of disinterest will result in loss of trust.

USE WRITTEN QUESTIONNAIRES FOR SENSITIVE QUESTIONS

Some adolescents find it easier to admit to risk behaviors on paper rather than out loud to an adult provider. It may be useful to use paper questionnaires in a busy office practice that does not allow time for lengthy "get-to-know-you" and rapport-building visits (see Appendix for list of free, online, adolescent risk-behavior screening tools). These forms can be completed while the patient is waiting to be seen and then quickly reviewed by the provider to identify areas on which to focus during the patient interview. Remember to provide a parent-free space for the adolescent to complete the questionnaire in privacy without fear of disclosure. The utility may be limited in patients who have limited literacy skills or in populations where there are language barriers.

INTERVIEWING TECHNIQUES

Obtaining pertinent information from an adolescent and engaging her in a comfortable conversation at the same time is an art. The following are several interview techniques that can aid the provider in leading an informative dialog with the adolescent patient.[4]

Open-Ended Questions

An adolescent, especially one with concrete thought, will be quick to answer "yes" or "no" in response to a specifically directed question. Avoid questions that yield yes or no responses. One might phrase the question, "How often do you use condoms? " rather than, "Do you use condoms all the time?"

Reflection Responses

Reflection responses mirror the adolescent's feelings and can help stimulate further conversation on a topic. "So, you feel it is difficult to get your partner to use condoms? Tell me about that."

Clarification Questions

Asking the adolescent to explain anything the practitioner does not understand is not insulting, and is in fact empowering to the adolescent, as now she is the expert teaching the practitioner, "What do you mean when you say.......?"

Restatement and Summation Responses

Restating and summarizing the relevant issues can clarify the question and encourage more dialog. "It seems like you want to tell your partner that you have chlamydia, but you are afraid he will blame you and get angry. Is that right?"

Reassuring Statements and Generalization

Reassuring statements validate the adolescent's feelings, reestablish the practitioner's role as an advocate, and can stimulate more dialog. "Many young women your age decide to wait to have sex until they are older, out of high school, or even married. Deciding what is right for you does not mean there is anything wrong with you, even if it is different than what your friends are doing."

Support and Empathy

A supportive and empathetic response during the conversation acknowledging the adolescent's difficult experience can stimulate more dialog and impart further trust. "It sounds like this has been difficult for you. I see this happen to a lot of my patients ...."

The Quiet Adolescent

For the noncommunicative adolescent, return to icebreakers; the goal is to get these patients to talk about anything. Ask her to discuss something that interests her, such as school, sports, or friends, to help her relax and feel comfortable.

Adolescent Sexuality, Culture, and Religion

In the next decade, the ethnic make up of adolescents in the United States will continue to diversify, bringing with it a mélange of cultural and religious traditions. Health care providers must be savvy to the varying cultural and religious beliefs of their patient population and demonstrate cultural sensitivity to different practices. For example, youth may be resistant to discussing the topic of sex regardless of their level of sexual experience, because sexual activity before marriage is shunned by many cultures and religions. Therefore, framing information about sexuality in the context of helping their peers and friends who may be or become sexually active is a nonthreatening and effective method to provide sexual education to all patients.

Caveats to Asking the Sex Questions—What Practitioners Need to Know About their Patient's Sexuality and How to do the Examination

The hidden agenda—if practitioners ask, patients will tell; if practitioners do not they will not

The hidden agenda is the phenomena of adolescents seeking care for a sensitive health issue (eg, STI symptoms) and assuming their provider will know what is wrong with them without actually verbalizing the problem. For example, an adolescent female presents with complaints of a belly ache; the provider works up the abdominal pain, but does not screen for sexual behaviors and treats the patient for presumed gastritis. The patient leaves the office reassured that she is not infected with an STI, because she believes the provider is omniscient and would have known if she were infected. To know whether an adolescent patient is having sex, providers must ask the patient; the adolescent will not always volunteer her true health concerns but is surprisingly candid when asked directly.

What Kind of Sex?

Oral, anal, and vaginal sex and whether condoms are used and used correctly result in varying levels of STI risk. As adolescents present in varying stages of cognitive development, sexual knowledge, and sexual experience, the general question of, "Are you sexually active?" will be interpreted differently by individual adolescents. Providers need to ask very direct and specific questions to yield the information needed to make an accurate risk assessment and determine the extent of STI screening required. "Have you had sex with guys, girls, or both? Have you ever had oral sex? Anal sex? Vaginal or regular sex?" If in doubt of a youth's understanding of the definitions of oral, anal, or vaginal sex, the provider should pose the questions to ensure they are discussing the same behavior. "Tell me what 'having sex' means to you." Most likely the adolescent will squirm, be embarrassed, and have difficulty answering the question. The provider then has the opportunity to provide the definitions. For example, "I want to make sure we are talking about the same thing: so oral sex means your partner kisses or puts his/her mouth on your vagina/penis; some people call it 'going down on each other;' have you ever done that?" (**Box 2**).

The Physical Examination

Foremost, the provider always should make the adolescent feel like she is in control. Providers should let the adolescent know what part of the examination will be performed next and that the physical examination will stop at any time if she is uncomfortable. Providers should explain that they are doing the examination to best take care of their patients' health and want to make sure that they are indeed healthy. Offer as many options as possible during the examination to empower the patient and make her feel as safe and comfortable as possible. For example, ask the adolescent if she would be more comfortable completely undressing and changing into a gown before the examination or would prefer to undress only the part of the body being examined at the time, so that she remains partially dressed throughout the examination. Younger adolescents may prefer the latter option, because they may feel insecure about their bodies. Another strategy for females who are resistant to undressing and only require an external genital examination is to allow them to

---

Box 2
Key topics to cover and sample questions for the sexual interview with adolescents

Introduce the topic and establish confidentiality

"I need to ask you some personal questions that I ask all of my patients so that I can best take care of your health. What we talk about is confidential from your family, which means I am not going to tell them what we talk about, unless I am worried that somebody is hurting you, you are hurting yourself, or you are hurting somebody else. You do not have to answer any question that you don't want to answer."

Sexual orientation

"You are at the age when people start to figure out who they like, are interested in or attracted to. Have you thought about that? Do you like guys, girls, or both?"

Sexual activity

"Have you ever been so close to a guy/girl that you held hands or kissed? What about touching your private areas, on top of or under your clothes? Have you ever had sex? By that I mean, have you had sex where a guy puts his penis inside a girl's vagina? What about oral sex where your partner puts his or her mouth on your vagina? What about anal sex, where a guy puts his penis inside your anus or bottom?"

Sexual abuse

"Have you ever had sex when you didn't really want to? Has anyone ever touched you in your private areas in a way that made you feel uncomfortable?"

Partners and concurrency

"How many people have you had sex with in the past 2 months? Past year? Your whole life?"

"Do you think your partner is having sex with anyone else? Are you?"

Sexually transmitted infections

"Has a doctor ever told you that you had a sexually transmitted infection like chlamydia? gonorrhea? trichomonas? herpes? genital warts? syphilis? HIV/AIDS? Have any of your partners ever had one"?

Pregnancy

"Have you ever been pregnant? What happened with that pregnancy? Are you trying to get pregnant right now?"

Condoms

"What do you do to keep yourself and your partner from getting a sexually transmitted disease? Do you use condoms? Did you use a condom the last time you had sex? How often do you think you use condoms? Have you ever had trouble using condoms? Did they ever break or slip off during sex?"

Hormonal contraception

"What do you do to keep yourself from getting pregnant? Are you on any hormonal contraception like the birth control pill? The shot? The patch? The ring? How is that going? Is it hard to remember to take your pills?"

---

continue wearing their underwear during the genital examination. For the examination, the provider can shift the underwear to one side, allowing full visibility of the genitalia.

The stage of secondary sexual characteristic development should be documented in any adolescent examination involving the genitalia. Tanner[16] classified the level of pubertal maturation into five levels based on breast and pubic hair development in females, and it is used as a measure of pubertal development. **Figs. 3** and **4** describe Tanner's classification of stages of pubertal development.

With new urine-based STI testing and revised Papanicolaou's test guidelines (recommending first adolescent test performed within 3 years after coitarche or by age 21 years), many asymptomatic adolescent females do not require a pelvic examination. Females presenting with genital symptoms and adolescents requiring their first Papanicolaou's test do need to have a pelvic examination performed. A first pelvic examination can be an anxiety-provoking experience. A reassuring and confident provider sets the tone for the examination. Providers should discuss what is going to occur and answer all questions before initiating the examination. Pelvic models or diagrams may be helpful to describe the procedure. Allowing a support person in the room, such as a friend, relative, or nurse, can ease the tension for the patient. As examination rooms are often cold, ensure that adolescent remains warm and as

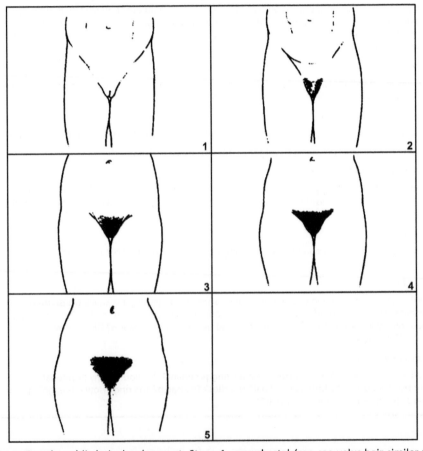

Fig. 3. Female public hair development. Stage 1: prepubertal (can see velus hair similar to abdominal wall). Stage 2: sparse growth of long, slightly pigmented hair, straight or curled, along labia. Stage 3: darker, coarser, and more curled hair, spreading sparsely over junction of pubes. Stage 4: hair adult in type, but covering smaller area than in adult; no spread to medial surface of thighs. Stage 5: adult in type and quantity, with horizontal distribution. (*From* Daniel WA, Paulshock BZ. A physician's guide to sexual maturity rating. Patient Care 1979:13;122.)

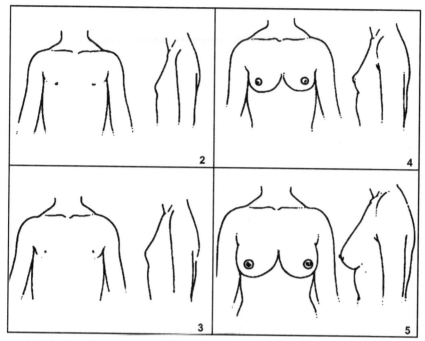

Fig. 4. Female breast development. Stage 1: prepubertal. Stage 2: breast bud stage with elevation of breast and papilla; enlargement of areola. Stage 3: further enlargement of breast and areola; no separation of their contour. Stage 4: areola and papilla form a secondary mound above level of breast. Stage 5: mature stage with projection of papilla only, related to recession of areola. (*From* Daniel WA, Paulshock BZ. A physician's guide to sexual maturity rating. Patient Care 1979:13;122.)

comfortable as possible with additional sheets or blankets. Visual imagery can help the adolescent relax during the examination and is performed easily by encouraging the adolescent to concentrate on imaging herself doing her favorite sport or activity in her favorite location. Visual imagery and focused breathing are helpful techniques to decrease anxiety and muscular tension, thereby facilitating the successful performance of the pelvic examination and a more positive experience for the adolescent. Some providers also place an interesting and hopefully distracting poster on the examination room ceiling for the patients to view during the examination.

Adolescent females may feel embarrassed and uncomfortable with male providers. If the adolescent demonstrates discomfort, every effort should be taken, if at all possible, to offer a choice in the provider gender. When there is discordant gender in the provider and patient, chaperones should be used (eg, nurse, medical assistant, or parent/guardian) as a measure of safety and comfort for the patient and to protect the provider against false impropriety claims.

Laboratory Tests

Sexually active adolescents are at high risk for acquiring STIs, such as gonorrhea and chlamydia. Current guidelines for delivery of adolescent primary care services recommend yearly STI screening for all sexually active adolescents.[17] Tests for chlamydia, gonorrhea, and trichomonas should be obtained routinely. Many experts recommend chlamydia screening every 6 months for sexually active adolescent females. The Centers for Disease Control and Prevention (CDC) recommend using a nucleic acid amplification test (NAAT), if resources permit, for diagnosing genital chlamydia and gonorrhea infections. NAATs are the most sensitive chlamydia tests available. In addition to testing endocervical and urethral specimens, NAATs allow for noninvasive STI testing by means of urine and self-collected vaginal swabs, thereby avoiding invasive pelvic examinations as a major obstacle to many adolescents seeking care. Studies demonstrate that gonorrhea and chlamydia NAATs also perform well on rectal and oropharyngeal specimens, but are not US Food and Drug Administration (FDA)-approved. More information on chlamydia NAATs is available at www.igh.org/castd/downloadable/chlamydia_testing_tables.pdf. Currently, CDC[17] recommends HIV screening all Americans 13 to 64 years at least once and more often as indicated by sexual risk behaviors.

TREATMENT

In all 50 states, adolescents may consent for reproductive health care without parental consent. States vary, however, in regards to the age minimum required to consent for health care related to STIs. Providers should check their state for age-specific guidelines. CDC-recommended adolescent STI management does not vary from that of adults, except with the caveat of ensuring completed treatment. Because adolescents are notorious for poor compliance with treatment and follow-up recommendations, single-dose therapy is recommended when available, and directly observed therapy is ideal.

Providers should verify that all sexual partners have been tested and treated. Ensuring partner treatment can be an arduous task but is imperative for public health. One strategy to increase partner treatment and decrease reinfection rates is expedited partner therapy (EPT); treating a partner of an STI-infected individual without requiring a prior clinical examination. EPT usually is practiced by patient-delivered partner therapy (PDPT). With PDPT, the provider gives the index patient medications or a prescription for medications to deliver to her partner(s). The medication usually is accompanied by a brochure describing the infection, the medication, and the need to see a clinician for a complete STI evaluation. As of February 2009, EPT is legal in 15 states as an option for providers when caring for heterosexual individuals infected with gonorrhea or chlamydia. For more information on EPT, including legal status, go to: www.dcd.gov/std/ept.

Follow-up

The no-show rate tends to be high for adolescent patients and is a perpetual challenge for providers. Phone calls the night before and even day of the appointment are advisable. Documenting which telephone number is acceptable to maintain confidentiality is important. For many adolescents, calling or texting them on their own cell phones is feasible. Having a dedicated nurse who the adolescent can access easily when she needs to promotes the usability of the practice and facilitates their return to care. Monthly follow-up is ideal when taking care of any high-risk adolescent.

There are many reasons why adolescents do not keep appointments, so alerting them to other options for care is useful: provide patients with a list of teen-friendly clinics and pharmacies where they can be tested and obtain condoms and contraception and may be able to access after hours and on weekends.

SUMMARY

Adolescence is an exciting yet challenging time of life. Among adolescents, rate of physical development surpasses their rate of cognitive development. Adolescents are physically able to engage in behaviors that place them at risk for STIs, but they have not yet fully developed the capabilities to judge when and how to protect themselves. Gynecologists are in the unique position and are a potentially valuable resource to educate adolescents about their health and their bodies in a private and safe environment where they can offer individualized information and strategies to guide adolescents and young adults toward physical and emotional health. As providers of health care for adolescents, it is the gynecologist's job to support patients to remain in good sexual health, despite their developmental dichotomy between judgment and action.

APPENDIX
THE FOLLOWING IS A LIST OF WEB SITES FOR PROVIDERS:

The Adolescent Health Working Group: http://ahwg.net/

The Adolescent Wellness through Access to Resources to Education (AWARE) Foundation: http://www.awarefoundation.org/

Advocates for Youth: http://www.advocatesforyouth.org/

American College of Preventive Medicine Adolescent Health Initiative: http://www.acpm.org/ah/default.htm

American College of Obstetrics and Gynecology Adolescent Health Care: http://www.acog.org/departments/dept_web.cfm?recno = 7

American Social Health Association (ASHA): www.ashastd.org

The California STD/HIV Prevention Training Center: www.stdhivtraining.org/educ/training_module/tools.html

Centers for Disease Control and Prevention: www.cdc.gov/std/treatment

The Center for Young Women's Health (CYWH): http://www.youngwomenshealth.org/

ETR Associates (patient brochures): www.etr.org

Gay and Lesbian Medical Association (GLMA): http://www.glma.org

The Guttmacher Institute: http://www.guttmacher.org/

Kaiser Family Foundation: http://www.kff.org/

The Massachusetts STD/HIV Prevention Training Center: http://www.mass.gov/dph/cdc/std/guidelines/chlamydia_toolkit.pdf

The National Campaign to Prevent Teen Pregnancy: http://www.teenpregnancy.org/

The North American Society for Pediatric and Adolescent Gynecology: http://www.naspag.org/

Pediatric Health Care Alliance Teen Growth: http://www.teengrowth.com/

Planned Parenthood Federation of America: http://www.plannedparenthood.org/index.htm

Rutgers, the State University of New Jersey, teen sexual health information Web site for parents and professionals at: http://sexetc.org/page/parents_professionals/

Society of Obstetricians and Gynecologists of Canada: www.sexualityandu.ca

ADOLESCENT RISK-SCREENING TOOLS FOR PROVIDERS INCLUDE:

American College of Obstetrics and Gynecology Tool Kit for Teen Care: http://www.acog.org/bookstore/Tool_Kit_for_Teen_Care_P348.cfm

Adolescent Health Working Group: http://ahwg.net/

American Medical Association Guidelines for Adolescent Preventive Services (GAPS): http://www.ama-assn.org/ama/pub/category/1980.html
New York State Department of Health Office of Managed Care Screener/Trigger questionnaire: http://www.urmc.rochester.edu/gchas/div/adol/leah/resources. HTM

THE LIST OF WEB SITES FOR ADOLESCENT PATIENTS INCLUDES:

Advocates for Youth "Youth Lounge" information: http://www.advocatesforyouth. org/youth/index.htm
Advocates for Youth Web site for gay, lesbian, bisexual, transgender, and questioning (GLBTQ): http://www.youthresource.com/
The Adolescent Wellness through Access to Resources to Education (AWARE) Foundation: http://www.awarefoundation.org/
The American Social Health Association adolescent sexual health information: http://www.iwannaknow.org
Atlantic Health System: http://www.teenhealthfx.com
Campaign for Our Children: http://www.cfoc.org/
Canadian Association for Adolescent Health: www.youngandhealthy.ca
The Center for Young Women's Health (CYWH): http://www.youngwomenshealth. org/
Columbia University's Health Promotion Program "Go Ask Alice" Web site for adolescents and young adults: http://www.goaskalice.columbia.edu/
DIPEx Web site (UK) at: http://www.youthhealthtalk.org/
MTV collaboration with Kaiser Family Foundation: http://www.itsyoursexlife.com/
The Nemours Foundation's Center for Children's Health Media: http://www. kidshealth.org/teen/sexual_health/
Palo Alto Medical Foundation (PAMF): http://www.pamf.org/teen/
Pediatric Health Care Alliance Teen Growth: www.TeenGrowth.com
Planned Parenthood Teens: http://www.teenwire.com/
Rutgers, the State University of New Jersey, teen sexual health: http://www.sexetc. org/
Society of Obstetricians and Gynecologists of Canada: www.sexualityandu.ca
Teenage Health Websites Ltd Web site at (UK): http://www.doctorann.org/
Youth Embassy Web site at: http://www.youthembassy.com/

THE LIST OF WEB SITES FOR PARENTS OR GUARDIANS OF ADOLESCENTS INCLUDES:

The Adolescent Wellness through Access to Resources to Education (AWARE) Foundation: http://www.awarefoundation.org/
Advocates for Youth: http://www.advocatesforyouth.org/
Advocates for Youth "Parents' Sex Ed Center": http://www.advocatesforyouth. org/parents/index.htm
The American Social Health Association adolescent sexual health: http://www. iwannaknow.org
Campaign for Our Children: http://www.cfoc.org/
Children Now: http://www.talkingwithkids.org/
Palo Alto Medical Foundation (PAMF) Web site for parents at: http://www.pamf. org/teen/parents/

Rutgers, the State University of New Jersey, teen sexual health information for parents and professionals: http://www.sexetc.org/page/parents_professionals/
Society of Obstetricians and Gynecologists of Canada: www.sexualityandu.ca
Youth Embassy (for parents): http://www.youthembassy.com/parents.asp

REFERENCES

1. Eaton DK, Kann L, Kinchen S, et al. Youth risk behavior surveillance—United States, 2007. MMWR Surveill Summ 2008;57(4):1–131.
2. Weinstock H, Berman S, Cates W Jr. Sexually transmitted diseases among American youth: incidence and prevalence estimates, 2000. Perspect Sex Reprod Health 2004;36(1):6–10.
3. CDC. Youth risk behavior surveillance—United States. MMWR Morb Mortal Wkly Rep 2003;53:1–29.
4. Neinstein L. Adolescent healthcare: a practical guide. New York: Lippincott Williams & Wilkins; 2002.
5. Ford K, Lepkowski JM. Characteristics of sexual partners and STD infection among American adolescents. Int J STD AIDS 2004;15(4):260–5.
6. Kirby D. Antecedents of adolescent initiation of sex, contraceptive use, and pregnancy. Am J Health Behav 2002;26(6):473–85.
7. Shafii T, Stovel K, Davis R, et al. Is condom use habit-forming? condom use at sexual debut and subsequent condom use. Sex Transm Dis 2004;31(6):366–72.
8. Upchurch DM, Mason WM, Kusunoki Y, et al. Social and behavioral determinants of self-reported STD among adolescents. Perspect Sex Reprod Health 2004;36(6):276–87.
9. Strassburger V, Brown RT, Braverman PK, et al. Adolescent medicine: a handbook of primary care. New York: Lippincott Williams & Wilkins; 2006.
10. Bar-Cohen A, Lia-Hoagberg B, Edwards L. First family planning visit in school-based clinics. J Sch Health 1990;60(8):418–22.
11. Finer LB, Zabin LS. Does the timing of the first family planning visit still matter? Fam Plann Perspect 1998;30(1):30–3 42.
12. McKee MD, Karasz A, Weber CM. Health care seeking among urban minority adolescent girls: the crisis at sexual debut. Ann Fam Med 2004;2(6):549–54.
13. Stone N, Ingham R. When and why do young people in the United Kingdom first use sexual health services? Perspect Sex Reprod Health 2003;35(3):114–20.
14. Zabin LS, Stark HA, Emerson MR. Reasons for delay in contraceptive clinic utilization. Adolescent clinic and nonclinic populations compared. J Adolesc Health 1991;12(3):225–32.
15. Mosher WD, Chandra A, Jones J. Sexual behavior and selected health measures: men and women 15-44 years of age, United States, 2002. Advanced data from vital health statistics; no 362. Hyattsville, MD: National Center for Health Statistics: p. 1–56.
16. Tanner J. Growth at adolescence. 2nd edition. Springfield (IL): Charles C Thomas; 1962.
17. Centers for Disease Control and Prevention Sexually transmitted diseases treatment guidelines, 2006. MMWR 2006;55(No.RR-11):1–95.

Update in Adolescent Contraception

Eduardo Lara-Torre, MD, FACOG

KEYWORDS

• Adolescent • Contraception • Long term methods

Despite a recent decrease in the pregnancy rate in the United States, the pregnancy rates in Europe and Canada remain close to 50% lower than that in the United States.[1] The use of appropriate contraception is especially important in adolescents. As this age group matures and becomes capable of reproduction, visits to a practitioner should include counseling on adequate methods of birth control to target adolescents' needs and ability to improve their compliance. Unfortunately, it is not uncommon to see adolescents months after their initiation of sexual activity, with some patients seeking contraception up to 12 months or later. The misconception that pregnancy cannot occur during your "first time" or during certain times of the month increases the risk for unintended pregnancy and provides false reassurance to teens. The 2007 Youth Risk Behavior Surveillance System, which tracks different health risk behaviors among high-school students, including sexual behaviors that contribute to unintended pregnancies, surveyed more than 14,000 high-school students from every state and the District of Columbia.[2] Important findings of this survey included the following:

- 47.8% of students reported ever having had sexual intercourse (46.8% in 2005)
- 7.1% of students reported having had sex before the age of 13 years (6.2% in 2005)
- 14.9% of students reported having had sex with four or more sexual partners (14.3% in 2005)
- 35.0% of students reported being currently sexually active, defined as having had sexual intercourse in the 3 months before the survey (33.9% in 2005)
- 61.5% of sexually active students reported that they or their partner had used a condom during last sex (62.8% in 2005)

These findings reinforce the importance of addressing contraception during an adolescent's initial health care evaluation.

Preventive visits are a great venue for discussing contraception even before the initiation of sexual activity provided that this information does not result in an increased rate of sexual activity, earlier age at first intercourse, or greater number of sexual

Department of Obstetrics and Gynecology, Carilion Clinic, Virginia Tech-Carilion School of Medicine, 102 Highland Avenue, Suite 303, Roanoke, VA 24013, USA
E-mail address: eltorre@carilion.com

Obstet Gynecol Clin N Am 36 (2009) 119–128
doi:10.1016/j.ogc.2008.12.003
0889-8545/08/$ – see front matter © 2009 Elsevier Inc. All rights reserved.

partners. On the contrary, if the adolescent perceives that there is an obstacle to obtaining contraception, he or she is more likely to experience negative outcomes related to sexual activity.[3] The American College of Obstetricians and Gynecologists (ACOG) has recently published recommendations for the first preventive visit with a gynecologist to be between the ages of 13 and 15 years.[4] The time spent with their provider allows adolescents the opportunity to identify risk factors and challenges that can be overcome before the initiation of hormonal or nonhormonal contraception, in addition to encouraging abstinence.

Many teens also perceive the pelvic examination to be a barrier for accessing contraceptive services; therefore, the physical examination may be deferred until after initiation of contraceptives if requested by the patient and judged appropriate by the clinician. One significant reason why adolescents hesitate or delay in obtaining family planning services or contraception is concern about confidentiality. Health care providers need to be familiar with current local statutes on the rights of minors to consent to health care services that affect confidentiality. For more information and up to-date reproductive health reproductive rights of adolescents, visit the Guttmacher Institute Web site.[5]

The purpose of this review is to provide some new developments of commonly used contraceptive methods as they apply to adolescents and some new information to the reader for use in his or her daily practice. A table from the World Health Organization (WHO) is provided, with updates on the changes for patients who have specific medical conditions for which certain contraceptive methods may be contraindicated **(Table 1)**. New absolute contraindications for contraception are limited to only two conditions: thromboembolic mutations and the use of estrogen-containing methods and current pelvic inflammatory disease or mucopurulent cervicitis and initial placement of an intrauterine device (IUD).

ABSTINENCE

Although abstinence is the most effective means of birth control, the lack of other contraception education has caused controversy and disagreement with the efforts of specialty societies. During the first part of the decade, the US administration placed an emphasis on abstinence-only education for pregnancy prevention. Unfortunately, recent data suggest that abstinence-only programs are not as effective as those in which other contraceptive options are offered at the same time.[6] The choice to remain or return to abstinence may be a difficult one for some adolescents, and adequate resources, such as support and chat rooms for counseling, may be required. Those who choose abstinence should be encouraged and reminded of the advantages of decreased risk for pregnancy and sexually transmitted infections (STIs).

BARRIER METHODS

Barrier methods include such devices as male condoms, female condoms, cervical caps, diaphragms, and spermicidal and contraceptive film and ovules. Although effective, the use of these devices by adolescents is not consistent, even when chosen by them as their method to protect against STIs.[7] The need for application before each sexual encounter decreases the use of the method by "decreasing the spontaneity" of the act, as some teens explain.

The male condom is the most commonly used barrier method by adolescents. The efficacy in preventing STIs and the HIV epidemic increased their use during the 1990s. Despite their widespread availability, however, the use of condoms is still not widespread. Many limitations, such as cost, personal beliefs, and the inability of adolescents to be good "planners," allows for inconsistency of use.

Female barrier methods, such as the female condom, have not received great popularity within the adolescent population. Discontinuation rates are as high as 55%, and when used,[8] it is common to have "accidents" secondary to the inappropriate use of the method. Practitioners should encourage the use of barrier methods, even when the teen is on another form of contraception.

COMBINED ORAL CONTRACEPTIVE PILLS

The combined oral contraceptive pill (OCP) is the most commonly used method of contraception in the adolescent group, with the rate of use approaching 50%.[9] A wide range of estrogen dosing and progestin products makes the choice of the best pill difficult. The contraceptive and noncontraceptive benefits (eg, light, predictable, regular pain-free menses) of the different combinations are about the same, and the brand should be chosen based on the side effect profile and practitioner's preference. In the quest for the best contraceptive method, adolescents look for safety, convenience, privacy, and efficacy as the most important factors in choosing a contraceptive method. Because the incidence and severity of side effects increase with age and smoking, the overall safety provided by OCPs in adolescents without thromboembolic disease risk factors may assist the practitioner in reassuring teens about the use of this method.[10]

Other indications of use may also influence the selection of this method in adolescents. In particular, the prevalence of acne and premenstrual dysphoric disorder (PMDD) may play an important role in selecting this method as the one of choice for many of our patients. Newer indications, such as PMDD with a low-dose (ethinyl estradiol, 20 µg) formulation containing drospirenone (3 mg), which has antiandrogenic and antimineralocorticoid properties, in a 24/4 regimen (24 days of active drug/4 days of placebo), have proved to be efficacious in reducing symptoms of PMDD.[11] By the same token, this formulation has been proved efficacious in the treatment of acne.[12] Information on the efficacy of some other formulations in reducing acne, including cyproterone, levonorgestrel, or desogestrel, may also favor the use of some combinations and allow the patient to obtain multiple benefits with one drug.[13]

Unfortunately, despite the wide use of the OCP, adolescent users have failure rates as high as 15% in the first year of use because of missed pills, with 28% of 15- to 17-year-old patients reporting that they have missed two or more pills in their most recent cycle (compared with 13% of those aged 18 years and older).[9,14] To prevent some of the noncompliance in adolescents, initiation of the pill on the same day (Quick Start) versus the traditional start initiation on a Sunday seems to improve compliance and still maintains an acceptable side effect profile without any teratogenic effects, even if the patient is pregnant. This innovative method may be yet another way to encourage adolescent patients to take their method of birth control even before they leave the office, with the hope of improving their compliance.[15]

Extended regimens, such as the available 84/7-day package (ethinyl estradiol [30 µg]/levonorgestrel [150 µg]), have shown similar efficacy and compliance, with only a mild increase in breakthrough bleeding in the adult population, and may be a good option for patients who desire less frequent menses, such as athletes and military personal, although studies in adolescents are lacking.[7]

OTHER COMBINED HORMONAL METHODS

The contraceptive transdermal patch uses the technology of a medicated adhesive that allows the skin to absorb and maintain a constant hormonal level without the

Table 1
WHO categories of safety for use of contraceptive methods: changes since 2002

Condition	COC	CIC	POP	DMPA NET-EN	LNG/ETG	Cu-IUD		LNG-IUD	
						I	C	I	C
Personal characteristics and reproductive history									
Obesity ≥30 kg/m² BMI	2	2	1	1	1	1		1	
Cardiovascular disease									
Known thrombogenic mutations (eg, factor V Leiden; prothrombin mutation; protein S, protein C, and antithrombin deficiencies)	4	4	2	2	2	1		2	
Depressive disorders									
Depressive disorders	1	1	1	1	1	1		1	
Reproductive tract infections and disorders									
Uterine fibroids									
(a) Without distortion of the uterine cavity	1	1	1	1	1	1		1	
(b) With distortion of the uterinecavity	1	1	1	1	1	4		4	
PID									
(a) Past PID (assuming no current risk factors for STIs)	—	—	—	—		I	C	I	C
(i) With subsequent pregnancy	1	1	1	1	1	1	1	1	1
(ii) Without subsequent pregnancy	1	1	1	1	1	2	2	2	2
(b) PID: current	1	1	1	1	1	4	2	4	2
STIs									
(a) Current purulent cervicitis or chlamydial infection or gonorrhoea	1	1	1	1	1	4	2	4	2
(b) Other STIs (excluding HIV and hepatitis)	1	1	1	1	1	2	2	2	2
(c) Vaginitis (including trichomonas vaginalis and bacterial vaginosis)	1	1	1	1	1	2	2	2	2
(d) Increased risk for STIs	1	1	1	1	1	2/3	2	2/3	2
HIV/AIDS									
High risk for HIV	1	1	1	1	1	2		2	

HIV-infected	1	1	1	1	2	2	2	2
AIDS	1	1	1	1	3	2	3	2
Clinically well on antiretroviral therapy	See antiretroviral therapy							
Drug interactions								
Drugs which affect liver enzymes								
(a) Rifampicin	3	2	3	3	3	1	1	1
(b) Certain anticonvulsants (phenytoin, carbamazepine, barbiturates, primidone, topiramate, oxcarbazepine)	3	2	3	2	3	1	1	1
Antibiotics (excluding rifampicin)								
(a) Griseofulvin	2	1	2	1	2	1	1	1
(b) Other antibiotics	1	1	1	1	1	1	1	1
Antiretroviral therapy	—/2	2	2	2	2	—/2	2/3	C/2	2

Conditions for which there was a classification change for one or more methods or a major modification to the condition description. Changed classifications are in bold.

Abbreviations: BMI, body mass index; C, continuation; CICs, combined injectable contraceptives; COCs, low-dose combined oral contraceptives; Cu-IUDs, copper intrauterine devices; DMPA, depot-medroxyprogesterone acetate; ETG, etonogestrel; I, initiation; LNG, levonorgestrel; LNG-IUDs, levonorgestrel-releasing IUDs; NET-EN, norethisterone enantate; PID, pelvic inflammatory disease; POPs, progestogen-only pills.

1. A condition for which there is no restriction for the use of the contraceptive method.
2. A condition where the advantages of using the method generally outweigh the theoretic or proved risks.
3. A condition where the theoretic or proved risks usually outweigh the advantages of using the method.
4. A condition which represents an unacceptable health risk if the contraceptive method is used.

Also,

1. Use method in any circumstances
2. Generally use the method
3. Use of method not usually recommended unless other more appropriate methods are not available or not acceptable
4. Method not to be used

From World Health Organization. Categories of safety for use of contraceptive methods. Changes since 2002. In: Medical eligibility criteria for contraceptive use. 3rd edition. Geneva (Switzerland): Reproductive Health Research, World Health Organization; 2004; with permission. Available at: www.who.org. Accessed August 1, 2008.

fluctuations seen with orally absorbed forms. In the adult population, failure rates and side effect profiles are similar to those of OCPs. In adolescents, 21% experienced a patch coming off completely and 32% experienced a patch peeling partially in the corner.[16] Given the weekly dosing, many adolescents find this method appealing. Good acceptance, cycle control, and adherence rates have been shown and are greater than those observed with the OCP.[16–19] Most adolescents were extremely or somewhat satisfied with the patch, and 93% would recommend it to a friend.[15] Recent safety data released by the manufacturer warn of an increased exposure to estrogen compared with the average-dose OCP, which may increase the risk for cardiovascular events.[20] Adolescents should be cautioned about these risks and counseled about the potential side effects before prescribing the method, remembering that the risk for thromboembolic or cardiovascular events associated with pregnancy is greater in an adolescent than that associated with the transdermal patch. For those noncompliant with the pill, the patch may be a good alternative.

The vaginal contraceptive ring (ethinyl estradiol [15 μg]/etonogestrel [120 μg]) is another approved method of birth control. This method requires motivation from the patient to insert and remove the contraceptive device from the vagina once a month and has not been well studied in adolescents. Adequate trials on adolescents are still underway and should provide additional information regarding other applications, such as extended regimens. Preliminary results indicate favorable acceptability when compared with the OCP.[21]

The transdermal patch and intravaginal ring methods have been used in a continuous fashion. They have shown promising results without affecting safety or effectiveness.[22,23]

The monthly injectable combination contraceptive that combines medroxyprogesterone acetate (25 mg) and estradiol cypionate (5 mg) has been recalled by the manufacturer and is not available for use in the United States. Previous studies of this product did show good efficacy, and the future release of a revised version of this method is predicted. The once-monthly dosing of the regimen may provide teens with another alternative to improve their compliance.

PROGESTIN-ONLY METHODS

The progestin-only contraceptive pill has been shown to have similar efficacy to the OCP. Unfortunately, given its short half-life, failure rates may be increased because of patient noncompliance with the proper timing of the pill, which requires taking it around the same time of day (within 3 hours) each day.[24] Extensive education regarding the irregular bleeding occurring in the first 3 months and need for compliance with pill dosing at a similar time each day is required to enhance adolescent compliance. Certain contraindications to these hormonal methods may include sensitivity to the agents, osteoporosis, undiagnosed vaginal bleeding, pregnancy, or severe liver disease.

Depot medroxyprogesterone acetate (DMPA) is a common contraceptive used by the adolescent population because of the minimal intervention on the part of the patient required to achieve compliance. This method is the choice for adolescents who are breastfeeding and those with contraindications to the use of estrogen, such as thrombophilias and certain medical conditions. The application of one intramuscular dose of 150 mg every 3 months increases convenience but still requires compliance to continue the method. Although its efficacy has been shown to be better than that of the OCP, most of its effect is probably related to compliance and ease of use. Weight gain and irregular bleeding are common and unpleasant side effects for adolescents. The product insert indicates an average weight gain of 2.5 kg after the first year of use, 3.7 kg after the second year of use, and 6.3 kg after the fourth year of use.[25] Conversely, amenorrhea occurs in 55% to 60% of DMPA users at 12 months and in up to 68% of users at greater then 1 year.[26] Many teenagers perceive this as an appealing feature of the medication, which may contribute to their compliance and request for this method.

A recent concern has been the effect of the hypoestrogenic state created by long-term use of DMPA on bone density in adolescents. The use of DMPA has been shown to decrease the bone mineral density of adolescent users when compared with the bone mineral density of normal menstrual controls and oral contraceptive users; however, the potential effect on future bone health is unknown.[27] The lack of long-term prospective trials on the bone health of adults who used DMPA as adolescents, in addition to the potential bone loss associated with pregnancy in the absence of contraception, makes DMPA a valid and reliable method to prevent pregnancy until further data are obtained. Those patients who are smokers and sedentary should be counseled on the detrimental implication regarding bone health and encouraged to quit smoking and get involved in exercise. Appropriate calcium intake (1200–1500 mg/d) and monitoring of bone density should be encouraged in those adolescents who use the method for more than 2 years, especially those who continue to be amenorrheic and have any of the other risk factors mentioned previously. The WHO suggests that the advantages of using DMPA generally outweigh the theoretic safety concerns regarding fracture risk in the adolescent population (younger than 18 years of age).[28]

Recent reports have shown the recovery of bone mineral density in those DMPA users who stop the method when compared with nonusers and should encourage its continuing use.[29] The addition of estrogen (oral or injectable) may be considered in these patients and may provide protection against bone mineral density loss.[30]

Progestin subdermal implants in the form of six levonorgestrel rods were previously commonly used in the adolescent population because of the long-term contraception provided (5 years) and a 12-month continuation rate of 91%.[13] The difficulty in removing the six rods, in addition to the voluntary recall of certain lots by the manufacturer during 1999, limited the use of this method, however.

In 1998, the introduction of a single etonogestrel implant, with a 3-year contraceptive duration and easy insertion and removal, has reopened subdermal implants as an alternative for adolescents looking for long-term contraception.[31] Unfortunately, menstrual irregularities are common and may deter teens from using this method or result in a request for removal after insertion.

EMERGENCY CONTRACEPTION

Emergency contraception (ECP), the use of nonabortifacient hormonal medications within 72 to 120 hours after unprotected or underprotected coitus for the prevention of unintended pregnancy, is an important part of contraception counseling in adolescents. Misconceptions regarding the effectiveness, availability, and mechanism of action make this method less used than its counterparts. Even when providers are trained in adolescent care, only 80% of them provide the method to their patients and believe that its efficacy is reserved to 48 hours.[13]

The use of ECP decreases the risk for pregnancy from 8% to 1% to 2% after a single episode of unprotected coitus.[32] The most efficient method consists of levonorgestrel, 1.5 mg, divided in two doses taken 12 hours apart. A recent Cochrane review showed that taking a single dose of levonorgestrel, 1.5 mg, may be as efficacious as when it is taken in divided doses, possibly increasing compliance.[33] Timing is of importance, but recent studies have shown that even if more than 72 hours have passed, either regimen is efficacious and should be offered, with the understanding that there may be a reduction in its efficacy the later it is taken. Advanced prescription of ECP has been shown to increase the likelihood of the use of ECP by young women and teens when needed and yet not to increase sexual or contraceptive risk-taking behavior when compared with those receiving only education about ECP.[34]

INTRAUTERINE DEVICES AND SYSTEMS

The experience with IUDs and intrauterine systems (IUSs) in adolescents is limited. Traditionally, use of an IUD or IUS has been avoided in adolescents, because this population has the highest rates for STIs. Age alone is not an absolute contraindication to the use of these devices. In fact, the WHO categorizes this forms of contraception as class 2 for individuals less than or equal to the age of 20 years. With proper counseling and condom use, an IUD or IUS may be a viable option for some teens, regardless of their gravidity and parity status, and should be considered as part of the available armamentarium for contraception.[35]

In recent studies, there has not been an increase in infertility or STI incidence with the use of these devices.[6] Most of the ascending infections are probably related to contracting the infection from lack of condom use rather than to the presence of the device facilitating it. The risk for ascending infection is probably related to the presence of an STI at the time of insertion, and screening patients before insertion should be encouraged. The use of STI prophylaxis at the time of insertion is currently not required but may be of value in those patients in whom the STI incidence is higher than 5% and there are no adequate screening tests.[36] In 2007, the Adolescent Healthcare Committee of the ACOG advocated for the increased use of an IUD or IUS in this population and has undertaken a full review on the topic.[37]

SUMMARY

The future of adolescent contraception requires the collaboration between providers, patients, and, sometimes, their parents. New contraceptive methods allow teens to choose from a variety of convenient, safe, reliable, and confidential options. Teen pregnancy prevention in the United States is a priority because of the implications for the patient and society as a whole. The ability to provide nondiscriminatory, confidential, accessible care and our role in the education and guidance of our patients are likely to determine the future of this generation of teens.

Long-term contraceptives, such as injectables and implantable devices or IUDs, are safe for use in young patients. As providers of adolescent health care, encouraging patients and other providers to use these methods should be part of our efforts to improve the health care of this population. Limiting access to comprehensive care, which includes abstinence and all contraceptive methods, and requiring pelvic examinations before the provision of services would be detrimental to the success of our prevention programs and should be discouraged.

REFERENCES

1. Darroch JE, Singh S, Frost JJ. Differences in teenage pregnancy rates among five developed countries: the roles of sexual activity and contraceptive use. Fam Plann Perspect 2001;33:244–50.

2. Centers for Disease Control and Prevention. Youth risk behavior surveillance—United States 2007. MMWR Surveill Summ 2008;57(4):1–131.
3. Smith CA. Factors associated with early sexual activity among urban adolescents. Soc Work 1997;42:334–46.
4. American College of Obstetricians and Gynecologists. The initial reproductive health visit. ACOG Committee Opinion No. 335. Obstet Gynecol 2006;107:745–7.
5. Available at: www.guthmacher.org. Accessed August 1, 2008.
6. Kohler PK, Manhart LE, Lafferty WE. Abstinence-only and comprehensive sex education and the initiation of sexual activity and teen pregnancy. J Adolesc Health 2008;42:344–51.
7. Stuart GS, Castano PM. Sexually transmitted infections and contraceptives: selective issues. Obstet Gynecol Clin North Am 2003;30:795–808.
8. Anderson FD, Hait H. A multicenter, randomized study of an extended cycle oral contraceptive. Contraception 2003;68:89–96.
9. Hewitt G, Cromer B. Update on adolescent contraception. Obstet Gynecol Clin North Am 2000;27:143–62.
10. Rimsza ME. Counseling the adolescent about contraception. Pediatr Rev 2003; 24:162–70.
11. Yonkers KA, Brown C, Pearlstein TB, et al. Efficacy of a new low-dose oral contraceptive with drospirenone in premenstrual dysphoric disorder. Obstet Gynecol 2005;106:492–501.
12. Batukan C, Muderris II, Ozcelik B, et al. Comparison of two oral contraceptives containing either drospirenone or cyproterone acetate in the treatment of hirsutism. Gynecol Endocrinol 2007;23:38–44.
13. Arowojolu AO, Gallo MF, Lopez LM, et al. Combined oral contraceptive pills for treatment of acne. Cochrane Database Syst Rev 2007:CD004425.
14. Polaneczky M. Adolescent contraception. Curr Opin Obstet Gynecol 1998;10:213–9.
15. Lara-Torre E, Schroeder B. Adolescent compliance and side effects with Quick Start initiation of oral contraceptive pills. Contraception 2002;66:81–5.
16. Harel Z, Riggs S, Vaz R, et al. Adolescents' experience with the combined estrogen and progestin transdermal contraceptive method Ortho Evra. J Pediatr Adolesc Gynecol 2005;18:85–90.
17. Gupta N. Advances in hormonal contraception. Adolesc Med Clin 2006;17: 653–71 [abstract xi].
18. Burkman RT. The transdermal contraceptive system. Am J Obstet Gynecol 2004; 190(4 Suppl):S49–53.
19. Archer DF, Bigrigg A, Smallwood GH, et al. Assessment of compliance with a weekly contraceptive patch (Ortho Evra/Evra) among North American women. Fertil Steril 2002;77(2 Suppl 2):S27–31.
20. FDA warning on the contraceptive patch. Available at: http://www.fda.gov/bbs/topics/news/2005/NEW01262.html. Accessed August 1, 2008.
21. Stewart FH, Brown BA, Raine TR, et al. Adolescent and young women's experience with the vaginal ring and oral contraceptive pills. J Pediatr Adolesc Gynecol 2007;20:345–51.
22. Stewart FH, Kaunitz AM, Laguardia KD, et al. Extended use of transdermal norelgestromin/ethinyl estradiol: a randomized trial. Obstet Gynecol 2005;105: 1389–96.
23. Miller L, Verhoeven CH, Hout J. Extended regimens of the contraceptive vaginal ring: a randomized trial. Obstet Gynecol 2005;106:473–82.
24. Graham S, Fraser IS. The progestogen-only mini-pill. Contraception 1982;26: 373–88.

25. Black A, Francoeur D, Rowe T, et al. Canadian contraception consensus. J Obstet Gynaecol Can 2004;26:347–87, 389–436.
26. Menstrual bleeding patterns in untreated women and with long-acting methods of contraception. Task Force on Long-Acting Systemic Agents for Fertility Regulation. Adv Contracept 1991;7:257–70.
27. Lara-Torre E, Edwards CP, Perlman SE, et al. Prospective study evaluating bone mineral density in adolescent females using Depo-Provera. J Pediatr Adolesc Gynecol 2004;17:17–21.
28. World Health Organization. WHO statement on hormonal contraception and bone health. Wkly Epidemiol Rec 2005;80:302–4.
29. Scholes D, LaCroix AZ, Ichikawa LE, et al. Change in bone mineral density among adolescent women using and discontinuing depot medroxyprogesterone acetate contraception. Arch Pediatr Adolesc Med 2005;159:139–44.
30. Cromer BA, Lazebnik R, Rome E, et al. Double-blinded randomized controlled trial of estrogen supplementation in adolescent girls who receive depot medroxyprogesterone acetate for contraception. Am J Obstet Gynecol 2005;192:42–7.
31. Le J, Tsourounis C. Implanon: a critical review. Ann Pharmacother 2001;35: 329–36.
32. Randomized controlled trial of levonorgestrel versus the Yuzpe regimen of combined oral contraceptives for emergency contraception. Task Force on Postovulatory Methods of Fertility Regulation. Lancet 1998;352:428–33.
33. Cheng L, Gulmezoglu AM, Oel CJ, et al. Interventions for emergency contraception. Cochrane Database Syst Rev 2004;(3):CD001324.
34. Belzer M, Uoshida E, Tejirian R, et al. Advanced supply of emergency contraception for adolescent mothers increased utilization without reducing condom or primary contraception use. J Adolesc Health 2003;32:122–3.
35. World Health Organization. Improving access to quality care in family planning: medical eligibility criteria for contraceptive use. 2nd edition. Geneva: WHO; 2001.
36. Grimes DA, Schulz KF. Prophylactic antibiotics for intrauterine device insertion: a metaanalysis of the randomized controlled trials. Contraception 1999;60:57–63.
37. American College of Obstetricians and Gynecologists. Intrauterine device and adolescents. ACOG Committee Opinion No. 392. Obstet Gynecol 2007;110: 1493–5.

Polycystic Ovary Syndrome in the Adolescent

Samantha M. Pfeifer, MD[a],*, Sari Kives, MD[b]

KEYWORDS

- Polycystic ovarian syndrome • Hirsutism • Insulin resistance
- Adolescent • Obesity • Acne

Polycystic ovary syndrome (PCOS), traditionally thought of as a triad of oligomenorrhea, hirsutism, and obesity, is now recognized as a heterogeneous disorder that results in overproduction of androgens, primarily from the ovary, and is associated with insulin resistance. The disorder is characterized by oligo- or amenorrhea and signs of hyperandrogenism. Because many women who have PCOS have the onset of symptoms during adolescence, it is important to be able to recognize and understand this disorder so as to facilitate treatment and prevention of long-term sequelae.

PATHOPHYSIOLOGY

The prevalence of PCOS in the general population has been estimated to be 5% to 10% of women of reproductive age.[1,2] Screening of an unselected population in the southwestern United States showed an incidence of 4%.[3] Studies in first-degree relatives of patients who have PCOS have shown that 24% of mothers and 32% of sisters are affected, suggesting a major genetic association.[4] Although candidate genes have been proposed, the gene or genes responsible for the syndrome have not been identified.

The cause of PCOS remains unknown, and this is an area of active investigation. Theories focus on the impact of luteinizing hormone (LH) stimulation and the role of insulin in the production of ovarian hyperandrogenism. Increased LH pulse amplitude and frequency have been demonstrated in women and adolescents who have PCOS, suggesting an aberrant pattern of hypothalamic gonadotropin-releasing hormone (GnRH) secretion as a causative factor.[5–8] This increase in LH leads to increased production of androgens from the theca cell of the ovary. Preferential LH secretion from GnRH pulsatility may be explained by observations in rats showing that variations of GnRH pulse frequencies result in differential expression of subunit genes.[9] A rapid

[a] University of Pennsylvania Medical Center, 3701 Market Street, Suite 800, Philadelphia, PA 19104, USA
[b] Hospital for Sick Children, Toronto, ON, Canada
* Corresponding author.
E-mail address: spfeifer@obgyn.upenn.edu (S.M. Pfeifer).

Obstet Gynecol Clin N Am 36 (2009) 129–152
doi:10.1016/j.ogc.2008.12.004
0889-8545/08/$ – see front matter © 2009 Elsevier Inc. All rights reserved.

frequency of GnRH leads to an increase in α and LHβ mRNA expression, thereby favoring LH secretion. Some nonobese patients who have PCOS have an elevated LH/follicle-stimulating hormone (FSH) ratio (>2).[10]

Insulin resistance has been implicated in the pathophysiology of PCOS because of the evidence that insulin stimulates androgen production from the ovary in hyperandrogenic women. Ovarian stroma obtained from hyperandrogenic women has been shown to produce high levels of androgens when exposed to insulin. Insulin had no effect on androgen production from ovarian stroma from nonhyperandrogenic women, however.[11] An observational study in five obese women who had PCOS demonstrated that administration of diazoxide, which decreases insulin secretion, resulted in a significant decrease in androgen levels after administration for 10 days.[12] In a case report of an adolescent female patient who had severe type II diabetes and hyperandrogenism, intravenous administration of insulin to control blood glucose was shown to increase serum androgen levels significantly. These androgen levels returned to baseline when the insulin infusion was stopped.[13]

Women who have PCOS have decreased sensitivity to insulin in muscle and adipose tissue, leading to a compensatory increase in insulin levels. Decreased insulin sensitivity has been demonstrated in lean and obese women, suggesting that the defect is intrinsic to PCOS.[14] Insulin resistance has been described in 20% to 60% of women who have PCOS.[15] It has also been proposed that all women who have PCOS have insulin resistance; however, because of differences in populations studied and the sensitivity and specificity of the methods used to measure insulin resistance, not all women who have PCOS manifest insulin resistance.[16]

In PCOS, insulin resistance is selective: insulin action on glucose transport and metabolic pathways is affected, whereas insulin's action on ovarian steroidogenesis is preserved. There are several theories to explain this apparent paradox. Insulin resistance in PCOS seems to be attributable to a postbinding defect in insulin receptor signaling.[17] Binding to the insulin receptor results in tyrosine phosphorylation before stimulating insulin action. If, however, serine phosphorylation occurs, insulin action is inhibited by decreasing its kinase activity.[1] In the ovary, serine phosphorylation stimulates 17,20 lyase activity, the enzyme responsible for converting 17-hydroxy progesterone to androstenedione, which results in increased production of androgens from the ovary.[18] Therefore, serine phosphorylation inhibits insulin action in the metabolic pathways and stimulates insulin action to produce androgens in the ovary.

There are several theories to explain how insulin stimulates release of androgens. Insulin stimulates ovarian androgen production by direct and indirect mechanisms.[1] Insulin has been shown to decrease secretion of sex hormone-binding globulin (SHBG), which, in turn, increases available and active androgens. Insulin directly increases production of LH and androgens by activating its own receptor on the ovary, adrenal, and pituitary. Insulin also binds to the insulin-like growth factor I (IGF-I) receptor on the ovary, thereby directly stimulating androgen production. Insulin indirectly stimulates the production of androgens by up-regulating IGF-I receptor number and decreasing insulin-like growth factor binding protein-1 (IGFBP-1), which, in turn leads, to an increase in IGF-I.

In summary, insulin postreceptor binding defects in PCOS explain how insulin can stimulate and suppress actions in metabolic pathways and in the ovary. Insulin binding to the pituitary results in release of LH hormones. Insulin-stimulated release of LH, in combination with direct and indirect stimulation to adrenal and ovary, results in release of androgens from the ovary and adrenal glands. The result is hyperandrogenism.

HEALTH CONSEQUENCES OF POLYCYSTIC OVARY SYNDROME

Health consequences of PCOS relate to insulin resistance and hyperandrogenism. They include diabetes, obesity, metabolic syndrome (MS), endometrial hyperplasia, anovulatory infertility, and depression.

Diabetes

The risk for diabetes has been shown to be higher in women and adolescents who have PCOS. Studies have shown that in women who have PCOS, 7.5% to 10% had type II diabetes and approximately 30% to 35% had impaired glucose tolerance.[19,20] The incidence of type II diabetes and impaired glucose tolerance in the control population was significantly lower at 0% and 14%, respectively.[19] Impaired glucose tolerance is known to be a significant risk factor for developing diabetes, as was shown in the Diabetes Prevention Trial.[21] In this study, more than 3000 people with impaired glucose tolerance were randomized to treatment or placebo. In the placebo group, 11% went on to develop diabetes, with a mean follow-up of 2.8 years. Detecting impaired glucose tolerance in women and adolescents who have PCOS is important so that treatment can be initiated to decrease the risk for developing type II diabetes. The most sensitive way to detect impaired glucose tolerance in women who have PCOS is the 2-hour glucose tolerance test. This test involves drawing serum glucose at baseline (fasting) and then again at 1 and 2 hours after a 75-g oral glucose load. In adults and adolescents, the 2-hour glucose tolerance test is more sensitive than the fasting glucose measurement. In adults and adolescents, the incidence of abnormal fasting glucose was 5% and 8%, respectively. The incidence of an abnormal 2-hour glucose tolerance test result was higher at 31% and 33%, respectively, reflecting the better sensitivity of the 2-hour glucose tolerance test.[19,22]

Obesity

Obesity is another significant health consequence of PCOS. Obesity is determined by a body mass index (BMI) greater than 30 kg/m^2. In women who have PCOS, the incidence of obesity is in the range of 50% to 75%. The weight accumulation is predominantly in the abdominal area and is reflected in an increased waist-to-hip ratio. In addition to health consequences of obesity later in life, obesity in adolescents is correlated inversely with obstructive sleep apnea, orthopedic disorders, fatty liver, and decreased quality of life.[23]

Metabolic Syndrome

MS is a constellation of cardiovascular disease risk factors associated with insulin resistance, including glucose intolerance, dyslipidemia, hypertension, and central obesity. The prevalence of MS in obese women who have PCOS has been shown to be significantly higher (33%–40%) compared with nonobese controls (10%–13%).[24] Adolescent girls who have PCOS have also been shown to have a higher incidence of MS compared with the general population. In one study, 49 adolescents who had PCOS were compared with 165 girls from the Third National Health and Nutrition Examination Survey (NHANES III).[25] Thirty-seven percent of girls who had PCOS had MS compared with 5% of girls from the NHANES III (P<.0001). MS in the girls who had PCOS was also associated with BMI. The incidence of MS in normal BMI, overweight, and obese PCOS girls was 0%, 11%, and 63%, respectively. In this study, hyperandrogenism was also found to be a risk factor for MS independent of obesity and insulin resistance. In contrast, a cross-sectional study of overweight and obese adolescents who had PCOS compared with BMI-matched controls showed that the incidence of MS was no different in the PCOS group compared with controls.[26] The investigators concluded that PCOS did not increase the risk for MS more than the risk associated with obesity alone. The group that had PCOS did demonstrate higher levels of total testosterone and free androgen index, increased incidence of glucose intolerance, and higher plasminogen activator inhibitor-1 (PAI-1). Further studies are needed to evaluate the association with MS and the diverse phenotypes of PCOS.

Cardiovascular Disease

PCOS is associated with many signs and symptoms that correlate with increased risk for cardiovascular disease. These include obesity, dyslipidemia, diabetes and insulin resistance, and hyperandrogenemia. PCOS has also been shown to be associated with increased carotid intima-media thickness and increased PAI-I, both of which are risk factors for cardiovascular disease. Although these risk factors are present in women who have PCOS, an increase in cardiovascular events has not been observed in this population.[27–29] Additional studies are needed to clarify the relation between observed risk factors and prevalence of cardiovascular disease.

Endometrial Hyperplasia

Endometrial hyperplasia is a potential consequence of the effect of unopposed estrogen stimulation on the endometrium. Endometrial hyperplasia is seen most frequently in perimenopausal women and historically in postmenopausal women treated with unopposed estrogen. Adolescents and reproductive-aged women who have PCOS are also at risk because of the chronic anovulation associated with this disorder, however. Endometrial hyperplasia, if left untreated, can progress to adeno-carcinoma. The risk is lowest for simple hyperplasia without atypia (1%) and highest for complex hyperplasia with atypia (29%).[30] The incidence of endometrial hyperplasia in a study of 56 women who had PCOS and anovulatory infertility (age range: 21–41 years) was found to be 36%.[31] Of the women who had endometrial hyperplasia, 25% were found to have cytologic atypia, which increases the risk for developing endometrial adenocarcinoma. The risk for having endometrial hyperplasia was significantly correlated with an intermenstrual interval of longer than 3 months and an endometrial thickness, measured by transvaginal ultrasound, of greater than 7 mm. The risk for endometrial hyperplasia in the adolescent population that had PCOS has not been determined, but it is probably quite low.

Infertility

Infertility in women who have PCOS seems to be caused by oligo- or anovulation. This condition is treatable. It is important to reassure the adolescent that pregnancy is possible with current treatments available, because many are left with the impression that they are never going to be able to conceive. Treatment options include weight reduction for obese individuals, because pregnancy rates are poorer in morbidly obese women.[32] In addition, pregnancy complications, such as gestational diabetes, pre-eclampsia, large-for-gestation infants, and neonatal death, are significantly increased in obese and morbidly obese individuals.[33,34] Clomiphene citrate is the first-line drug for treatment of anovulation. Approximately 75% to 80% of women ovulate in response to clomiphene citrate.[35] Cumulative pregnancy rates have been reported as 40% to 50% for 6 or fewer months and 70% to 75% for 6 to 9 months.[36–38] Conception rates per cycle with clomiphene citrate have been reported to be 22%, which is comparable to normal cycle fecundity.[35] Metformin is not recommended as a first-line therapy for anovulatory infertility, because success rates are not as good as with clomiphene citrate.[39,40] The use of metformin as an adjunct to other therapies in subsets of women who have PCOS with infertility has yet to be determined. Gonadotropin therapy and in vitro fertilization are also valuable techniques to treat anovulatory infertility in women who have failed to ovulate or conceive with clomiphene citrate. The pregnancy rate with gonadotropin therapy is approximately 22% per cycle, but there is a risk for high-order multiple gestations because of multifollicular development.[35] Clinical pregnancy rates with in vitro fertilization and embryo transfer are similar for women with PCOS compared with women who do not have PCOS.[35]

Impaired Quality of Life

Depression and decreased quality of life have been reported in women who have PCOS more frequently than in controls. It seems that increased weight is the largest contributor to poor quality of life in women who have PCOS.[41] Quality-of-life scores in adolescents and women who have PCOS have also been shown to be inversely correlated to BMI.[42,43] In a study of 104 women diagnosed with PCOS, the relative risk for depressive disorder compared with control women was 4.23 (95% confidence interval [CI]: 1.49–11.98) and was independent of obesity and infertility.[44]

DIAGNOSTIC CONSIDERATIONS

PCOS is the most common cause of androgen excess, with a suspected incidence of 3% in the adolescent population.[45] There are no good estimates of the prevalence of the disorder in this age group, however. The classic presentation of PCOS is a heterogeneous syndrome characterized by features of anovulation amenorrhea, oligomenorrhea, or irregular cycles in combination with signs of androgen excess acne, hirsutism, or alopecia.[46] Some researchers think that PCOS is a maladaptation of the evolutionary phenomenon that is adrenarche. During pubertal development, adolescents typically have relative androgenemia, insulin resistance, cystic ovaries, and anovulatory cycles, which transition into an estrogenic state later in puberty. Failure to make this transition may result in PCOS secondary to abnormal pubertal development.[47] The path to PCOS remains unknown, however. Persistent menstrual irregularity seems to be a better predictor compared with biochemical parameters in predicting PCOS.[48]

The American Society for Reproductive Medicine and the European Society of Human Reproduction and Embryology have developed a consensus called the 2003 Rotterdam criteria to diagnose PCOS.[49] The diagnosis depends on the presence of two of the three following features: chronic anovulation characterized by persistent menstrual irregularities for more than 6 months, ultrasonographic appearance of the polycystic ovary (of at least one ovary greater than 10 cm^3 [10 mL] or polycystic ovarian morphology with 12 or more peripheral follicles 2–9 mm in diameter), and androgen excess (clinical or laboratory), with the exclusion of other etiologies.[49]

There has been some debate about the Rotterdam criteria because they include women with polycystic ovaries and anovulation but no clinical or biochemical evidence of hyperandrogenism. The general practice is to include all subgroups within the spectrum of PCOS. Some investigators have found that the different subgroups arising from the Rotterdam criteria have varying significance with respect to developing metabolic disturbances and the long-term consequences, such as type 2 diabetes mellitus, which occurs in women who have PCOS.[50–52] The nonhyperandrogenic phenotype may represent a form of PCOS associated with a milder metabolic profile.[53]

Some researchers have proposed an alternative method for diagnosis of PCOS in the adolescent, which includes four of the following five criteria: (1) oligo- or amenorrhea 2 years after menarche, (2) clinical hyperandrogenism, (3) biologic hyperandrogenism (eg, elevated plasma testosterone, LH/FSH ratio >2), (4) insulin resistance or hyperinsulinemia (eg, acanthosis nigricans, abdominal obesity, glucose intolerance), and (5) polycystic ovaries.[54] This set of diagnostic criteria is suggested as a way to avoid mislabeling an adolescent with transitional functional hyperandrogenism and menstrual disorders as having PCOS. Some researchers think that the Rotterdam criteria may overestimate the diagnosis in the adolescent; however, currently, the definition of PCOS is the same for adolescents and adults.

Using menstrual irregularity to diagnosis PCOS in the adolescent population is difficult, because a history of menstrual irregularity is considered normal in the first few years after menarche secondary to anovulation.[50] Persistent irregularity of cycles for longer than 2 years after menarche is a strong predictor of continued irregularity and PCOS, because most adolescent have regular cycles 2 years after menarche.[55–57] Furthermore, adolescents with irregular cycles within the first 3 years of menarche and no evidence of clinical hyperandrogenism may, in fact, have biochemical evidence of hyperandrogenism similar to that found in PCOS.[58] Hyperandrogenism can occasionally be found in the postmenarchal years without significant sequelae in adolescents with anovulatory regular cycles.[59]

Rarely, an adolescent who has PCOS presents with primary amenorrhea as the first manifestation. Depending on the literature, primary amenorrhea as the initial feature occurs in 1.4% to 14% of all adolescents.[60–62] This group of adolescents exhibits more features of the MS and has higher androstenedione levels, which may represent a more severe spectrum of this common condition.[63] In addition, this group of adolescents may be less likely to respond to a progesterone challenge because of a persistently decidualized endometrium in response to the high levels of androgens.[63]

PCOS may also present before menarche in the form of androgen excess. Premature pubarche and adrenarche are manifestations of androgen excess and may predispose adolescents to PCOS.[57,64] The correlation found between androgen levels at the time of presentation of premature pubarche and the development of PCOS in adolescence is thought to be compatible with an inborn dysregulation of steroidogenesis in the ovary and the adrenal gland.[57]

In addition to menstrual irregularity, adolescents have a physiologic increase in insulin resistance and androgen levels in response to growth hormone (GH).[65,66] The GH may lead to an increase in insulin levels and a decrease in circulating SHBG.[65,66] Both of these features are cardinal to the diagnosis of PCOS but may also represent a normal variation in many adolescents. Hirsutism, hyperandrogenism, and ultrasonographic evidence of polycystic ovaries are often not evident in the adolescent who has PCOS.

Recent literature has identified a specific biochemical marker (adiopentin), which is significantly lower in concentration in the daughters of women who have PCOS before the onset of hyperandrogenism and may be an early marker of metabolic derangement in adolescent girls.[67]

PHYSICAL FINDINGS
Hirsutism

Hirsutism tends to be less marked in adolescents, because the duration of exposure to excess androgens is much shorter than in their adult counterparts. Adolescents may also hide their excess hair by shaving or laser treatment, and therefore should be specifically asked about excess hair on their upper lip, chin, neck, or abdomen. In addition, ethnicity, sensitivity of the hair follicles, and levels of androgens can all cause variations in the extent of the hirsutism.[68] The Ferriman-Gallwey score may not be as useful in the adolescent who may only exhibit upper lip hair. Furthermore, this grading system was standardized in white women older than 24 years of age.[69]

Acne

Acne affects fewer adolescents who have PCOS and has been correlated with an increase in dehydroepiandrosterone sulfate (DHEAS) rather than free testosterone.[56] It is often the first sign of hyperandrogenism in the adolescent.[70]

Obesity

Although obesity is common in women who have PCOS, it is not necessary to make the diagnosis. In fact, the prevalence of obesity varies, and many patients who have PCOS have a normal BMI. The presence of obesity does, however, amplify the severity of PCOS and increase the risk for metabolic dysfunction.[46] For most patients, there is an increased upper body adiposity or central distribution that gives rise to an increased waist-to-hip ratio.[56] In addition, insulin resistance is worsened by obesity. Acanthosis nigricans, a marker of insulin resistance, is more common in the obese adolescent who has PCOS. Common areas involve the dorsal surface of the neck and intertriginous areas, such as the upper thigh and axilla. More children today are overweight, which puts more adolescents who have PCOS at risk for an increase in the severity of their symptoms. In fact, with the rising tide of childhood obesity, children who may have never displayed symptoms of PCOS, with the exception of irregular cycles, may now experience symptoms of anovulation and androgen excess.[46] Obesity exacerbates the PCOS phenotype in previously asymptomatic individuals.[71] Weight reduction in adults has been shown to improve free androgen levels, insulin sensitivity, and ovulatory function.[72]

DIAGNOSIS

As with adults, the Rotterdam criteria should be used to make the diagnosis of PCOS in adolescents. A history of persistent oligomenorrhea or secondary amenorrhea should be evaluated, and other conditions that could cause these symptoms should be excluded. Blood tests for FSH, estradiol, thyroid-stimulating hormone, and prolactin should be performed to rule out premature ovarian failure, thyroid disease, and hyperprolactinemia. The adolescent should be examined for signs and symptoms of hyperandrogenism, and blood tests for total and free testosterone, and possibly for androstenedione, should be obtained. An ultrasound scan is indicated to evaluate for polycystic ovarian morphology. Height and weight should be obtained, and the adolescent should be examined for signs of insulin resistance (acanthosis nigricans), virilization, and other endocrinopathies (eg, Cushing's syndrome).

Role of Luteinizing Hormone/Follicle-Stimulating Hormone Ratio

It is important to check FSH and estradiol levels when evaluating for PCOS to exclude the diagnosis of premature ovarian failure. Obtaining the LH/FSH ratio is not necessary. Multiple studies support the finding that an elevation of the plasma LH concentration, or an LH/FSH ratio greater than 2, is not required for the diagnosis of hyperandrogenism.[73–75] In one recent study, only 11 of the 24 patients who had female hyperandrogenism had elevated baseline LH levels, suggesting a primary hypothalamic-pituitary abnormality.[74] The remaining 13 had ovarian hyperandrogenism independent of an elevation in LH, suggesting abnormal modulation of ovarian androgen responsiveness to normal levels of LH. Similar to adults who have PCOS, however, some adolescents have an increased LH concentration and elevated LH/FSH ratio.[76]

Testosterone, Dehydroepiandrosterone Sulfate, and Androstenedione Measurements

Androgen levels are traditionally ordered to exclude more serious causes of androgen excess, such as an ovarian or adrenal tumor. Total testosterone greater than 200 ng/dL and DHEAS greater than 6000 ng/mL are suggestive of ovarian and adrenal tumors and require further evaluation. Rapid onset and progression of hyperandrogenic symptoms also suggest tumor or drug exposure rather than PCOS and should be investigated. In PCOS, total testosterone can be normal or slightly elevated, but free testosterone is thought to be a more sensitive test for androgen excess. Free testosterone has been reported to be elevated in 60% to 80% of adult women who have PCOS (>10 pg/mL), whereas DHEAS is elevated in only 25% of patients.[77] The difficulty often encountered with androgen measurements is in interpreting the results, because there is a tendency for significant variation among laboratories.[68] Furthermore, in adolescents, the range of normal testosterone levels is generally lower than that observed in adults. Free testosterone is the most specific because it has been demonstrated to reach adult levels by midpuberty in normal girls.[78]

Ultrasound

The Rotterdam criteria include polycystic ovaries demonstrated by ultrasound as one of the key features of the syndrome.[49] The ultrasound definition of polycystic ovarian morphology is the presence of 12 or more follicles with a 2- to 9-mm diameter on the ovary. An increased ovarian volume of greater than 10 mL is also suggestive. Only one ovary consistent with polycystic ovarian morphology is sufficient for the diagnosis. Transvaginal ultrasound is the preferred technique over the transabdominal approach to detect polycystic morphology, but in a virginal adolescent, it is not reasonable to perform transvaginal ultrasound. In addition, transabdominal ultrasound may underestimate the presence of PCOS.[68] Although the ultrasound appearance of ovaries is included in the diagnosis of PCOS, recent studies in hyperandrogenic women do not confirm the consistency of transvaginal ultrasound accuracy in detecting all patients who have female hyperandrogenism.[73] In one study of 42 adolescents, pelvic ultrasound failed to detect 46% of patients who had female ovarian hyperandrogenism.[45] The role of ultrasound in the adolescent population is further complicated by the mere fact that many controls have polycystic ovaries that are not pathologic. In one study, 48% of controls with no evidence of PCOS (regular cycles, no hirsutism, normal oral glucose tolerance) had polycystic ovaries.[49] Similarly, ultrasound imaging has shown that 25% of healthy adolescent volunteers develop multifollicular ovaries, defined as 6 to 10 follicles 4 to 10 mm in diameter without increased stroma.[77,79] The prevalence of polycystic ovaries seems to occur at a rate of 10% in regular menstruating adolescents.[71] The presence of polycystic ovaries in asymptomatic adolescents may represent a subclinical PCOS type of ovarian dysfunction.[80] In women who have PCOS, polycystic ovaries occur as frequently as 95% of the time, suggesting that these ultrasound findings are usually abnormal.[81]

The typical ovarian findings of polycystic morphology or ovarian volume are related to increased stroma. The volume of the ovary is much less specific than the morphology of the ovary in detecting individuals who have PCOS. In one series, neither the morphology nor the size of the ovaries was helpful in identifying distinctive metabolic or reproductive abnormalities in women who had PCOS.[81] In another series, however, adolescents who had PCOS or irregular cycles for longer than 3 years more frequently had an increased ovarian volume as compared with multiple cysts.[58]

At present, the role of ultrasound in women with a history of anovulation and hyperandrogenism is uncertain when a diagnosis of PCOS is already made.[45,82] Ultrasound may help to screen for anatomic abnormalities (ie, polyps), but in the adolescent, routine ultrasound may be unnecessary. In addition, in the adolescent population, pelvic ultrasound is usually performed transabdominally rather than transvaginally, which can make counting follicles more problematic and underestimates the prevalence of polycystic ovaries.[68] MRI has been used in this setting to confirm PCOS morphology, particularly in an obese girl with hirsutism and oligomenorrhea.[83] Alternatively, three-dimensional transrectal ultrasound may improve the precision of the diagnosis of PCOS in the adolescent.[84]

Role of 17-OH Progesterone

17-OH progesterone (17-OHP) is a good screening test for the detection of nonclassic adrenal hyperplasia (NCAH). Blood samples should be drawn in the early morning, when adrenal secretion of hormones is highest, and in the follicular phase of the menstrual cycle in cycling women to avoid confusion with ovarian production of 17-OHP in the luteal phase. A follicular phase/morning 17-OHP level of 2 ng/mL or less is normal, suggesting that NCAH is not present with a specificity of 100%.[85] If the 17-OHP level is greater than 2 ng/mL, the diagnosis of NCAH should be confirmed by a corticotropin stimulation test.

Many patients who have PCOS exhibit exaggerated 17-OHP responses to adrenal stimulation but not high enough to be consistent with NCAH.[74] Previous researchers have suggested that this elevation in 17-OHP may, in fact, be a mild homozygous or heterozygous form of nonclassic congenital adrenal hyperplasia, whereas others suggest that it is simply generalized overactivity to corticotropin stimulation by the adrenal gland, and the carrier status for 21-OH deficiency may be an incidental finding.[86]

Oral Glucose Screen

Adolescents who are obese and have a diagnosis of PCOS should undergo a 2-hour 75-g oral glucose tolerance test (OGTT).[46] This is a more sensitive test than a fasting glucose test to detect diabetes and impaired glucose tolerance, a significant risk factor for diabetes.[22] Adolescent girls with premature pubarche during childhood who develop functional ovarian hyperandrogenism show increased mean serum insulin in response to an OGTT, which correlates with evidence of ovarian hyperandrogenism.[87] The significance of hyperinsulinemia diagnosed at such at early age is unknown, but it may act as a marker for the development of functional ovarian hyperandrogenism.[87]

Insulin Testing

There is no accurate way to measure insulin resistance. Fasting insulin levels are not reliable, because 25% of normal patients have insulin values that overlap with those of patients with insulin resistance.[1] The most accurate tests for insulin resistance are the euglycemic clamp technique and the frequently sampled intravenous glucose tolerance test. Both of these require inpatient hospitalization, however, and are not practical for screening. A fasting glucose/insulin ratio has been proposed as a rapid and easy screening alternative. In obese adult women, a fasting glucose/insulin ratio less than 4.5 suggests insulin resistance, whereas in the adolescent, a ratio less than 7 is suggestive.[88,89] The clinical recognition of insulin resistance is based on the associated physical features of acanthosis nigricans and obesity.[56] Evidence of insulin resistance in the adolescent with menstrual irregularities may be consistent with a diagnosis of PCOS.

Stimulation Tests

The leuprolide acetate stimulation test may be a reliable tool for identification of the ovary as the cause of ovarian excess. In one study of 42 adolescents, more than half (58%) of hyperandrogenic adolescents had an abnormal response to leuprolide acetate testing suggestive of functional ovarian hyperandrogenism.[45] The rapid GnRH pulse frequency favors the pituitary synthesis and secretion of LH over FSH, resulting in the abnormal LH/FSH ratios seen in these individuals. This test is not frequently performed.

Metabolic Syndrome

The incidence of MS is increasing in the obese adolescent and occurs frequently in the adolescent who has PCOS. The incidence of MS has been shown to be increased significantly in adolescents with increasing BMI, insulin resistance, and hyperandrogenemia as compared with adolescents in the general population.[25] Adolescent phenotypes with hyperandrogenemia are also at increased risk for elevated triglycerides and low-density lipoprotein cholesterol.[90] Any adolescent with androgen excess should be monitored for evidence of hypertension and hypertriglyceridemia (MS) regardless of body weight, because the risk for MS in women who have PCOS seems to be independent of BMI.[25] Obesity is thought to be a stronger predictor of MS than is PCOS, however.[26]

TREATMENT

Treatment options for PCOS in the adolescent include weight loss for obese individuals, symptom-directed therapy to address the main symptoms noted by the adolescent, and metabolic correction of the underlying insulin resistance using insulin-sensitizing medications. For the adolescent, the goal should be addressing the most distressing symptoms while stressing a healthy lifestyle with reduction of risks for long-term sequelae of PCOS.

Weight Loss

Weight loss should be the first-line treatment, or at least an important component of treatment, for all adolescents who are overweight or obese. Weight loss of approximately 5% to 10% has been shown to result in reduction in testosterone, increase in SHBG, resumption of menses, and improved reproductive outcome in women who have PCOS.[91–97] Other advantages of weight loss include low cost, few negative side effects, and avoidance of use of long-term medications. Weight loss in women who have PCOS is difficult, however.

Lifestyle Modification

The emphasis of weight loss should be lifestyle modification, with a program encompassing calorie restriction and an increase in formal exercise. Regular physical exercise is essential for weight loss and long-term weight management. A minimum of 30 minutes of moderately intense exercise at least 3 days per week is recommended.[98] Women participating in structured weight loss programs that include a behavioral modification component do better than women attempting weight loss on their own.[99] One study evaluated patients who had PCOS and were enrolled in a calorie restriction and exercise program over 6 months.[95] The mean weight loss was 2% to 5%. Decreased abdominal fat and improved insulin sensitivity were observed. Nine of the 15 anovulatory patients became ovulatory. Another study evaluated a structured weight loss program, including calorie restriction and exercise, of 6 months' duration in anovulatory infertile women.[92,94] The average weight loss was 15 lb. The spontaneous ovulation rate was 92%, and there was a 33% to 45% spontaneous pregnancy rate.

Dietary interventions should focus on restricting calories and increasing energy expenditure. A low-calorie diet is considered to be 1000 to 1200 kcal/d, which should reduce total body weight by average loss of 10% over 6 months.[100] A 500- to 1000-kcal/d reduction from usual intake should result in weight loss of 1 to 2 lb/wk. Calorie restriction is the most important factor for weight loss. It does not seem to matter what the dietary composition is. Theoretically, low-fat high-carbohydrate diets should not be beneficial in women who have PCOS, because carbohydrates induce insulin secretion. In obese women who have PCOS, however, low-carbohydrate low-fat diets result in a similar decrease in weight and abdominal fat in addition to improvements in insulin sensitivity.[97] In obese individuals, a low-carbohydrate diet causes greater weight loss at 6 months when compared with a low-fat diet; however, at 12 months, both diets result in the same weight loss.[101] Comparison of the Atkins, Ornish, Weight Watchers, and Zone diets over a 1-year period show that all result in similar weight reduction.[102] Greater weight loss was associated with dietary adherence. Decreases in insulin, total cholesterol, and C-reactive protein were associated with weight loss and did not differ among diets. The difficulty is finding a "diet" that the individual can maintain and making a change in lifestyle.

Unfortunately, like all chronic conditions, lifestyle changes must be continued or women regain weight. This is particularly difficult for the adolescent, who may not be offered healthy food choices at home and who also may have difficulty in dealing with peers. Diet and behavioral therapies have been shown to fail within 3 years of follow-up, with weight regain of 60% to 86 % at 3.5 years and 75% to 121% at 5 years reported.[103]

Bariatric Surgery

For those who are unable to lose weight despite multiple attempts, bariatric surgery may offer the only hope for significant weight loss. Bariatric surgery is being used with increasing frequency to treat morbid obesity. From 1990 to 2000, there was a sixfold increase in the national annual rate of bariatric surgery performed, from 2.4 to 14.1 per 100,000 adults ($P = .001$).[104] Bariatric surgical procedures currently in use can be classified as restrictive procedures or combined restrictive/malabsorptive procedures. Restrictive procedures, such as vertical banded gastroplasty, adjustable gastric banding, and intragastric balloon, involve the creation of a small gastric pouch, which fills rapidly, leading to early satiety. Restrictive/malabsorptive procedures, such as the Roux-en-Y bypass, involve reducing the size of the gastric pouch in addition to bypassing a large section of the small bowel, thereby reducing the surface area for absorption. The introduction of high osmolar material into the jejunum leads to a dumping syndrome and avoidance of food. Currently, gastric bypass (Roux-en-Y gastric bypass) procedures are performed most commonly, with more than half performed laparoscopically.

The 1991, a National Institutes of Health Consensus Development Panel recommended that surgical treatment be considered for any adult patient with a BMI of

40 kg/m^2 or greater or for those with a BMI of 35 kg/m^2 or greater who have serious coexisting medical problems worsened by obesity.[105] Additional selection criteria for bariatric surgery include failed dietary therapy, psychologic stability, knowledge about the operation and sequelae, highly motivated patient, and medical problems that do not preclude likely survival from the operation.

Improvement of obesity-related medical problems is the primary goal of bariatric surgery. Two large meta-analyses have shown that in patients who have a BMI of 40 kg/m^2 or greater, surgery results in a mean weight loss of 20 to 40 kg over 2 years, which was maintained for up to 10 years.[106,107] Overall mortality from all procedures is less than 1%.[106] In addition to weight loss, significant improvement in diabetes, hypertension, dyslipidemia, and sleep apnea has been observed.[106,107] Bariatric surgery also results in improved menstrual regularity and fertility in women.[108]

Despite much information about bariatric surgery in obese adults, there is a lack of studies on bariatric surgery in adolescents, much less adolescent girls who have PCOS.[23,109,110] What is the impact on adolescent growth and development? Should the recommendations for performing bariatric surgery in adolescents be the same as for adults? There are few long-term data evaluating the effect of bariatric surgery on the adolescent decades later in adulthood. Further research is needed before this procedure is widely used in this population.

When considering bariatric surgery in a young adolescent female patient, consequences for future pregnancy must be considered. One large population-based study found that previous bariatric surgery was not associated with an adverse perinatal outcome.[111] Additional studies of pregnancies after bariatric surgery have found that the pregnancies were uncomplicated and well tolerated by the mothers.[112,113] Although there is a higher incidence of anemia and nutritional deficiencies, weight loss from bariatric surgery decreases the risk of pregnancy complications compared with these risks in the obese pregnant population.

Symptom-Directed Therapy for Polycystic Ovary Syndrome

Hirsutism or acne

Hirsutism is a significant issue for the adolescent. Abnormal hair growth attributable to excess androgens is progressive; therefore, the sooner it is treated, the better is the success. The approach to treating hirsutism involves suppression and removal of current hair in addition to prevention of new hair growth. This is best accomplished by using many methods simultaneously: hair removal techniques should be combined with medical suppression of current and new hair growth. It is advisable to institute therapy in a young adolescent with minimal hirsutism, because early intervention can prevent significant accumulation of excess hair. Because of the growth cycle of hair, it is important to allow 6 months of therapy before judging the efficacy of treatment.

Hair removal techniques

The first-line treatment for addressing excess body or facial hair is hair removal techniques. These include waxing, plucking, shaving, depilation, electrolysis, and laser hair removal techniques. Contrary to popular belief, shaving does not make hair grow back faster and it avoids the folliculitis seen with waxing and plucking. Electrolysis results in permanent hair removal, but it is time-consuming and costly and results depend on the ability of the individual performing the electrolysis. Laser techniques are best suited to individuals with pale skin and dark hair, limiting this technique in treating dark-skinned individuals.

Combined hormonal contraceptive

The most common treatment offered for PCOS is the combined hormonal contraceptive because it effectively controls symptoms of PCOS. This refers to medication containing estrogen and progestin. The most common form is the combined oral contraceptive, but transdermal and vaginal ring systems are also now available. The advantages of the combined hormonal contraceptive include regulation of menstruation, prevention of endometrial hyperplasia, and control of hirsutism or acne. The mechanism of action is primarily decreased production of androgens from the ovary and increased production of SHBG from the liver. The result is a decrease in free, or active, androgens. A study in women who had PCOS compared with controls demonstrated that use of a combined oral contraceptive resulted in significant decreases in androgens and gonadotropins in the women who had PCOS and in controls.[114] In the women who had PCOS, however, there was a significant decrease in LH, total testosterone, and androstenedione, whereas FSH levels did not change. In a similar fashion, it has been demonstrated that SHBG serum levels increased significantly after administration of combined oral contraceptives containing ethinyl estradiol and desogestrel or norethindrone.[115] Combined oral contraceptives have also been shown to increase insulin resistance;[116] however, this effect is not thought to be clinically significant when compared with the therapeutic benefits derived from their use.

The progestin component of the older combined hormonal contraceptives is a testosterone derivative and has some androgenic activity in vitro. There is no difference in clinical efficacy in suppression of androgenic symptoms between the available hormonal contraceptives containing the more androgenic progestins (norethindrone or levonorgestrel) and the newer less androgenic progestins (desogestrel, norgestimate, or drospirenone), however.[117] Low-dose oral contraceptives containing ethinyl estradiol, 20 μg, have also been shown to be effective in the management of acne.[118] Therefore, in deciding on a combined hormonal contraceptive, it is best to use the one that has the fewest side effects, best efficacy, and best compliance for that individual.

Antiandrogens

These medications work at the level of the hair follicle to block androgen binding to the androgen receptor or inhibit 5α-reductase, the enzyme that converts testosterone to the active androgen dihydrotestosterone (DHT). Several antiandrogen medications are available in the United States. The most commonly used antiandrogen is spironolactone. Its mechanism of action is primarily competitive binding at the level of the androgen receptor. It also has some inhibitory effect on 5α-reductase and decreases testosterone production. The recommended dosage is 100 to 200 mg/d usually given in divided doses. Side effects include urinary frequency and postural hypotension. Because it is a potassium-sparing diuretic, use of this medication can result in hyperkalemia; thus, potassium levels should be checked after initiation of therapy. Flutamide is commonly used in adolescents in Europe. It is an androgen receptor blocker that inhibits DHT binding. It also decreases adrenal 17,20 lyase activity, resulting in decreased androgen production. The recommended dosage is 250 to 500 mg/d. Hepatic failure is a rare complication of this medication. Finasteride is a 5α-reductase inhibitor. It is rarely used for treatment of hirsutism in women. The recommended dosage is 5 mg/d.

Spironolactone, flutamide, and finasteride are all equally effective in the treatment of hirsutism. A randomized placebo-controlled trial over 6 months in hirsute women showed equivalent and significant decreases in Ferriman-Gallwey hirsutism scores for all three medications compared with placebo.[119] Flutamide has been studied in adolescents in Europe for the treatment of hirsutism. In an observational study in a group of 18 adolescent female subjects aged 14 to 18 years of age, 18-month treatment with flutamide resulted in a significant decrease in Ferriman-Gallwey scores and free androgen index.[120] In the United States, spironolactone is the most widely used antiandrogen because of its effectiveness, lower cost, and side-effect profile. None of these medications are approved by the US Food and Drug Administration for the treatment of hirsutism. In addition, these medications are potential teratogens and should be used with caution in women of reproductive age, especially teenagers, who may not be forthcoming about their sexual activity and need for contraception. Antiandrogens are frequently used in combination with combined hormonal contraceptives because their mechanism of action is different and their combined effect is additive.[121,122]

Gonadotropin-releasing hormone agonists

GnRH agonists represent a modification of the natural GnRH decapeptide, which results in an increase in the half-life. GnRH agonists, when used continuously, result in down-regulation of the pituitary with a resulting decrease in hormone production from the ovary, including estrogen and androgens. When used alone, the resulting hypoestrogenism leads to significant bone loss that is believed to be reversible after therapy for 6 months or less. A randomized placebo-controlled study in 64 patients who had PCOS evaluated the GnRH agonist nafarelin alone or in combination with the combined oral contraceptive pill for 6 months.[123] Although total testosterone and free testosterone were seen to decrease significantly with nafarelin and the combined hormonal contraceptive, the combination of these two medications resulted in a more significant decrease in total testosterone and increase in SHBG. Although this medication has been shown to be effective in the short term, its long-term use in adolescent girls is not advisable because of a potential detrimental effect on bone density and the availability of alternative medications with fewer side effects.

Abnormal bleeding

The goals of treating abnormal bleeding are to regulate menstrual cycle bleeding, thereby preventing anemia, and menstrual bleeding accidents, which can be embarrassing for the adolescent, and also to prevent long-term risk for endometrial hyperplasia. Standard treatments to regulate menses include combined hormonal contraceptives as discussed previously. These medications afford excellent cycle regulation and decreased menstrual flow. Another option to regulate bleeding is the use of progestins. Progestins can be administered on a cyclic or continuous schedule. Cyclic options include medroxyprogesterone acetate, 5 to 10 mg; norethindrone acetate, 5 mg; or oral micronized progesterone, 100 to 200 mg. These medications should be given monthly for 10 to 14 days to achieve the greatest reduction in development of endometrial hyperplasia.[30] Some have suggested that these medications can be given every 3 months to induce menses four times a year, however.[124] Another option is to use the progestin-only pill. This pill contains norethindrone at a dose of 0.35 μg/d. The incidence of abnormal spotting is higher with this pill compared with the combined hormonal contraceptive, although the contraceptive benefit is similar. Depo-medroxy progesterone acetate can also be used in women who have PCOS, although weight gain is a concern for overweight and obese individuals. In addition, with Depo-Provera and any of the progestin-only alternatives, the effect on hirsutism and acne is not as significant as with the combined hormonal contraceptives, because progestin alone does not increase SHBG and does not suppress ovarian function as well.

Metabolic Correction with Insulin-Sensitizing Agents

With emerging evidence that insulin resistance plays a significant role in the pathophysiology of PCOS, insulin-sensitizing agents have been proposed as treatment for this disorder. Metformin and thiazolidinediones are the two classes of insulin-sensitizing medications that have been studied. Thiazolidinediones have been associated with liver failure and should not be used in the adolescent until their efficacy and safety in this population have been studied. Metformin, the most widely studied of all the insulin-sensitizing drugs, inhibits hepatic glucose production and increases peripheral tissue sensitivity to insulin.[125] At a dosage of 1500 to 2000 mg/d, metformin has been shown to decrease androgens, decrease insulin, improve ovulatory rates, and resume menstrual cyclicity.[126–128] A meta-analysis of the use of metformin versus placebo revealed that the odds ratio of ovulating on metformin compared with placebo for women who have PCOS was 3.88 (95% CI: 2.25–6.69).[129] Metformin alone does not reliably lead to weight loss in patients who have PCOS.[127,130,131] When metformin is combined with a restricted calorie diet, however, significant weight loss is observed.[132,133]

Although the use of metformin seems promising, several issues remain. Most published studies evaluating metformin in women who have PCOS involve a small number of select patients, are observational in design, and are of short duration (12–26 weeks). There are few randomized controlled studies comparing metformin with established therapies. The effect of metformin on hirsutism has not been adequately studied, and results are conflicting.[120,130] In addition, there are few studies evaluating the use of metformin in adolescents.[134] Metformin use in obese and nonobese adolescent girls who have PCOS has shown resumption of menses in 91% to 100% of subjects[133,135] and ovulation in 78% of subjects.[136] In sexually active adolescents taking metformin, contraception is necessary, and there are no contraindications to using hormonal contraception with this drug.

The use of metformin compared with other therapies has been evaluated in a few studies. One prospective randomized trial in adolescents who had hyperinsulinemia and PCOS compared metformin (750 mg given twice daily) with placebo in conjunction with healthy lifestyle counseling over 12 weeks.[137] The use of metformin was found to be associated with a significant decrease in testosterone and an increased relative risk for menses of 2.5 (95% CI: 1.12–5.58) when compared with placebo. There was no significant change in BMI, total cholesterol, or insulin sensitivity.

A randomized placebo-controlled trial in 43 obese adolescent female subjects who had PCOS evaluated the effect of four treatment arms over 6 months: placebo, metformin, oral contraceptive, or lifestyle management.[138] In the oral contraceptive and lifestyle modification groups, SHBG was increased and total and free androgens were decreased. Those who lost weight showed greater increases in SHBG. Metformin was associated with increased menstrual frequency but not with a change in weight.

Another randomized placebo-controlled trial was performed in 36 obese adolescent subjects who had PCOS and were placed on lifestyle modification and oral contraceptives and randomized to metformin, 1500 mg/d, or placebo over 6 months.[138] BMI was reduced in the placebo and metformin groups but did not differ between groups. Waist circumference was reduced significantly in the metformin-only group. Free androgen index was equally decreased in the placebo and metformin groups, but suppression of total testosterone was greater in the metformin group. The investigators concluded that there may be a beneficial impact of a lifestyle program in combination with oral contraceptives. Metformin, when combined with lifestyle modification and oral contraceptives, may enhance reduction in central adiposity and androgen suppression. Larger prospective randomized studies are needed.

Surgical Therapy

Stein and Leventhal[139] first described ovarian wedge resection as a treatment for anovulation in seven amenorrheic women who had PCOS in 1935. This procedure involved removal of one half to three fourths of each ovary at laparotomy. In a subsequent series of 108 women who had PCOS published in 1966, ovarian wedge resection was shown to result in a resumption of menses in 95% and pregnancy in 86.7%.[140] This technique is no longer used because of invasiveness, risk for significant periovarian adhesions leading to infertility, and ovarian failure. Laparoscopic ovarian drilling was introduced as a less invasive alternative to wedge resection in women with infertility. This procedure involves drilling holes into the ovary at laparoscopy using monopolar cautery, bipolar cautery, or laser. Three to five holes per ovary are sufficient to achieve resumption of ovulation.[141] A greater number of holes and more energy may be associated with ovarian failure. Review of the literature reveals this technique to result in decreased serum testosterone and LH and resumption of spontaneous ovulation in 50% to 100% of patients.[140] The mechanism of action is not understood, but theories suggest that destruction of follicles results in decreased local concentration of androgens. Laparoscopic ovarian drilling is a procedure to correct anovulation and infertility and should not be used as a treatment for adolescents who have PCOS.

Treatment Approach

Treatment of the adolescent should be instituted early. Early intervention has the advantage of treating distressing symptoms in the adolescent, such as hirsutism, acne, and weight gain, with the goal of improving self-esteem and quality of life. This strategy may also prevent long-term sequelae of PCOS by controlling symptoms at a younger age. A symptom-directed treatment strategy should be used. For the obese or overweight adolescent, counseling or enrollment in programs for healthy diet and exercise regimens should be instituted. Manual hair removal techniques, including electrolysis or laser, should be considered for hirsutism, in addition to referral to a dermatologist for treatment of acne. Hormonal contraceptives should be considered as first-line medical treatment. This therapy offers the advantage of regulating menses and treating hirsutism and acne while preventing new hair growth. Hormonal contraceptives do not lead to earlier sexual activity in the adolescent, which is often a concern of the parent. Antiandrogen therapy, usually with spironolactone, can be added to hormonal contraceptives for treatment of hirsutism or acne. Metformin should be reserved for those adolescents with insulin resistance or who are not responding or do not tolerate other therapies. Metformin is not a weight loss drug. Some patients have less hunger on metformin, however, and are better able to sustain a healthy diet. Adolescents should be reassured about their ability to have children in the future using medical therapy or assisted reproductive technologies if necessary.

SUMMARY

PCOS is a heterogeneous endocrinologic disorder that is characterized by oligo- or amenorrhea and signs of hyperandrogenism. The cause of PCOS is unknown, but the syndrome is associated with insulin resistance, which, in turn, leads to hyperandrogenism. Long-term health consequences of PCOS are significant and include obesity, diabetes, MS, and anovulatory infertility. The symptoms of PCOS can be disturbing to an adolescent girl. Early diagnosis and intervention are important to treat these symptoms and prevent long-term sequelae. The Rotterdam criteria for PCOS should be used for diagnosis in the adolescent. Current treatment regimens target the specific symptoms of PCOS. These include weight management and reduction programs for obese adolescents and hormonal contraceptives and antiandrogens for menstrual irregularity, hirsutism, and acne. Insulin-sensitizing agents are promising in the treatment of this disorder, especially in those with insulin resistance, but randomized controlled trials are needed to determine the long-term risks and benefits in addition to efficacy over traditional therapies before using them as first-line therapy.

REFERENCES

1. Dunaif A. Insulin resistance and the polycystic ovary syndrome: mechanism and implications for pathogenesis. Endocr Rev 1997;18:774–800.
2. Azziz R, Woods KS, Reyna R, et al. The prevalence and features of the polycystic ovary syndrome in an unselected population. J Clin Endocrinol Metab 2004;89: 2745–9.
3. Knochenhauer ES, Key TJ, Kahsar-Miller M, et al. Prevalence of the polycystic ovary syndrome in unselected black and white women of the southeastern United States: a prospective study. J Clin Endocrinol Metab 1998;83:3078–82.
4. Kahsar-Miller MD, Nixon C, Boots LR, et al. Prevalence of polycystic ovary syndrome (PCOS) in first-degree relatives of patients with PCOS. Fertil Steril 2001;75:53–8.
5. Waldstreicher J, Santoro NF, Hall JE, et al. Hyperfunction of the hypothalamic-pituitary axis in women with polycystic ovarian disease: indirect evidence for partial gonadotroph desensitization. J Clin Endocrinol Metab 1988;66:165–72.
6. Apter D, Butzow T, Laughlin GA, et al. Accelerated 24 h luteinizing hormone pulsatile activity in adolescent girls with ovarian hyperandrogenism: relevance to the developmental phase of polycystic ovarian disease. J Clin Endocrinol Metab 1994;79:99–125.
7. Apter D, Butzow T, Laughlin GA, et al. Metabolic features of polycystic ovary syndrome are found in adolescent girls with hyperandrogenism. J Pediatr Endocrinol Metab 1995;80(10):2966–73.
8. Veldhuis JD, Pincus M, Garcia-Rudaz MC, et al. Disruption of the joint synchrony of luteinizing hormone, testosterone, and androstenedione secretion in adolescents with polycystic ovarian syndrome. J Clin Endocrinol Metab 2001;86:72–9.
9. Yasin M, Dalkin AC, Haisenleder DJ, et al. Testosterone is required for gonadotropin-releasing hormone stimulation of luteinizing hormone-P messenger ribonucleic acid expression in female rats. Endocrinology 1996;137:1265–71.
10. Azziz R. The time has come to simplify the evaluation of the hirsute patient. Fertil Steril 2000;74:870–2.
11. Barbieri RL, Makris A, Randall RW, et al. Insulin stimulates androgen accumulation in incubations of ovarian stroma obtained from women with hyperandrogenism. J Clin Endocrinol Metab 1986;62:904–10.
12. Nestler JE, Barlascini CO, Matt DW, et al. Suppression of serum insulin by diazoxide reduces serum testosterone levels in obese women with polycystic ovary syndrome. J Clin Endocrinol Metab 1989;68:1027–32.
13. DeClue TJ, Shah SC, Marchese M, et al. Insulin resistance and hyperinsulinemia induce hyperandrogenism in a young type B insulin-resistant female. J Clin Endocrinol Metab 1991;72:1308–11.
14. Dunaif A, Segal KR, Futterweit W, et al. Profound peripheral insulin resistance, independent of obesity, in the polycystic ovary syndrome. Diabetes 1989; 38(9):1165–74.

15. Azziz R. Androgen excess is the key element in polycystic ovary syndrome. Fertil Steril 2003;80:252–4.
16. Dunaif A. Hyperandrogenemia is necessary but not sufficient for polycystic ovary syndrome. Fertil Steril 2003;80:262–3.
17. Dunaif A, Thomas A. Current concepts in the polycystic ovary syndrome. Ann Rev Med 2001;52:401–19.
18. Zhang L, Rodriguez H, Ohno S, et al. Serine phosphorylation of human P450c17 increases 17,20-lyase activity: implications for adrenarche and the polycystic ovary syndrome. Proc Natl Acad Sci USA 1995;92:10619–23.
19. Legro RS, Kunselman AR, Dodson WC, et al. Prevalence and predictors of risk for type 2 diabetes mellitus and impaired glucose tolerance in polycystic ovary syndrome: a prospective, controlled study in 254 affected women. J Clin Endocrinol Metab 1999;84:165–9.
20. Ehrmann DA, Barnes RB, Rosenfeld RL, et al. Prevalence of impaired glucose tolerance and diabetes in women with polycystic ovary syndrome. Diabetes Care 1999;22:141–6.
21. Knowler WC, Barrett-Connor E, Fowler SE, et al, for the Diabetes Prevention Program Research Group. Reduction in the incidence of type 2 diabetes with lifestyle intervention of metformin. N Engl J Med 2002;346:393–403.
22. Palmert MR, Gordon CM, Kartashov AI, et al. Screening for abnormal glucose tolerance in adolescents with polycystic ovary syndrome. J Clin Endocrinol Metab 2002;87:1017–23.
23. Helmrath MA, Brandt ML, Inge TH. Adolescent obesity and bariatric surgery. Surg Clin North Am 2006;86:441–54.
24. Cussons AJ, Watts GF, Burke V, et al. Cardiometabolic risk in polycystic ovary syndrome: a comparison of different approaches to defining the metabolic syndrome. Hum Reprod 2008;23:2532–58.
25. Coviello AD, Legro RS, Dunaif A. Adolescent girls with polycystic ovary syndrome have an increased risk of the metabolic syndrome associated with increasing androgen levels independent of obesity and insulin resistance. J Clin Endocrinol Metab 2006;91:492–7.
26. Rossi B, Sukalich S, Droz J, et al. Prevalence of metabolic syndrome and related characteristics in obese adolescents with and without polycystic ovary syndrome. J Clin Endocrinol Metab 2008 Sep 23; [Epub ahead of print].
27. Pierpoint T, McKeigue PM, Isaacs AJ, et al. Mortality of women with polycystic ovary syndrome at long-term follow-up. J Clin Epidemiol 1998;51:581–6.
28. Wild S, Pierpoint T, McKeigue P, et al. Cardiovascular disease in women with polycystic ovary syndrome at long-term follow-up: a retrospective cohort study. Clin Endocrinol (Oxf) 2000;52:595–600.
29. Legro RS. Polycystic ovary syndrome and cardiovascular disease: a premature association? Endocr Rev 2003;24:302–12.
30. Montgomery BE, Daum GS, Dunton CJ. Endometrial hyperplasia: a review. Obstet Gynecol Surv 2004;59:368–78.
31. Cheung AP. Ultrasound and menstrual history in predicting endometrial hyperplasia in polycystic ovary syndrome. Obstet Gynecol 2001;98:325–31.
32. Jungheim ES, Lanzendorf SE, Odem RR, et al. Morbid obesity is associated with lower clinical pregnancy rates after in vitro fertilization in women with polycystic ovary syndrome. Fertil Steril 2008 Aug 8; [Epub ahead of print].
33. Weiss JL, Malone FD, Emig D, et al. Obesity, obstetric complications and cesarean delivery rate—a population-based screening study. Am J Obstet Gynecol 2004;190:1091–7.

34. Cedergren MI. Maternal morbid obesity and the risk of adverse pregnancy outcome. Obstet Gynecol 2004;103:219–24.
35. The Thessaloniki ESHRE/ASRM-Sponsored PCOS Consensus Workshop Group. Consensus on infertility treatment related to polycystic ovary syndrome. Hum Reprod 2008;23:462–77.
36. Hammond MG, Halme JK, Talbert LM. Factors affecting the pregnancy rate in clomiphene citrate induction of ovulation. Obstet Gynecol 1983;62:196–202.
37. Imani B, Eijkemans MJ, te Velde ER, et al. Predictors of chances to conceive in ovulatory patients during clomiphene citrate induction of ovulation in normogonadotropic oligoamenorrheic infertility. J Clin Endocrinol Metab 1999;84:1617–22.
38. Imani B, Eijkemans MJ, te Velde ER, et al. A nomogram to predict the probability of live birth after clomiphene citrate induction of ovulation in normogonadotropic oligoamenorrheic infertility. Fertil Steril 2002;77:91–7.
39. Legro RS, Barnhart HX, Schlaff WD, et al, for the Cooperative Multicenter Reproductive Medicine Network. Clomiphene, metformin, or both for infertility in the polycystic ovary syndrome. N Engl J Med 2007;356:551–66.
40. Palomba S, Orio F, Falbo A, et al. Clomiphene citrate versus metformin as first-line approach for the treatment of anovulation in infertile patients with polycystic ovary syndrome. J Clin Endocrinol Metab 2007;92:3498–503.
41. Barnard L, Ferriday D, Guenther M, et al. Quality of life and psychological well being in polycystic ovary syndrome. Hum Reprod 2007;22:2279–86.
42. Ching HL, Burke V, Stuckey BG. Quality of life and psychological morbidity in women with polycystic ovary syndrome: body mass index, age and the provision of patient information are significant modifiers. Clin Endocrinol (Oxf) 2007;66:373–9.
43. Trent M, Austin SB, Rich M, et al. Overweight status of adolescent girls with polycystic ovary syndrome: body mass index as mediator of quality of life. Ambul Pediatr 2005;5:107–11.
44. Hollinrake E, Abreu A, Maifeld M, et al. Increased risk of depressive disorders in women with polycystic ovary syndrome. Fertil Steril 2007;87:1369–76.
45. Ibanez L, Potau N, Zampolli M, et al. Source localization of androgen excess in adolescent girls. J Clin Endocrinol Metab 1994;79:1778–84.
46. Franks S. Polycystic ovary syndrome in adolescents. Int J Obes (Lond) 2008;32:1035–41.
47. Nader S. Adrenarche and polycystic ovary syndrome: a tale of two hypotheses. J Pediatr Adolesc Gynecol 2007;20:353–60.
48. Fernandes AR, de Sa Rosa e Silva AC, Romao GS, et al. Insulin resistance in adolescents with menstrual irregularities. J Pediatr Adolesc Gynecol 2005;18:269–74.
49. The Rotterdam ESHRE/ASRM-Sponsored PCOS consensus workshop group. Revised 2003 consensus on diagnostic criteria and long-term health risks related to polycystic ovary syndrome (PCOS). Hum Reprod 2004;19:41–7.
50. Dewailly D, Catteau-Jonard S, Reyss AC, et al. Oligoanovulation with polycystic ovaries but not overt hyperandrogenism. J Clin Endocrinol Metab 2006;91:3922–7.
51. Welt CK, Gudmundsson JA, Arason G, et al. Characterizing discrete subsets of polycystic ovary syndrome as defined by the Rotterdam criteria: the impact of weight on phenotype and metabolic features. J Clin Endocrinol Metab 2006;91:4842–8.
52. Barber TM, Wass JA, McCarthy MI, et al. Metabolic characteristics of women with polycystic ovaries and oligo-amenorrhoea but normal androgen

levels: implications for the management of polycystic ovary syndrome. Clin Endocrinol (Oxf) 2007;66:513–7.

53. Shroff R, Syrop CH, Davis W, et al. Risk of metabolic complications in the new PCOS phenotypes based on the Rotterdam criteria. Fertil Steril 2007;88:1389–95.

54. Sultan C, Paris F. Clinical expression of polycystic ovary syndrome in adolescent girls. Fertil Steril 2006;86(Suppl 1):S6.

55. Pasquali R, Gambineri A. Polycystic ovary syndrome: a multifaceted disease from adolescence to adult age. Ann N Y Acad Sci 2006;1092:158–74.

56. Chang JR, Coffler MS. Polycystic ovary syndrome: early detection in the adolescent. Clin Obstet Gynecol 2007;50:178–87.

57. Rosenfield RL. Clinical review: identifying children at risk for polycystic ovary syndrome. J Clin Endocrinol Metab 2007;92:787–96.

58. Avvad CK, Holeuwerger R, Silva VC, et al. Menstrual irregularity in the first postmenarchal years: an early clinical sign of polycystic ovary syndrome in adolescence. Gynecol Endocrinol 2001;15:170–7.

59. Apter D. Serum steroids and pituitary hormones in female puberty: a partly longitudinal study. Clin Endocrinol (Oxf) 1980;12:107–20.

60. Obhrai M, Lynch SS, Holder G, et al. Hormonal studies on women with polycystic ovaries diagnosed by ultrasound. Clin Endocrinol (Oxf) 1990;32:467–74.

61. Dramusic V, Rajan U, Chan P, et al. Adolescent polycystic ovary syndrome. Ann N Y Acad Sci 1997;816:194–208.

62. Dramusic V, Goh VH, Rajan U, et al. Clinical, endocrinologic, and ultrasonographic features of polycystic ovary syndrome in Singaporean adolescents. J Pediatr Adolesc Gynecol 1997;10:125–32.

63. Rachmiel M, Kives S, Atenafu E, et al. Primary amenorrhea as a manifestation of polycystic ovarian syndrome in adolescents: a unique subgroup? Arch Pediatr Adolesc Med 2008;162:521–5.

64. Ibanez L, Potau N, Francois I, et al. Precocious pubarche, hyperinsulinism, and ovarian hyperandrogenism in girls: relation to reduced fetal growth. J Clin Endocrinol Metab 1998;83:3558–62.

65. Hannon TS, Janosky J, Arslanian SA. Longitudinal study of physiologic insulin resistance and metabolic changes of puberty. Pediatr Res 2006;60:759–63.

66. Caprio S, Plewe G, Diamond MP, et al. Increased insulin secretion in puberty: a compensatory response to reductions in insulin sensitivity. J Pediatr 1989; 114:963–7.

67. Sir-Petermann T, Maliqueo M, Codner E, et al. Early metabolic derangements in daughters of women with polycystic ovary syndrome. J Clin Endocrinol Metab 2007;92:4637–42.

68. Biro FM, Emans SJ. Whither PCOS? The challenges of establishing hyperandrogenism in adolescent girls. J Adolesc Health 2008;43:103–5.

69. Lucky AW, Biro FM, Daniels SR, et al. The prevalence of upper lip hair in black and white girls during puberty: a new standard. J Pediatr 2001;138:134–6.

70. Slayden SM, Moran C, Sams WM, et al. Hyperandrogenemia in patients presenting with acne. Fertil Steril 2001;75:889–92.

71. Blank SK, Helm KD, McCartney CR, et al. Polycystic ovary syndrome in adolescence. Ann N Y Acad Sci 2008;1135:76–84.

72. Ankarberg C, Norjavaara E. Diurnal rhythm of testosterone secretion before and throughout puberty in healthy girls: correlation with 17beta-estradiol and dehydroepiandrosterone sulfate. J Clin Endocrinol Metab 1999;84:975–84.

73. Ehrmann DA, Rosenfield RL, Barnes RB, et al. Detection of functional ovarian hyperandrogenism in women with androgen excess. N Engl J Med 1992;327:157–62.

74. Barnes R, Rosenfield RL. The polycystic ovary syndrome: pathogenesis and treatment. Ann Intern Med 1989;110:386–99.
75. Stewart PM, Shackleton CH, Beastall GH, et al. 5 Alpha-reductase activity in polycystic ovary syndrome. Lancet 1990;335:431–3.
76. Venturoli S, Porcu E, Fabbri R, et al. Longitudinal evaluation of the different gonadotropin pulsatile patterns in anovulatory cycles of young girls. J Clin Endocrinol Metab 1992;74:836–41.
77. Azziz R, Carmina E, Dewailly D, et al. Positions statement: criteria for defining polycystic ovary syndrome as a predominantly hyperandrogenic syndrome: an Androgen Excess Society guideline. J Clin Endocrinol Metab 2006;91: 4237–45.
78. Moll GW Jr, Rosenfield RL. Plasma free testosterone in the diagnosis of adolescent polycystic ovary syndrome. J Pediatr 1983;102:461–4.
79. Zimmermann S, Phillips RA, Dunaif A, et al. Polycystic ovary syndrome: lack of hypertension despite profound insulin resistance. J Clin Endocrinol Metab 1992; 75:508–13.
80. Mortensen M, Rosenfield RL, Littlejohn E. Functional significance of polycystic-size ovaries in healthy adolescents. J Clin Endocrinol Metab 2006;91:3786–90.
81. Legro RS, Chiu P, Kunselman AR, et al. Polycystic ovaries are common in women with hyperandrogenic chronic anovulation but do not predict metabolic or reproductive phenotype. J Clin Endocrinol Metab 2005;90:2571–9.
82. Lachelin GC, Barnett M, Hopper BR, et al. Adrenal function in normal women and women with the polycystic ovary syndrome. J Clin Endocrinol Metab 1979;49:892–8.
83. Yoo RY, Sirlin CB, Gottschalk M, et al. Ovarian imaging by magnetic resonance in obese adolescent girls with polycystic ovary syndrome: a pilot study. Fertil Steril 2005;84:985–95.
84. Sun L, Fu Q. Three-dimensional transrectal ultrasonography in adolescent patients with polycystic ovarian syndrome. Int J Gynaecol Obstet 2007;98:34–8.
85. Azziz R, Hincapie LA, Knochenhauer ES, et al. Screening for 21-hydroxylase-deficient nonclassic adrenal hyperplasia among hyperandrogenic women: a prospective study. Fertil Steril 1999;72:915–25.
86. Azziz R, Wells G, Zacur HA, et al. Abnormalities of 21-hydroxylase gene ratio and adrenal steroidogenesis in hyperandrogenic women with an exaggerated 17-hydroxyprogesterone response to acute adrenal stimulation. J Clin Endocrinol Metab 1991;73:1327–31.
87. Ibanez L, Potau N, Zampolli M, et al. Hyperinsulinemia in postpubertal girls with a history of premature pubarche and functional ovarian hyperandrogenism. J Clin Endocrinol Metab 1996;81:1237–43.
88. Legro RS, Finegood D, Dunaif A. A fasting glucose to insulin ratio is a useful measure of insulin sensitivity in women with polycystic ovary syndrome. J Clin Endocrinol Metab 1998;83:2694–8.
89. Legro RS. Detection of insulin resistance and its treatment in adolescents with polycystic ovary syndrome. J Pediatr Endocrinol Metab 2002;15(Suppl 5): 1367–78.
90. Fruzzetti F, Perini D, Lazzarini V, et al. Adolescent girls with polycystic ovary syndrome showing different phenotypes have a different metabolic profile associated with increasing androgen levels. Fertil Steril 2008 Aug 13. [Epub ahead of print]
91. Kiddy DS, Hamilton-Fairley D, Bush A, et al. Improvement in endocrine and ovarian function during dietary treatment of obese women with polycystic ovary syndrome. Clin Endocrinol 1992;36:105–11.

92. Clark AM, Ledger W, Galletly C, et al. Weight loss results in significant improvement in pregnancy and ovulation rates in anovulatory obese women. Hum Reprod 1995;10:2705–12.

93. Holte J, Bergh T, Berne C, et al. Restored insulin sensitivity but persistently increased early insulin secretion after weight loss in obese women with polycystic ovary syndrome. J Clin Endocrinol Metab 1995;80:2586–93.

94. Clark AM, Thornley B, Tomlinson L, et al. Weight loss in obese infertile women results in improvement in reproductive outcome for all forms of fertility treatment. Hum Reprod 1998;13:1502–5.

95. Huber-Buchholz MM, Carey DGP, Norman RJ. Restoration of reproductive potential by lifestyle modification in obese polycystic ovary syndrome: role of insulin sensitivity and luteinizing hormone. J Clin Endocrinol Metab 1999;84:1470–4.

96. Crosignani PG, Colombo M, Vegetti W, et al. Overweight and obese anovulatory patients with polycystic ovaries: parallel improvements in anthropomorphic indices, ovarian physiology and fertility rate induced by diet. Hum Reprod 2003;18:1928–32.

97. Moran LJ, Noakes M, Clifton PM, et al. Dietary composition in restoring reproductive and metabolic physiology in overweight women with polycystic ovary syndrome. J Clin Endocrinol Metab 2003;88:812–9.

98. Pate RR, Pratt M, Blair SN, et al. Physical activity and public health. A recommendation from the Centers for Disease Control and Prevention and the American College of Sports Medicine. JAMA 1995;273:402–7.

99. Wadden TA, et al. Behavioral treatment of obesity. Med Clin North Am 2000;84:441–61.

100. National Institutes of Health. Clinical guidelines on the identification, evaluation, and treatment of overweight and obesity in adults—the evidence report. Obes Res 1998;6(Suppl 2):51S–209S.

101. Foster GD, Wyatt HR, Hill JO, et al. A randomized trial of a low-carbohydrate diet for obesity. N Engl J Med 2003;348:2082–90.

102. Dansinger ML, Gleason JA, Griffith JL, et al. Comparison of the Atkins, Ornish, Weight Watchers, and Zone diets for weight loss and heart disease risk reduction. JAMA 2005;293:43–53.

103. Bray GA. Uses and misuses of the new pharmacotherapy of obesity. Ann Med 1999;31(1):1–3.

104. Trus TL, Pope GD, Finlayson SRG. National trends in utilization and outcomes of bariatric surgery. Surg Endosc 2005;19:616–20.

105. National Institutes of Health Consensus Development Panel. Gastrointestinal surgery for severe obesity. Ann Intern Med 1991;115:956–61.

106. Buchwald H, Avidor Y, Braunwald E, et al. Bariatric surgery a systematic review and meta-analysis. JAMA 2004;292:1724–37.

107. Maggard MA, Shugarman LR, Suttorp M, et al. Meta-analysis: surgical treatment of obesity. Ann Intern Med 2005;142:547–59.

108. Deitel M, Stone E, Kassam HA, et al. Gynecologic-obstetric changes after loss of massive excess weight following bariatric surgery. J Am Coll Nutr 1988;7:147–53.

109. Sugerman HJ, Sugerman EL, DeMaria EJ, et al. Bariatric surgery for severely obese adolescents. J Gastrointest Surg 2003;7:102–8.

110. Nadler EP, Youn HA, Ren CJ, et al. An update on 73 US obese pediatric patients treated with laparoscopic adjustable gastric banding: comorbidity resolution and compliance data. J Pediatr Surg 2008;43:141–6.

111. Sheiner E, et al. Pregnancy after bariatric surgery is not associated with adverse perinatal outcome. Am J Obstet Gynecol 2004;190:1335–40.

112. Printen KJ, Scott D, et al. Pregnancy following gastric bypass for the treatment of morbid obesity. Am Surg 1982;48:363–5.
113. Marceau P, Kaufman D, Biron S, et al. Outcome of pregnancies after bilio-pancreatic diversion. Obes Surg 2004;14:318–24.
114. Korytkowski MT, Mokan M, Horwitz MJ, et al. Metabolic effects of oral contraceptives in women with polycystic ovary syndrome. J Clin Endocrinol Metab 1995;80:3327–34.
115. Jung-Hoffmann C, Kuhl H. Divergent effects of two low-dose oral contraceptives on sex hormone-binding globulin and free testosterone. Am J Obstet Gynecol 1987;156:199–203.
116. Mastorakos G, Koliopoulos C, Deligeoroglou E, et al. Effects of two forms of combined oral contraceptives on carbohydrate metabolism in adolescents with polycystic ovary syndrome. Fertil Steril 2006;85:420–7.
117. Burkman RT. The role of oral contraceptives in the treatment of hyperandrogenic disorders. Am J Med 1995;98(1A):130S–6S.
118. Thorneycroft IH, Stanczyk FZ, Bradshaw KD, et al. Effect of low-dose oral contraceptives on androgenic markers and acne. Contraception 1999;60:255–62.
119. Moghetti P, Tosi F, Tosti A, et al. Comparison of spironolactone, flutamide, and finasteride efficacy in the treatment of hirsutism: a randomized double blind, placebo-controlled trial. J Clin Endocrinol Metab 2000;85:89–94.
120. Ibanez L, Potau N, Marcos MV, et al. Treatment of hirsutism, hyperandrogenism, oligomenorrhea, dyslipidemia, and hyperinsulinism in nonobese, adolescent girls: effect of flutamide. J Clin Endocrinol Metab 2000;85(9):3251–5.
121. Cusan L, Dupont A, Gomex J, et al. Comparison of flutamide and spironolactone n the treatment of hirsutism: a randomized controlled trial. Fertil Steril 1994;61:281–7.
122. Tartagni M, Schonauer LM, De Salvia MA, et al. Comparison of Diane 35 and Diane 35 plus finasteride in the treatment of hirsutism. Fertil Steril 2000;73:718–23.
123. Heiner JS, Greendale GA, Kawakami AK, et al. Comparison of a gonadotropin-releasing hormone agonist and a low dose oral contraceptive given alone or together in the treatment of hirsutism. J Clin Endocrinol Metab 1995;80: 3412–8.
124. Ettinger B, Selby J, Citron JT, et al. Cyclic hormone replacement therapy using quarterly progestin. Obstet Gynecol 1994;83:693–700.
125. Inzucchi SE, Maggs DG, Spollett GR, et al. Efficacy and metabolic effects of metformin and troglitazone in type II diabetes mellitus. N Engl J Med 1998; 338(13):867–72.
126. Sattar N, Hopkinson ZE, Greer IA. Insulin-sensitizing agents in polycystic ovary syndrome. Lancet 1998;351:305–7.
127. Moghetti P, Castello R, Negri C, et al. Metformin effects on clinical features, endocrine and metabolic profiles, and insulin sensitivity in polycystic ovary syndrome: a randomized, double-blind, placebo-controlled 6-month trial, followed by open, long-term clinical evaluation. J Clin Endocrinol Metab 2000; 85:139–46.
128. Fleming R, Hopkinson ZE, Wallace AM, et al. Ovarian function and metabolic factors in women with oligomenorrhea treated with metformin in a randomized double blind placebo controlled trial. J Clin Endocrinol Metab 2002;87:569–74.
129. Lord JM, Flight IH, Norman RJ. Metformin in polycystic ovary syndrome: systematic review and meta-analysis. BMJ 2003;327:951–3.
130. Diamanti-Kandarakis E, Kouli C, Tsianateli T, et al. Therapeutic effects of metformin on insulin resistance and hyperandrogenism in polycystic ovary syndrome. Eur J Endocrinol 1998;138(3):269–74.

131. Morin-Papunen LC, Koivunen RM, Roukonen A, et al. Metformin therapy improves the menstrual pattern with minimal endocrine and metabolic effects in women with polycystic ovary syndrome. Fertil Steril 1998;69:691–6.
132. Pasquali R, Gambineri A, Biscotti D, et al. Effect of long-term treatment with metformin added to hypocaloric diet on body composition, fat distribution and androgen and insulin levels in abdominally obese women with and without the polycystic ovary syndrome. J Clin Endocrinol Metab 2000;85(8):2767–74.
133. Glueck CJ, Wang P, Fontaine R, et al. Metformin to restore normal menses in oligo-amenorrheic teenage girls with polycystic ovary syndrome (PCOS). J Adolesc Health 2001;29:160–9.
134. Costello MF, Eden JA. A systematic review of the reproductive system effects of metformin in patients with polycystic ovary syndrome. Fertil Steril 2003;79:1–13.
135. Ibanez L, Valls C, Potau N, et al. Sensitization to insulin in adolescent girls to normalize hirsutism, hyperandrogenism, oligomenorrhea, dyslipidemia, and hyperinsulinism after precocious pubarche. J Clin Endocrinol Metab 2000;85: 3526–30.
136. Ibanez L, Valls C, Ferrer A, et al. Sensitization to insulin induces ovulation in non-obese adolescents with anovulatory hyperandrogenism. J Clin Endocrinol Metab 2001;86:3595–8.
137. Bridger T, MacDonald S, Baltzer F, et al. Randomized placebo-controlled trial of metformin for adolescents with polycystic ovary syndrome. Arch Pediatr Adolesc Med 2006;160:241–6.
138. Hoeger K, Davidson K, Kochman L, et al. The impact of metformin, oral contraceptives and lifestyle modification on polycystic ovary syndrome in obese adolescent women in two randomized, placebo-controlled clinical trials. J Clin Endocrinol Metab 2008;93:4299–306 [Epub 2008 Aug 26].
139. Stein IF, Leventhal ML. Amenorrhea associated with bilateral polycystic ovaries. Am J Obstet Gynecol 1935;29:181–91.
140. Seow K, Juan C, Hwang J, et al. Laparoscopic surgery in polycystic ovary syndrome: reproductive and metabolic effects. Semin Reprod Med 2008;26: 101–10.
141. Armar NA, McGarrigle HH, Honour J, et al. Laparoscopic ovarian diathermy in the management of anovulatory infertility in women with polycystic ovaries: endocrine changes and clinical outcome. Fertil Steril 1990;53:45–9.

Bleeding Disorders in Adolescents

Andra H. James, MD, MPH

KEYWORDS

- Menorrhagia • Adolescent • Bleeding disorder
- Von Willebrand disease • Hemorrhagic ovarian cyst

Normal hemostasis requires a normal number of platelets, normal platelet function, normal collagen in the subendothelium, and normal levels of clotting factors. Abnormal bleeding can result from thrombocytopenia; disorders of platelet function; abnormal collagen (eg, Ehlers-Danlos syndrome); and clotting factor deficiencies, including deficiency of von Willebrand factor (VWF), which is required to adhere platelets to exposed subendothelium and protect factor VIII from proteolysis in the circulation.

Bleeding disorders may be inherited or acquired. Disorders of platelet function are probably more common than von Willebrand disease (VWD), but VWD is the most common inherited bleeding disorder. VWD results from a deficiency of VWF (type 1), abnormal VWF (type 2), or absence of VWF (type 3). Based on studies of individuals with bleeding symptoms, a family history of bleeding, and low levels of VWF, VWD affects as many as 1 in 100 individuals.[1] Based on the numbers of individuals enrolled at hemophilia treatment centers, however, VWD affects only 1 in 10,000 individuals.[1] Nonetheless, there are probably many people who have mild type 1 VWD and other mild bleeding disorders who have never been diagnosed. In general, mild bleeding disorders are common, and severe bleeding disorders (eg, type 3 VWD) are rare, affecting as few as 1 in 10,000 to 1 in 1 million people.[2]

Signs and symptoms of VWD and other bleeding disorders include the following:

- Prolonged bleeding from wounds
- Heavy, prolonged, or recurrent bleeding after surgery
- Bruising with minimal or no trauma, especially bruising resulting in a lump
- Nosebleeds that last more than 10 minutes or require medical attention to stop
- Heavy, prolonged, or recurrent bleeding after dental procedures or tooth extraction
- Unexplained bleeding from the gastrointestinal tract
- Anemia requiring iron therapy or transfusion
- Heavy menstrual bleeding or menorrhagia

Division of Maternal-Fetal Medicine, Department of Obstetrics and Gynecology, Duke University Medical Center, Box 3967, Durham, NC 27710, USA
E-mail address: andra.james@duke.edu

Obstet Gynecol Clin N Am 36 (2009) 153–162
doi:10.1016/j.ogc.2008.12.002
0889-8545/08/$ – see front matter © 2009 Elsevier Inc. All rights reserved.

MENORRHAGIA

Heavy menstrual bleeding, or menorrhagia, is the most common symptom that women who have bleeding disorders experience. Most data about the prevalence of menorrhagia in women who have bleeding disorders comes from reports of women who have VWD. The prevalence of menorrhagia in these reports ranges from 32% to 100%.[3] In a survey of 102 women who had VWD compared with controls conducted by the US Centers for Disease Control and Prevention (CDC), 95% of the women who had VWD reported a history of menorrhagia compared with 61% of controls.[4] Sramek and colleagues[5] found that women who had VWD were five times more likely to experience menorrhagia than women who did not have the condition. With respect to the prevalence of menorrhagia in women who have other bleeding disorders, the prevalence in women who have severe platelet dysfunction has been reported to be 51% in women who have Bernard-Soulier syndrome[6] and 98% in women who have Glanzmann's thrombasthenia;[7] the prevalence in women who have factor XI deficiency, an inherited bleeding disorder of varying severity, has been reported to be 59%;[8] the prevalence in hemophilia carriers, who have variably reduced levels of factor VIII or factor IX, has been reported to be 10% to 57%;[9–12] and the prevalence in women with rare factor deficiencies has been reported to be 35% to 70%.[13–16]

Not only is menorrhagia more prevalent among women who have bleeding disorders but bleeding disorders are more prevalent among women who have menorrhagia. Among women who have menorrhagia, the prevalence of VWD has been reported to be 5% to 20%;[17] the prevalence of platelet dysfunction, depending on how it its defined, has been reported to be less than 1% to 47%;[3] the prevalence of factor XI deficiency has been reported to be less than 1% to 4%;[3] the prevalence of hemophilia carriage has been reported to be less than 1% to 4%;[3] and the prevalence of rare factor deficiencies has been reported to be less than 1%.[3]

There are limited data regarding the prevalence of bleeding disorders among adolescents who have menorrhagia, but they are at least as likely to have an underlying bleeding disorder as adult women with heavy menstrual bleeding. Among adolescents who have menorrhagia, the prevalence of VWD has been reported to be 5% to 36%; the prevalence of platelet dysfunction, depending on how it is defined, has been reported to be 2% to 44%; the prevalence of clotting factor deficiency has been reported to be 8%;[18] and the prevalence of thrombocytopenia has been reported to be 13% to 20% (**Table 1**).

Recently, the American College of Obstetrics and Gynecology[19] Committee on Adolescent Health Care and the American Academy of Pediatrics Committee on Adolescence came to a consensus on what constitutes normal menstruation in girls and adolescents. Their report was issued in the form of a committee opinion published by the American College of Obstetricians and Gynecologists in November of 2006. The title of the document was "Menstruation in Girls and Adolescents: Using the Menstrual Cycle as a Vital Sign." The committee agreed that normal menstruation begins at 11 to 14 years of age, the normal cycle length is 21 to 45 days, the length of the period is 7 days or less, and product use is no more than three to six pads or tampons per day.

Menorrhagia is defined as heavy menstrual bleeding that lasts for more than 7 days[20] or results in the loss of more than 80 mL of blood per menstrual cycle.[20] The clinical definition of 80 mL or more was formulated after a study by Hallberg and colleagues[21,22] found that the 95th percentile of blood loss per menstrual cycle among 183 normal women was 76 mL and that the prevalence of impaired iron status was higher among women with blood loss of more than 60 mL. These investigators concluded that that the upper limit of normal menstrual blood loss was between 60

Table 1
Bleeding disorders associated with menorrhagia in adolescents

	N	Site	% VWD	% Platelet Dysfxn	% Low Factor	% LowPlatelets
Claessens and Cowell, 1981[54]	59	Inpatient	5	2	—	—
Smith et al, 1998[55]	46	Inpatient	11	—	—	—
Oral et al, 2002[56]	25	Inpatient	8	—	—	20
Bevan et al, 2001[57]	71	ED, inpatient	8	3	—	13
Philipp et al, 2005[18]	25	Outpatient	4	44	8	—
Jayasinghe et al, 2005[58]	106	Inpatient, outpatient	5	6	—	—
Mikhail et al, 2007[59]	61	HTC	36	7	—	—

Abbreviations: ED, Emergency department; HTC, Hemophilia treatment center; Plt Dysfxn, Platelet dysfunction.

and 80 mL.[21] Subsequently, the upper limit of 80 mL per cycle has been adopted as the threshold for menorrhagia.[23]

Because measuring actual menstrual blood loss is unfeasible in clinical practice, Higham and colleagues[24] devised a pictorial blood assessment chart (PBAC) as an alternative. In their original study, women compared the degree of saturation of their pads and tampons with those depicted on a chart. Lightly stained pads or tampons obtained a score of 1, moderately stained pads or tampons obtained a score of 5, and soaked pads or tampons obtained a score of 20. The scores were summed, and a total score of greater than 100 per cycle was associated with menstrual blood loss of greater than 80 mL. A drawback of the use of the chart is that it must be completed prospectively and results are not available at the time of an initial evaluation. Additionally, the validity of the chart remains uncertain.[25,26]

Therefore, the practitioner must rely on a menstrual history and clinical impression. Warner and colleagues[27] attempted to assess the volume of blood loss by means of specific clinical features. In a logistic regression model, the variables that predicted menstrual blood loss of more than 80 mL were clots greater than a 50-pence coin in size (approximately 1 inch in diameter), low ferritin (according to the investigators' laboratory reference), or changing a pad or tampon more than hourly (flooding). The presence of these features may help the practitioner to determine which adolescents truly have heavy menstrual bleeding.

SCREENING FOR BLEEDING DISORDERS IN ADOLESCENTS WHO HAVE MENORRHAGIA

Philipp and colleagues[28] studied strategies for screening women with menorrhagia for an underlying bleeding disorder. A woman's bleeding history (the "screening tool") was considered positive if (1) her duration of menses was greater than or equal to 7 days and she experienced flooding or impairment of daily activities with most periods; (2) she had a history of treatment for anemia; (3) she had a family history of a diagnosed bleeding disorder; or (4) she had a history of excessive bleeding with tooth extraction, delivery, miscarriage, or surgery. A positive bleeding history alone had a sensitivity for detecting any bleeding disorder (including VWD, platelet function defect, or clotting factor deficiency) of 82%. The negative predictive value was 93% for VWD, 45% for platelet function defect, and 38% for any bleeding disorder. Sensitivity increased to

84% by the addition of the results of platelet function assessment, using an automated platelet function analyzer, to 94% by the addition of a PBAC score of greater than 100, and to 95% by the addition of both.

Based on these data, an evaluation for an underlying bleeding disorder should be considered if an adolescent has a positive bleeding history as described by Philipp and colleagues.[28] Conversely, if an adolescent has a negative bleeding history as described by Philipp and colleagues,[28] VWD or a serious bleeding disorder is unlikely. The patient who is suspected of having a bleeding disorder can be referred to a hemophilia treatment center or hematologist with expertise in bleeding disorders before or after an initial laboratory evaluation. The initial laboratory evaluation should include a complete blood cell count to assess the hemoglobin level and to exclude thrombocytopenia and a prothrombin time, activated partial thromboplastin time (aPTT), and fibrinogen or thrombin clot time to exclude a clotting factor deficiency. Although these tests are useful for excluding clotting factor deficiencies, the aPTT should be normal in patients with platelet dysfunction and may be normal in patients who have VWD. The next series of tests includes specific tests for VWD. If VWD is excluded, other categories of bleeding disorders that should be considered are platelet function defects; abnormalities of fibrinolysis; and, rarely, collagen defects, such as Ehlers-Danlos syndrome.

HEMORRHAGIC OVARIAN CYSTS

Although menorrhagia is the most common manifestation of reproductive tract bleeding that women who have bleeding disorders experience, it is not the only manifestation. In the same survey of 102 women who had VWD compared with controls conducted by the CDC, the next most common reproductive tract abnormality that women who had VWD reported, after menorrhagia, was a history of ovarian cysts (52% among cases compared with 22% among controls). Although ovulation is not normally accompanied by any significant amount of bleeding, in women who have VWD or other bleeding disorders, ovulation can result in bleeding into the follicular sac, the peritoneum, the broad ligament, and the retroperitoneum. In a case series of patients who had VWD, Silwer[29] found the incidence of hemorrhagic ovarian cysts in women to be 6.8%. Hemorrhagic ovarian cysts have also been reported in women who have hemophilia carriage, afibrinogenemia, factor X deficiency, factor XIII deficiency, and platelet defects.[3] Acutely, surgical therapy, tranexamic acid, and factor replacement have been used to manage hemorrhagic ovarian cysts.[11,30,31] Oral contraceptives, which suppress ovulation and may increase clotting factors, have been used to prevent recurrences.[31–33]

ENDOMETRIOSIS

In the same CDC survey, 30% of women who had VWD reported a history of endometriosis compared with 13% of controls.[4] There are several possible reasons why women who have VWD and other bleeding disorders would be more likely to be diagnosed with endometriosis. Although there is disagreement regarding the etiology of endometriosis, the prevailing theory is that it results from retrograde menstruation.[34] Heavy menstrual bleeding is a risk factor for retrograde menstruation and endometriosis.[35] Women who have bleeding disorders have heavier menstrual bleeding, more retrograde menstruation, and, possibly, more endometriosis. Another possible explanation is that women who have bleeding disorders are more likely to experience symptomatic bleeding from extrauterine endometrial implants. A third possibility is that women who have bleeding disorders are more likely to experience hemorrhagic ovarian cysts or intraperitoneal bleeding that is misdiagnosed as endometriosis.

GYNECOLOGIC MANAGEMENT OF MENORRHAGIA IN ADOLESCENTS WHO HAVE BLEEDING DISORDERS

There are data regarding the management of menorrhagia in women and adolescents who have bleeding disorders. Oral contraceptives reduce menstrual blood loss[36] in women with VWD, and possibly increase VWF and factor VIII levels.[37–39] The levonorgestrel intrauterine device (IUD) is effective at reducing menstrual blood loss.[40] Kingman and colleagues[40] reported a significant decrease in PBAC scores and a significant increase in hemoglobin concentration (g/dL) in 16 women who had bleeding disorders after the insertion of the levonorgestrel IUD. There are unpublished reports of the levonorgestrel IUD being used successfully in adolescents who have bleeding disorders to reduce menstrual blood loss. Although there are no accumulated data in women who have bleeding disorders regarding the use of other hormonal therapies, there is no reason to believe that other combined hormonal contraceptives, such as patches and rings, would not also be useful.

The extended-use and continuous-use oral contraceptives offer an additional possibility of reducing menstrual blood loss. Edelman and colleagues randomized subjects to receive levonorgestrel (100 µg)/ethinyl estradiol (20 µg), levonorgestrel (100 µg)/ethinyl estradiol (30 µg), norethindrone acetate (1000 µg)/ethinyl estradiol (20 µg), or norethindrone acetate (1000 µg)/ethinyl (30 µg) continuously for 180 days. Subjects who received formulations with norethindrone, 1000 µg, experienced less bleeding than subjects who received formulations with levonorgestrel, 100 µg. Additional ethinyl estradiol (10 µg) did not improve bleeding patterns, suggesting that a formulation with norethindrone acetate (1000 µg)/ethinyl estradiol (20 µg) would be preferred in a continuous regimen.[41]

Other progestin-only contraceptives, such as medroxyprogesterone acetate injections, progestin-only pills, and the progestin implant should also reduce endometrial proliferation and reduce menstrual blood loss. Medroxyprogesterone acetate is now available in a subcutaneous formulation, providing an alternative to the intramuscular formulation that might result in intramuscular bleeding in a patient who has a severe bleeding disorder. Insertion of the progestin implant could cause bleeding in a patient who has a severe bleeding disorder and might require pretreatment with a hemostatic agent.

HEMOSTATIC MANAGEMENT OF MENORRHAGIA IN ADOLESCENTS WHO HAVE BLEEDING DISORDERS

Adolescents who have had a proper gynecologic evaluation and fail hormonal management should be referred for consideration of hemostatic therapies, which have been reported to be effective in controlling menorrhagia in women and adolescents with bleeding disorders. These hemostatic therapies include 1-desamino-8-D-arginine vasopressin (DDAVP), antifibrinolytic medications (aminocaproic acid and tranexamic acid), and clotting factor concentrates.

DDAVP is a synthetic vasopressin that stimulates the release of VWF from endothelial cells. DDAVP is useful in the treatment of type 1 VWD, some cases of type 2 VWD, and some cases of platelet dysfunction and can be administered intranasally or intravenously. DDAVP causes some water retention and can reduce sodium levels. For this reason, and also because DDAVP relies on the release of stored VWF, DDAVP use should be limited to 48 hours. In a retrospective study, Amesse and colleagues[42] found that intranasal DDAVP was no more effective than oral contraceptives in controlling menorrhagia but was associated with severe headaches and flushing.

Aminocaproic acid and tranexamic acid inhibit fibrinolysis. The use of aminocaproic acid is limited by its gastrointestinal side effects. Tranexamic acid is better tolerated but is not currently available in the United States, although it is expected to be reintroduced in the next few years.

A recent multisite, prospective, crossover study demonstrated that DDAVP and tranexamic acid reduce menstrual blood flow in women who have bleeding disorders. Inclusion criteria were heavy menstrual bleeding and a PBAC score of greater than 100 with a negative gynecologic evaluation and abnormal laboratory hemostasis. The investigators enrolled 117 women aged 18 to 50 years: 62% had platelet dysfunction, 15% had VWD, and 23% had some other coagulation defect. Subjects were randomly assigned to DDAVP or tranexamic acid for two menstrual cycles, followed by crossover to the second study drug for an additional two cycles. The PBAC score and quality-of-life instruments were used to assess outcomes. With DDAVP, there was a decrease in the PBAC score from a baseline of −66.0, and with tranexamic acid, there was a decrease in the PBAC score from a baseline of −107.8. This difference of 41.8 was statistically significant, although both treatments improved quality of life.[43]

Clotting factor concentrates may be required at the time of surgery, peripartum, at the time of serious injury, and in episodes of severe acute bleeding (eg, severe acute menorrhagia). VWD can be treated with VWF concentrates, hemophilia carriers can be treated with recombinant factor VIII and factor IX products, and other factor deficiencies may be treated with fresh-frozen plasma or cryoprecipitate. Whenever possible, clotting factor concentrates, which are purified and carry an extremely low risk for viral transmission, should be administered as opposed to fresh-frozen plasma or cryoprecipitate, neither of which is purified. In Europe, there are specific clotting factor concentrates for fibrinogen, factor XI, and factor XIII deficiency, but these products are not available in the United States.

MANAGEMENT OF ACUTE SEVERE MENORRHAGIA

In the management of acute severe menorrhagia, every effort is made to preserve future fertility. In addition to clotting factor concentrates and intravenous antifibrinolytic medication, recombinant factor VIIa can be tried and has been used successfully in two cases of Bernard Soulier syndrome.[44] Platelet transfusions have been used in cases of severe thrombocytopenia.[45] Additionally, a single intravenous 25-mg dose of conjugated equine estrogen has been shown to be effective in the treatment of acute menorrhagia.[46] In women whose bleeding has not stopped within 3 hours, a second dose may be administered.[46] The duration of the effect of this treatment in healthy women is unknown, but in patients with renal failure, the effect lasted 2 to 3 weeks.[47] Although there have been no randomized trials, oral conjugated equine estrogen has been used successfully.[48] Treatment with conjugated equine estrogen is followed by treatment with progestins or combined oral contraceptives. Leuprolide acetate has been used to induce amenorrhea in patients at risk for severe acute menorrhagia attributable to thrombocytopenia.[49,50]

Surgical therapies have also been used to treat acute severe menorrhagia. Dilation and curettage (D & C), although occasionally necessary to diagnose intrauterine pathologic findings, is not particularly effective in controlling heavy menstrual bleeding in women who have bleeding disorders. In two cases of women who had VWD reported by Greer and colleagues[11] and two cases reported by Kadir and colleagues,[9] D & C resulted in further blood loss. In the absence of significant endometrial proliferation, D & C should be avoided.

Nonhormonal gynecologic therapies have been used successfully to control acute severe menorrhagia in adolescents. Rouhani and colleagues[51] reported using a Foley balloon to tamponade the endometrial cavity of a 12-year-old female patient with plasminogen activator inhibitor during her second menstrual period; Bowkley and colleagues[52] reported using uterine artery embolization with plasminogen activator inhibitor in a 12-year-old female patient during her first menstrual period; and Markovitch and collegues[53] reported packing the uterus of a 14-year-old female patient who had Glanzmann's thrombasthenia during her second menstrual period.

GENERAL ISSUES

Girls and adolescents with known bleeding disorders should be counseled before menarche and have a plan in place for the possibility of acute severe menorrhagia, which could occur with their first or any subsequent menstrual period. The plan should be made by the patient's gynecologist and hematologist in conjunction with the patient's family. Because of the increased risk of transfusion, girls and adolescents who have not already been immunized against hepatitis A and hepatitis B should be immunized. If they have not already done so, adolescents who have inherited bleeding disorders and their families should have the opportunity to speak with a knowledgeable genetic counselor.

SUMMARY

Adolescents who have bleeding disorders come to the attention of the gynecologist when menarche is anticipated or they develop reproductive tract bleeding. Menorrhagia is the most common symptom that adolescents who have bleeding disorders experience. Not only is menorrhagia more prevalent among adolescents who have bleeding disorders but bleeding disorders are more prevalent among adolescents who have menorrhagia. Adolescents who have bleeding disorders are probably also at an increased risk for hemorrhagic ovarian cysts and endometriosis. The patient who is suspected of having a bleeding disorder can be referred to a hemophilia treatment center or hematologist with expertise in bleeding disorders for evaluation. Adolescents and their parents need to understand and accept that hormonal contraception is the first-line treatment for menorrhagia. Adolescents who have a bleeding disorder, have had a proper gynecologic evaluation, and fail hormonal management should be considered for possible hemostatic therapy. Successful management of reproductive tract bleeding in adolescents requires the combined expertise of knowledgeable hematologists and gynecologists.

REFERENCES

1. Nichols W, Hultin M, James A, et al. The diagnosis, evaluation and management of von Willebrand disease. Bethesda (MD): National Heart Lung and Blood Institute, National Institutes of Health; 2007.
2. Roberts H, Escobar M. Other clotting factor deficiencies. In: Hoffman R, editor. Hematology: basic principles and practice. 4th edition. 3rd edition. New York: Churchill Livingstone; 2005.
3. James AH. More than menorrhagia: a review of the obstetric and gynaecological manifestations of bleeding disorders. Haemophilia 2005;11(4):295–307.

4. Kirtava A, Drews C, Lally C, et al. Medical, reproductive and psychosocial experiences of women diagnosed with von Willebrand's disease receiving care in haemophilia treatment centres: a case-control study. Haemophilia 2003;9(3):292–7.

5. Sramek A, Eikenboom JC, Briet E, et al. Usefulness of patient interview in bleeding disorders. Arch Intern Med 1995;155(13):1409–15.

6. Lopez JA, Andrews RK, Afshar-Kharghan V, et al. Bernard-Soulier syndrome. Blood 1998;91(12):4397–418.

7. George JN, Caen JP, Nurden AT. Glanzmann's thrombasthenia: the spectrum of clinical disease. Blood 1990;75(7):1383–95.

8. Kadir RA, Economides DL, Lee CA. Factor XI deficiency in women. Am J Hematol 1999;60(1):48–54.

9. Kadir RA, Economides DL, Sabin CA, et al. Assessment of menstrual blood loss and gynaecological problems in patients with inherited bleeding disorders. Haemophilia 1999;5(1):40–8.

10. Mauser Bunschoten EP, van Houwelingen JC, Sjamsoedin Visser EJ, et al. Bleeding symptoms in carriers of hemophilia A and B. Thromb Haemost 1988; 59(3):349–52.

11. Greer IA, Lowe GD, Walker JJ, et al. Haemorrhagic problems in obstetrics and gynaecology in patients with congenital coagulopathies. Br J Obstet Gynaecol 1991;98(9):909–18.

12. Yang J, Hartmann KE, Savitz DA, et al. Vaginal bleeding during pregnancy and preterm birth. Am J Epidemiol 2004;160(2):118–25.

13. Burrows RF, Ray JG, Burrows EA. Bleeding risk and reproductive capacity among patients with factor XIII deficiency: a case presentation and review of the literature. Obstet Gynecol Surv 2000;55(2):103–8.

14. Lak M, Keihani M, Elahi F, et al. Bleeding and thrombosis in 55 patients with inherited afibrinogenaemia. Br J Haematol 1999;107(1):204–6.

15. Lak M, Peyvandi F, Ali Sharifian A, et al. Pattern of symptoms in 93 Iranian patients with severe factor XIII deficiency. J Thromb Haemost 2003;1(8):1852–3.

16. Shetty S, Madkaikar M, Nair S, et al. Combined factor V and VIII deficiency in Indian population. Haemophilia 2000;6(5):504–7.

17. James A, Matchar DB, Myers ER. Testing for von Willebrand disease in women with menorrhagia: a systematic review. Obstet Gynecol 2004;104(2):381–8.

18. Philipp CS, Faiz A, Dowling N, et al. Age and the prevalence of bleeding disorders in women with menorrhagia. Obstet Gynecol 2005;105(1):61–6.

19. ACOG. Menstruation in girls and adolescents: using the menstrual cycle as a vital sign. Washington, DC: American College of Obstetricians and Gynecologists; 2006.

20. ACOG. Management of anovulatory bleeding. Washington, DC: American College of Obstetricians and Gynecologists; 2000.

21. Hallberg L, Hogdahl AM, Nilsson L, et al. Menstrual blood loss—a population study. Variation at different ages and attempts to define normality. Acta Obstet Gynecol Scand 1966;45(3):320–51.

22. Hallberg L, Hogdahl AM, Nilsson L, et al. Menstrual blood loss and iron deficiency. Acta Med Scand 1966;180(5):639–50.

23. Warner PE, Critchley HO, Lumsden MA, et al. Menorrhagia II: is the 80-mL blood loss criterion useful in management of complaint of menorrhagia? Am J Obstet Gynecol 2004;190(5):1224–9.

24. Higham JM, O'Brien PM, Shaw RW. Assessment of menstrual blood loss using a pictorial chart. Br J Obstet Gynaecol 1990;97(8):734–9.

25. Janssen CA, Scholten PC, Heintz AP. A simple visual assessment technique to discriminate between menorrhagia and normal menstrual blood loss. Obstet Gynecol 1995;85(6):977–82.
26. Reid PC, Coker A, Coltart R. Assessment of menstrual blood loss using a pictorial chart: a validation study. BJOG 2000;107(3):320–2.
27. Warner PE, Critchley HO, Lumsden MA, et al. Menorrhagia I: measured blood loss, clinical features, and outcome in women with heavy periods: a survey with follow-up data. Am J Obstet Gynecol 2004;190(5):1216–23.
28. Philipp CS, Faiz A, Dowling NF, et al. Development of a screening tool for identifying women with menorrhagia for hemostatic evaluation. Am J Obstet Gynecol 2008;198(2):163 e161–8.
29. Silwer J. von Willebrand's disease in Sweden. Acta Paediatr Scand Suppl 1973; 238:1–159.
30. Gomez A, Lucia JF, Perella M, et al. Haemoperitoneum caused by haemorrhagic corpus luteum in a patient with type 3 von Willebrand's disease. Haemophilia 1998;4(1):60–2.
31. Jarvis RR, Olsen ME. Type I von Willebrand's disease presenting as recurrent corpus hemorrhagicum. Obstet Gynecol 2002;99(5 Pt 2):887–8.
32. Ghosh K, Mohanty D, Pathare AV, et al. Recurrent haemoperitoneum in a female patient with type III von Willebrand's disease responded to administration of oral contraceptive. Haemophilia 1998;4(5):767–8.
33. Bottini E, Pareti FI, Mari D, et al. Prevention of hemoperitoneum during ovulation by oral contraceptives in women with type III von Willebrand disease and afibrinogenemia. Case reports. Haematologica 1991;76(5):431–3.
34. Lobo RA. Endometriosis: etiology, pathology, diagnosis, management. In: Katz V, Lentz G, Lobo R, et al, editors. Katz: comprehensive gynecology. 5th edition. Philadelphia: Mosby; 2007. p. 473–95.
35. Vercellini P, De Giorgi O, Aimi G, et al. Menstrual characteristics in women with and without endometriosis. Obstet Gynecol 1997;90(2):264–8.
36. Foster PA. The reproductive health of women with von Willebrand disease unresponsive to DDAVP: results of an international survey. On behalf of the Subcommittee on von Willebrand Factor of the Scientific and Standardization Committee of the ISTH. Thromb Haemost 1995;74(2):784–90.
37. Beller FK, Ebert C. Effects of oral contraceptives on blood coagulation. A review. Obstet Gynecol Surv 1985;40(7):425–36.
38. Kadir RA, Economides DL, Sabin CA, et al. Variations in coagulation factors in women: effects of age, ethnicity, menstrual cycle and combined oral contraceptive. Thromb Haemost 1999;82(5):1456–61.
39. Middeldorp S, Meijers JC, van den Ende AE, et al. Effects on coagulation of levonorgestrel- and desogestrel-containing low dose oral contraceptives: a crossover study. Thromb Haemost 2000;84(1):4–8.
40. Kingman CE, Kadir RA, Lee CA, et al. The use of levonorgestrel-releasing intrauterine system for treatment of menorrhagia in women with inherited bleeding disorders. BJOG 2004;111(12):1425–8.
41. Edelman AB, Koontz SL, Nichols MD, et al. Continuous oral contraceptives: are bleeding patterns dependent on the hormones given? Obstet Gynecol 2006; 107(3):657–65.
42. Amesse LS, Pfaff-Amesse T, Leonardi R, et al. Oral contraceptives and DDAVP nasal spray: patterns of use in managing vWD-associated menorrhagia: a single-institution study. J Pediatr Hematol Oncol 2005;27(7):357–63.

43. Kouides PA, Heit JA, Philipp CS, et al. A multi-site, prospective, cross-over study of intranasal desmopressin and oral tranexamic acid in women with menorrhagia and abnormal laboratory hemostasis. Blood 2007;110:711 [ASH Annual Meeting Abstracts].

44. Ozelo MC, Svirin P, Larina L. Use of recombinant factor VIIa in the management of severe bleeding episodes in patients with Bernard-Soulier syndrome. Ann Hematol 2005;84(12):816–22.

45. Levens ED, Scheinberg P, DeCherney AH. Severe menorrhagia associated with thrombocytopenia. Obstet Gynecol 2007;110(4):913–7.

46. DeVore GR, Owens O, Kase N. Use of intravenous Premarin in the treatment of dysfunctional uterine bleeding—a double-blind randomized control study. Obstet Gynecol 1982;59(3):285–91.

47. Livio M, Mannucci PM, Vigano G, et al. Conjugated estrogens for the management of bleeding associated with renal failure. N Engl J Med 1986;315(12):731–5.

48. Lobo RA. Abnormal uterine bleeding. In: Katz V, Lentz G, Lobo R, et al, editors. Katz: comprehensive gynecology. 5th edition. Philadelphia: Mosby; 2007. p. 915–29.

49. Laufer MR, Townsend NL, Parsons KE, et al. Inducing amenorrhea during bone marrow transplantation. A pilot study of leuprolide acetate. J Reprod Med 1997;42(9):537–41.

50. Amsterdam A, Jakubowski A, Castro-Malaspina H, et al. Treatment of menorrhagia in women undergoing hematopoietic stem cell transplantation. Bone Marrow Transplant 2004;34(4):363–6.

51. Rouhani G, Menon S, Burgis J, et al. An unusual method to manage a rare blood dyscrasia. J Pediatr Adolesc Gynecol 2003;20(2):S123–4.

52. Bowkley CW, Dubel GJ, Haas RA, et al. Uterine artery embolization for control of life-threatening hemorrhage at menarche: brief report. J Vasc Interv Radiol 2007; 18(1 Pt 1):127–31.

53. Markovitch O, Ellis M, Holzinger M, et al. Severe juvenile vaginal bleeding due to Glanzmann's thrombasthenia: case report and review of the literature. Am J Hematol 1998;57(3):225–7.

54. Claessens EA, Cowell CA. Acute adolescent menorrhagia. Am J Obstet Gynecol 1981;139(3):277–80.

55. Smith YR, Quint EH, Hertzberg RB. Menorrhagia in adolescents requiring hospitalization. J Pediatr Adolesc Gynecol 1998;11(1):13–5.

56. Oral E, Cagdas A, Gezer A, et al. Hematological abnormalities in adolescent menorrhagia. Arch Gynecol Obstet 2002;266(2):72–4.

57. Bevan JA, Maloney KW, Hillery CA, et al. Bleeding disorders: a common cause of menorrhagia in adolescents. J Pediatr 2001;138(6):856–61.

58. Jayasinghe Y, Moore P, Donath S, et al. Bleeding disorders in teenagers presenting with menorrhagia. Aust N Z J Obstet Gynaecol 2005;45(5):439–43.

59. Mikhail S, Varadarajan R, Kouides P. The prevalence of disorders of haemostasis in adolescents with menorrhagia referred to a haemophilia treatment centre. Haemophilia 2007;13(5):627–32.

Thrombophilic Conditions in the Adolescent: The Gynecologic Impact

Jennifer E. Dietrich, MD, MSc[a,b,*], Donald L. Yee, MD, MS[b]

KEYWORDS

- Thrombophilia • Combined hormonal contraception
- Progesterone-only methods • Thrombosis risk • Adolescent

Adolescent girls frequently present to providers with gynecologic concerns, ranging from routine health education about pubertal development and sexual activity to more acute disorders, such as ovarian cysts, dysfunctional uterine bleeding, dysmenorrhea, and many other common problems. Adolescent girls are a main population seeking benefit from contraceptive hormones,[1] because contraceptives are a primary treatment for many gynecologic problems and an effective means of birth control. Nonetheless, contraceptive hormone use has been linked conclusively to an increased risk for thrombosis. As conditions predisposing to thrombosis are being increasingly recognized and thrombosis in teenagers is increasingly diagnosed, the practitioner of adolescent gynecology must be knowledgeable about thrombophilic conditions and their potential interaction with such important components of the therapeutic armamentarium. This article provides a basic overview of the hemostatic system and the main thrombophilic conditions currently recognized, in addition to a discussion of the specific risks imposed by these conditions and a review of the primary therapeutic options available for affected patients who have gynecologic problems.

THE HEMOSTATIC SYSTEM: AN OVERVIEW

A detailed comprehensive review of the hemostatic system[2] is beyond the scope of this article; however, the physiology underlying hemostasis and thrombosis can be considered in terms of several constituent processes (**Fig. 1**). Primary hemostasis refers to the initial sequence of events leading to the formation of a platelet plug at

[a] Department of Obstetrics and Gynecology, Baylor College of Medicine, 6620 Main Street, Suite 1450, Houston, TX 77030, USA
[b] Department of Pediatrics, Baylor College of Medicine, 6621 Fannin Street, MC3-3320, Houston, TX 77030, USA
* Corresponding author.
E-mail address: jedietri@bcm.edu (J.E. Dietrich).

Obstet Gynecol Clin N Am 36 (2009) 163–175
doi:10.1016/j.ogc.2008.12.001
0889-8545/08/$ – see front matter © 2009 Elsevier Inc. All rights reserved.

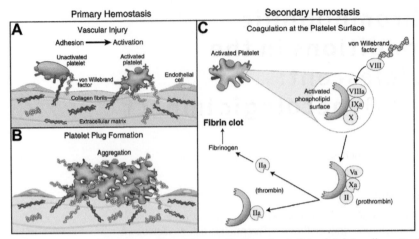

Fig. 1. Components of hemostasis. (*A*) With vessel injury, circulating platelets adhere to sites of injury. (*B*) With progressive adhesion, platelets undergo activation, culminating in formation of the platelet plug. (*C*) At the activated platelet surface, phosphatidylserine (a coagulation cofactor) is preferentially exposed at the outer membrane leaflet, thereby potentiating the activation of factor X to factor Xa and factor II (prothrombin) to factor IIa (thrombin). Thrombin is the critical enzyme that allows formation of the fibrin clot. (*From* Yee DL. Platelets as modifiers of clinical phenotype in hemophilia. Scientific World Journal 2006;6:661–8; with permission.)

the site of vascular injury. Platelets and von Willebrand factor are the major contributors to this process. Although distinct from the prothrombotic risk factors that are the focus of this review, "loss-of-function" abnormalities in primary hemostasis (eg, thrombocytopenia, platelet hypofunction, von Willebrand factor deficiency) are of special importance to obstetricians and gynecologists because they can manifest as menorrhagia, menometrorrhagia, or postpartum hemorrhage. In contrast, secondary hemostasis (ie, coagulation) is the series of catalytic reactions involving plasma serine proteases and their cofactors that culminates in thrombin generation and the formation of a stable fibrin clot at the site of the platelet plug. Elevated levels of these circulating plasma proteins and mutated versions of them that resist inactivation (eg, factor V Leiden [FVL]) contribute to increased thrombotic risk. Natural anticoagulants (eg, protein C, protein S, antithrombin, tissue factor pathway inhibitor) serve primarily as checks on key portions of the coagulation cascade. Deficiencies in these natural anticoagulants have long been recognized as prothrombotic risk factors and are discussed further elsewhere in this article. Circulating components of the fibrinolytic system include plasminogen, tissue type plasminogen activator, and plasminogen activator inhibitor-1. This system breaks down clots and is a key regulator of the fine line between appropriate hemostasis and pathologic thrombosis. Each of the systems and processes described here must be appropriately balanced to achieve vascular homeostasis. When the delicate balance shifts toward hemostatic hyperfunction or inadequate fibrinolysis, thrombophilia can result.

THROMBOPHILIC CONDITIONS

The terms *thrombophilia*, *hypercoagulable state*, and *prothrombotic state* have each been used to describe conditions of increased risk for thromboembolic events (TEs). Many clinicians use these terms solely to signify laboratory-based findings that have been linked with increased thrombotic risk (**Table 1**). Many risk factors that are not based on laboratory testing are extremely important to consider in any determination of an individual patient's risk for thrombosis, however. Many of these clinical risk factors even supersede laboratory-based factors in terms of their effect on risk (see **Table 1**). Although much of this discussion pertains to patients with identified laboratory-based prothrombotic risk factors, it should be emphasized that clinical risk factors may be most important; indeed, a history of thrombosis is perhaps the most significant risk factor to consider.[3]

Following is a brief review of several of the more widely recognized laboratory-based prothrombotic risk factors and their relevant epidemiology. Most of these currently recognized risk factors involve abnormalities of the natural anticoagulant system or secondary hemostasis. Given the critical role of primary hemostasis and the fibrinolytic system in forming and maintaining a thrombus, however, additional prothrombotic abnormalities involving these systems are likely to be identified in the future.[4,5]

- Activated protein C resistance and FVL: a mutation (G1691A) in the gene encoding factor V leads to the substitution of glutamine for arginine at position 506 of the factor V molecule, accounting for FVL.[6] Approximately 3% to 8% of white individuals are heterozygotes for FVL, which renders the activated factor V molecule resistant to cleavage by the natural anticoagulant-activated protein C (APC), leading to persistence of the activated procoagulant molecule. The condition (which can involve a heterozygous or homozygous state) is the most common cause for the laboratory finding of increased resistance to APC, which can also be caused by oral contraceptive use, a lupus anticoagulant, and other less common genetic variants of factor V.
- The prothrombin G20210A mutation (G20210A) in the 3′ untranslated region of the prothrombin gene was described in 1996,[7] and 2% to 3% of whites are

Table 1
Risk factors for thrombosis

Clinical	Laboratory Based
Personal or family history of thrombosis	FVL
Pregnancy and puerperium	Activated protein C resistance without FVL
Hormonal therapy	Prothrombin gene mutation
Obesity	Antithrombin deficiency
Intravascular access devices	Protein C deficiency
Immobility	Protein S deficiency
Infection	Tissue factor pathway inhibitor deficiency
Inflammation	Elevated factor VIII
Autoimmune disorders	Elevated factor IX
Dehydration	Elevated factor XI
Surgery or trauma	Elevated fibrinogen
Spinal cord injury	APS
Acute medical illness	Plasminogen deficiency
Cancer	Elevated homocysteine
Congenital heart disease	Elevated lipoprotein A
Prosthetic heart valves	Dysfibrinogenemia
Nephrotic syndrome	Myeloproliferative disorders

heterozygotes. This mutation leads to increased levels of prothrombin (factor II) and enhanced thrombin generation.

- The lupus anticoagulant and antiphospholipid antibodies are distinct classes of autoantibodies detected by a clot-based assay and ELISA-based assay, respectively. Each is a diagnostic criterion for antiphospholipid syndrome (APS), a disorder characterized by recurrent thrombotic complications. Although most of the thrombophilias are linked to recurrent fetal loss and other obstetric complications related to placental vascular insufficiency, such outcomes actually serve as diagnostic criteria for APS.[8] The mechanism underlying thrombosis in APS remains an active area of study, but inhibition of the protein C pathway and altered platelet/endothelial balance are primary considerations.[9] Reliable population-based data on the prevalence of this acquired form of thrombophilia in adolescents are not available, but the reported prevalence of the antibodies among children who have thrombosis is as high as 24%.[10]

- Congenital deficiencies of antithrombin, protein C, and protein S are less prevalent ($\sim$1 in 500)[11,12] than the thrombophilias described previously, but because of the critical role that these natural anticoagulants play in regulating activated procoagulant moieties, even mild deficiencies (ie, heterozygous state leading to levels approximating 50% or more of normal) lead to increased thrombotic risk. Homozygous/compound heterozygous states are incompatible with life or are associated with severe thrombotic disease early in life. Many conditions (eg, liver disease, disseminated intravascular coagulation, acute thrombosis) can lead to acquired deficiency of these proteins, complicating the diagnosis of hereditary deficiency states. In particular, protein S levels decline significantly with pregnancy and oral contraceptive use.

- Elevated factor levels are associated with increased thrombotic risk, with high levels of factors VIII, IX, and XI cited as risk factors for venous thrombosis.[13–15]

- Elevated homocysteine levels are a risk factor for venous and arterial thrombosis, although recent prospective studies have failed to show that therapy that successfully lowers these levels also reduces thrombotic risk.[16,17] Testing for the presence of a distinct polymorphism (at nucleotide 677) in the gene encoding methylenetetrahydrofolate reductase is a common component of many "hypercoagulation panels." The less common allele of this polymorphism renders the enzyme thermolabile with an associated loss of enzyme activity and mild to moderate homocystinemia in the presence of dietary folate depletion. The utility of testing for this variant is likely low, however, especially when compared with direct testing of homocysteine levels.

Additional prothrombotic risk factors are listed in **Table 1**. Any of these risk factors may occur in combination with any of the others (including homozygosity or compound heterozygosity for a single prothrombotic trait). The combination of such plasma-based factors with each other and with other clinical risk factors comprises the gene-gene and gene-environment interactions that dictate why an individual develops a clot at a given point in time.[18] Therefore, a careful individualized assessment of all such factors must occur to guide clinical decision making relevant to a patient's thrombotic risk.

HORMONAL THERAPY: AN IMPORTANT ACQUIRED RISK FACTOR FOR THROMBOSIS

One of the most significant prothrombotic risk factors to consider is hormonal therapy. Hormones are some of the most commonly prescribed drugs in adolescent girls, and combined oral contraceptives (COCs; estrogen and progestagen) are the most common class of these. A variety of studies in adults show that COCs induce resistance to APC;[19] increase levels of procoagulant proteins (factors II, VII, VIII, and fibrinogen);[20] decrease levels of antithrombin, protein S, tissue factor pathway inhibitor, and fibrinolytic proteins; and increase markers of coagulation and fibrinolysis activation.[21,22]

The thrombotic risk associated with oral contraceptive use varies with the time interval since starting treatment but is highest in the first year of use, especially in women who have a prothrombotic defect.[23,24] The dose of estrogen[25] and the type of progestagen used in the combination also influence thrombotic risk. Third-generation COCs containing the progestagen component gestodene or desogestrel have been associated with a roughly doubled risk for venous thrombosis compared with second-generation pills containing levonorgestrel.[23,24] Recent studies have identified differences in APC resistance, protein S, and tissue factor pathway inhibitor levels among the various formulations that differ by the progestagen component, thus providing a mechanistic rationale for the clinical observations.[19,26]

Although some have suggested that progestagens counteract the prothrombotic effect of estrogens[27] and raise protein S levels,[28] data are relatively scarce regarding the thrombotic risk associated with progesterone-only oral contraceptives. The available evidence, however, does not suggest that there is increased risk.[29,30]

ABSOLUTE AND RELATIVE RISKS FOR THROMBOSIS

To provide a more meaningful context for this discussion, a consideration of the absolute risk for thrombosis in adolescents and the relative risks imposed by the described risk factors is in order. Thrombosis risk increases with age (**Table 2**),[31] such that this risk is fairly minimal for adolescents compared with more senescent adults. Adolescents do constitute the second highest risk age group for thrombosis among pediatric patients, however.[32] Although specific population-based incidence data are not available for adolescents, a reasonable conservative estimate for the absolute thrombotic risk for this age group would be between those rates reported for the pediatric age group and young adults as listed in **Table 2** (estimate italicized). Inherited and acquired thrombophilic risk factors (eg, FVL, lupus anticoagulant) and prothrombotic clinical risk factors (eg, oral contraceptive use, pregnancy, obesity) increase this risk further (**Table 3**). The magnitude of these risks, how they may be modified, and their interaction with other aspects of the clinical scenario must be carefully weighed when making clinical decisions that have an impact on thrombotic risk. Often, decision making may be enhanced through involvement of a hematologist or other consultant experienced in dealing with disorders of hemostasis and thrombosis.

Table 2 Absolute thrombotic risk by age	
Age Group	**Incidence (Cases per 10,000 per Year)**
All children and adolescents (age ≤18 years)	0.07–0.14[32,68]
Adolescents	Estimated 0.5–1
Young adults (age ≤40 years)	1–2[69,70]
All adults	10–20[31,71]
Elderly adults (age ≤85 years)	~100[31]

Table 3
Risk for venous thrombosis associated with various prothrombotic conditions

Prothrombotic Condition	Relative Risk
Pregnancy	4–12[72–74]
Postpartum state	20–25[72]
Low-dose COC	3–4[74]
High-dose COC	6–10[74]
FVL (heterozygous)	8[75]
FVL (homozygous)	50–100[39]
FVL and COC use	35[75]
Elevated factor VIII (>150 IU/dL)	4[76,a]
Elevated factor VIII and COC use	10[76,a]

Defined control groups varied with the different studies but, in all cases, comprised girls or women unexposed to the risk factor being assessed.
[a] Reported as odds ratio.

It must be emphasized that thrombotic risk is further modified by the combination of multiple risk factors, including the use of COCs in the setting of inherited or acquired thrombophilic traits. For example, the combination of FVL (heterozygous state) with COC use increases the apparent thrombotic risk far beyond that which would be observed with either risk factor alone (see **Table 3**). Although such synergism seems to be the rule, the magnitude of effect seems to vary with the prothrombotic risk factor involved; a recent systematic review summarizes results for other thrombophilias.[33] Finally, it should be mentioned that in addition to overt thrombosis, thrombophilic conditions have been linked to a variety of adverse pregnancy outcomes, including pre-eclampsia, intrauterine growth retardation, placental abruption, and recurrent fetal loss.[34,35]

SHOULD SCREENING FOR THROMBOPHILIA BE PERFORMED?

Thrombophilia testing has become widely available, and the increased thrombotic risk imposed by oral contraceptive pill (OCP) use raises the important question of whether patients should be screened for thrombophilic traits before initiating such therapy. Although OCP use is associated with an increased relative risk for thrombosis, the absolute risk remains low and universal screening of patients before starting OCP therapy is not indicated. A cost-effectiveness study published in 1999 reported that more than 92,000 carriers of FVL would need to be identified and stopped from using COCs to prevent a single death attributable to COC use and the coexistence of this trait, at a charge exceeding $300 million.[36] A more recent analysis reported that screening for thrombophilic defects before initiating COC use would incur an additional £200,402 to prevent one additional case of venous thrombosis.[37] This figure dropped to £79,085 in the model in which screening was restricted to women who had a personal or family history of thrombosis. Of several screening strategies analyzed in this study, including screening with onset of pregnancy, before hormone replacement therapy, and before orthopedic surgery, thrombophilia screening before initiating COC use was the least cost-effective strategy evaluated.[37] Based largely on such cost-effectiveness data, the clear consensus is that screening before COC use in adolescents should not be universal but that careful evaluation for a personal or family history of thrombosis should be performed and directed screening should be considered on an individualized basis.[38,39] **Box 1** lists specific questions that may be helpful to the clinician in eliciting such histories.

INDICATIONS FOR HORMONAL THERAPY

Managing common gynecologic problems or recommending contraception can be challenging in adolescents, especially in light of recent teen statistics.[1] In the United States, approximately 800,000 teen pregnancies occur annually, with nearly 80% being unintended and one third ending in abortion. Sexual activity is not only seen among older adolescents, but current statistics demonstrate that 7% of teens become sexually active before the age of 12 years.[1,40,41] Negative consequences from early sexual activity abound, because 25% of all teens have had or currently have a sexually transmitted infection, with high-risk behavior demonstrated across all socioeconomic groups. Because adolescents are a sexually active group as a whole, there is clearly a need for contraception and sex education.[41–43]

Sexual activity and contraception are not the only reasons for prescribing hormonal contraception in adolescents. Acute gynecologic concerns are common among this population; therefore, many noncontraceptive benefits are gained from hormone pills. For example, ovarian cysts are present in approximately 20% of teens 12 to 17 years of age, and they are frequently benign in this age group.[44] Such cysts may be functional, be hemorrhagic, have cystic or solid components, and may vary in size. Menstrual cycle irregularity is also common in this age group, occurring in 75% of adolescents within the first few years of menarche.[44] Other reasons why an adolescent may present to a gynecologist include dysmenorrhea, premenstrual syndrome, endometriosis, outflow tract obstruction, pelvic pain, hyperandrogenism, and acne. Hormonal contraception may play a role in the treatment of each of these conditions.[45]

Adolescent girls who have coexisting conditions, such as systemic lupus erythematosus, APS, sickle cell disease, a history of TE, or other thrombophilic conditions (see **Table 1**), have relative contraindications to combination hormonal contraceptive methods, however, because these medications place them at higher risk for TE.[46–49] Therefore, decisions regarding contraception or noncontraceptive medical management for adolescents who have such coexisting conditions may be more difficult.[40,47,50,51]

First-Line Hormonal Options for Contraception and Noncontraceptive Medical Therapy

Presently, there are many options for teens with thrombophilic conditions, which allow individuals to choose an alternative that fits their lifestyle.[30,52–54] Progesterone-only

---

Box 1
Screening questions for personal or family history of thrombosis

Have you or a close family member ever had blood clots in the legs or lungs?

Have you or a close family member ever been hospitalized for blood clots in the legs or lungs?

What were the circumstances in which the blood clot took place (eg, cancer, airline travel, obesity, immobility, postpartum)?

Did you or your family member require blood thinning medication?

From Sass AE, Neufeld EJ. Risk factors for thromboembolism in teens: when should I test? Curr Opin Pediatr 2002;14:374–5; with permission.

methods have become a primary choice because of their ease of use and apparent lack of thromboembolic side effects.[30] Contraceptive progestagens have two important effects. First, they thicken cervical mucus, leading to endometrial atrophy. Numerous studies have demonstrated that failure rates for progesterone-only methods are less than 1% when taken correctly. Second, progesterone methods may lower TE risk by up-regulating free and total protein S, making this cofactor to protein C more available for anticoagulant effect.[55] The relative risk for a TE while using a contraceptive progestin has been previously reported as no more than 1.[30,40,56]

Pills

Contraceptive progestin pills are currently limited to norethindrone in the United States. These pills are taken daily and are available at a dose of 0.35 mg. Because this agent has a short half-life, follicular function can still persist. Pills are administered daily without a placebo week. Progestin pills are well tolerated by teens but can result in difficulties with compliance because of the need for daily administration[54,57] and the frequent side effect of breakthrough bleeding.

Injectables

There are two forms available for contraceptive administration. Depomedroxyprogesterone acetate (DMPA) is available for subcutaneous or intramuscular use. The intramuscular dose of 150 mg is administered once every 3 months. The subcutaneous dose of 104 mg is also administered once every 3 months. Both are options for the adolescent who may be less compliant with daily pills.[58] Important side effects include breakthrough bleeding, weight gain, loss of bone mineral density, and, rarely, episodes of depression. For management of other gynecologic conditions, such as endometriosis, or uncontrolled menorrhagia, gonadotropin-releasing hormone analogues may be used without increased risk for thrombosis. There are several different formulations available for use, but patients can choose to have administration of this medication monthly or once every 3 months.[52,58]

Implantables

The etonogestrel implant is the most recent method of contraception approved by the US Food and Drug Administration. Approximately 22% of patients achieve amenorrhea, and 33.6% report infrequent bleeding episodes. Bleeding irregularity was still the most common reason for method discontinuation.[53,59] Use of an implant with etonogestrel has also been associated with down-regulation of the coagulation cascade and subsequent thrombin generation, suggesting that this method may reduce TE risk.[60]

Intrauterine devices

Newer evidence suggests that intrauterine device (IUD) use in adolescents may be appropriate in certain situations. The levonorgestrel IUD is reversible, lasts 5 years, and induces amenorrhea in 20% of patients after 1 year of use. Irregular bleeding remains a concern, however, and may occur for 3 to 6 months after insertion. Candidates for IUD insertion include individuals who cannot receive estrogens and those who wish to use a long-acting progestin.[61-63]

Emergency contraception

Adolescents who are sexually active may inquire about options for pregnancy prevention in the setting of recent exposure. Progesterone-only emergency contraception is available and can be administered without increasing TE risk. Levonorgestrel in the form of 0.75-mg tablets is available for administration in two divided doses, but even when taken as one combined dose, efficacy rates are similar.[64]

Nonhormonal Options

There are several natural family planning methods available for adolescents who have known thrombophilias. The natural methods can be effective in the compliant adolescent with regular menstrual cycles. Using menstrual calendars or cycle beads may be helpful to remind adolescents when their most fertile period is and when to avoid sexual contact for pregnancy prevention. Because many adolescents are anovulatory and have irregular cycles, however, natural family planning cannot be used by everyone. Failure rates for menstrual calendar and cycle bead methods approach 20%, which is similar to using the withdrawal method.[45] Another option for pregnancy prevention in sexually active adolescent girls who have thrombophilias is barrier contraception. Barrier options include condoms, spermicides, sponges, cervical caps, and diaphragms. These methods are effective if used correctly, but typical failure rates range between 10% and 30%. Finally, a copper IUD is an effective method for pregnancy prevention, with failure rates of less than 1%; however, this may not be an option for an adolescent who has a history of pelvic inflammatory disease at the time of insertion, who is not currently in a monogamous relationship, or who desires a decrease in menstrual flow.[45]

ANTITHROMBOTIC TREATMENT AND PROPHYLAXIS IN ADOLESCENT GIRLS

For the adolescent who requires antithrombotic therapy or prophylaxis, several options are available. These include unfractionated heparin, low molecular weight heparin, and vitamin K antagonists (eg, warfarin). Although unfractionated heparin and low molecular weight heparin do not cross the placenta, adolescents taking warfarin must be warned about the potential for adverse fetal effects, and effective contraception must be undertaken. In patients who require warfarin, concomitant use of a low-dose COC or DMPA may be a reasonable choice to consider, given the teratogenic risks, the risk for intraperitoneal bleeding associated with ovulation, and the expected benefit of reduced menstrual flow.[56,65] Other antithrombotic strategies include use of graduated compression stockings or sequential compression devices after surgery or during other periods of risk (eg, prolonged immobilization). For specific details regarding thrombosis treatment and prophylaxis, the American College of Chest Physicians has published formal treatment guidelines for adolescents,[66] but close consultation with a hematologist is strongly recommended.

Any anticoagulant therapy carries a risk for severe bleeding, including menorrhagia. Appropriate management of acute and chronic menorrhagia requires knowledge of current anticoagulation status and a clear understanding of the underlying thrombophilia. A gonadotropin-releasing hormone agonist may be a useful adjunct in managing heavy menses in anticoagulated patients because it does not seem to increase thrombotic risk.[67] For acute management of severe menorrhagia or other severe bleeding, it may be necessary to withhold, or even reverse, anticoagulation. Such decisions should also involve close hematologic consultation, however.

SUMMARY

Thrombophilias, hereditary and acquired, encompass a wide-ranging array of conditions and traits that lead to increased thrombotic risk among those affected. It is of particular importance for clinicians to assess for TE risk in individuals seeking hormonal contraception or in those who are candidates for hormonal therapy for other indications. Universal laboratory screening of such patients for thrombophilia is not recommended. A careful evaluation of each patient's personal and family history is critical for identifying individuals who may (1) be at increased risk for thrombosis, (2) not be suitable for standard hormonal therapy, or (3) benefit from more directed thrombophilic testing, however. Furthermore, consultation with a hematologist is crucial for effective management of patients at increased risk for thrombosis. Finally, adolescent girls identified with a thrombophilic condition should fully understand the impact on their future gynecologic health.

REFERENCES

1. Klein JD. Adolescent pregnancy: current trends and issues. Pediatrics 2005; 116(1):281–6.
2. Colman RW, Clowes AW, George JN, et al. Overview of hemostasis. In: Colman RW, Hirsh J, Marder VJ, et al, editors. Hemostasis and thrombosis: basic principles and clinical practice. 4th edition. Hagerstown, MD: Lippincott, Williams and Wilkins; 2001. p. 3–16.
3. Sandoval JA, Sheehan MP, Stonerock CE, et al. Incidence, risk factors, and treatment patterns for deep venous thrombosis in hospitalized children: an increasing population at risk. J Vasc Surg 2008;47(4):837–43.
4. Yee DL, Sun CW, Bergeron AL, et al. Aggregometry detects platelet hyperreactivity in healthy individuals. Blood 2005;106(8):2723–9.
5. Lisman T, de Groot PG, Meijers JC, et al. Reduced plasma fibrinolytic potential is a risk factor for venous thrombosis. Blood 2005;105(3):1102–5.
6. Zoller B, Dahlback B. Linkage between inherited resistance to activated protein C and factor V gene mutation in venous thrombosis. Lancet 1994;343(8912): 1536–8.
7. Poort SR, Rosendaal FR, Reitsma PH, et al. A common genetic variation in the 3'-untranslated region of the prothrombin gene is associated with elevated plasma prothrombin levels and an increase in venous thrombosis. Blood 1996;88(10): 3698–703.
8. Miyakis S, Lockshin MD, Atsumi T, et al. International consensus statement on an update of the classification criteria for definite antiphospholipid syndrome (APS). J Thromb Haemost 2006;4(2):295–306.
9. de Laat B, Mertens K, de Groot PG. Mechanisms of disease: antiphospholipid antibodies—from clinical association to pathologic mechanism. Nat Clin Pract Rheumatol 2008;4(4):192–9.
10. Revel-Vilk S, Kenet G. Thrombophilia in children with venous thromboembolic disease. Thromb Res 2006;118(1):59–65.
11. Tait RC, Walker ID, Reitsma PH, et al. Prevalence of protein C deficiency in the healthy population. Thromb Haemost 1995;73(1):87–93.
12. Tait RC, Walker ID, Perry DJ, et al. Prevalence of antithrombin deficiency in the healthy population. Br J Haematol 1994;87(1):106–12.
13. Kraaijenhagen RA, in't Anker PS, Koopman MM, et al. High plasma concentration of factor VIIIc is a major risk factor for venous thromboembolism. Thromb Haemost 2000;83(1):5–9.
14. Van HV, van dL I, Bertina RM, et al. High levels of factor IX increase the risk of venous thrombosis. Blood 2000;95(12):3678–82.
15. Meijers JC, Tekelenburg WL, Bouma BN, et al. High levels of coagulation factor XI as a risk factor for venous thrombosis. N Engl J Med 2000;342(10):696–701.

16. Ray JG, Kearon C, Yi Q, et al. Homocysteine-lowering therapy and risk for venous thromboembolism: a randomized trial. Ann Intern Med 2007;146(11):761–7.
17. den Heijer M, Willems HP, Blom HJ, et al. Homocysteine lowering by B vitamins and the secondary prevention of deep vein thrombosis and pulmonary embolism: a randomized, placebo-controlled, double-blind trial. Blood 2007;109(1):139–44.
18. Rosendaal FR. Venous thrombosis: a multicausal disease. Lancet 1999; 353(9159):1167–73.
19. van Vliet HA, Bertina RM, Dahm AE, et al. Different effects of oral contraceptives containing different progestogens on protein S and tissue factor pathway inhibitor. J Thromb Haemost 2008;6(2):346–51.
20. Bloemenkamp KW, Rosendaal FR, Helmerhorst FM, et al. Hemostatic effects of oral contraceptives in women who developed deep-vein thrombosis while using oral contraceptives. Thromb Haemost 1998;80(3):382–7.
21. Kluft C, Lansink M. Effect of oral contraceptives on haemostasis variables. Thromb Haemost 1997;78(1):315–26.
22. Winkler UH. Blood coagulation and oral contraceptives. A critical review. Contraception 1998;57(3):203–9.
23. Rosendaal FR, Helmerhorst FM, Vandenbroucke JP. Female hormones and thrombosis. Arterioscler Thromb Vasc Biol 2002;22(2):201–10.
24. Blickstein D, Blickstein I. Oral contraception and thrombophilia. Curr Opin Obstet Gynecol 2007;19(4):370–6.
25. Gerstman BB, Piper JM, Tomita DK, et al. Oral contraceptive estrogen dose and the risk of deep venous thromboembolic disease. Am J Epidemiol 1991;133(1): 32–7.
26. Alhenc-Gelas M, Plu-Bureau, Guillonneau S, et al. Impact of progestagens on activated protein C (APC) resistance among users of oral contraceptives. J Thromb Haemost 2004;2(9):1594–600.
27. Battaglioli T, Martinelli I. Hormone therapy and thromboembolic disease. Curr Opin Hematol 2007;14(5):488–93.
28. Kemmeren JM, Algra A, Meijers JC, et al. Effect of second- and third-generation oral contraceptives on the protein C system in the absence or presence of the factor V Leiden mutation: a randomized trial. Blood 2004;103(3):927–33.
29. Vasilakis C, Jick H, del MM-M. Risk of idiopathic venous thromboembolism in users of progestagens alone. Lancet 1999;354(9190):1610–1.
30. Conard J, Plu-Bureau, Bahi N, et al. Progestogen-only contraception in women at high risk of venous thromboembolism. Contraception 2004;70(6):437–41.
31. Heit JA, Silverstein MD, Mohr DN, et al. The epidemiology of venous thromboembolism in the community. Thromb Haemost 2001;86(1):452–63.
32. Andrew M, David M, Adams M, et al. Venous thromboembolic complications (VTE) in children: first analyses of the Canadian Registry of VTE. Blood 1994; 83(5):1251–7.
33. Wu O, Robertson L, Langhorne P, et al. Oral contraceptives, hormone replacement therapy, thrombophilias and risk of venous thromboembolism: a systematic review. The Thrombosis Risk and Economic Assessment of Thrombophilia Screening (TREATS) study. Thromb Haemost 2005;94(1):17–25.
34. Robertson L, Wu O, Langhorne P, et al. Thrombophilia in pregnancy: a systematic review. Br J Haematol 2006;132(2):171–96.
35. Hoffman R, Brenner B. Thrombophilia related issues in women and children. Semin Thromb Hemost 2005;31(1):97–103.
36. Creinin MD, Lisman R, Strickler RC. Screening for factor V Leiden mutation before prescribing combination oral contraceptives. Fertil Steril 1999;72(4):646–51.

37. Wu O, Robertson L, Twaddle S, et al. Screening for thrombophilia in high-risk situations: a meta-analysis and cost-effectiveness analysis. Br J Haematol 2005; 131(1):80–90.
38. Dietrich JE, Hertweck SP. Thrombophilias in adolescents: the past, present and future. Curr Opin Obstet Gynecol 2008;20(5):470–4.
39. Sass AE, Neufeld EJ. Risk factors for thromboembolism in teens: when should I test? Curr Opin Pediatr 2002;14(4):370–8.
40. ACOG Committee on Practice Bulletins, Gynecology. ACOG practice bulletin No. 73. Use of hormonal contraception in women with coexisting medical conditions. Obstet Gynecol 2006;107(6):1453–72.
41. CDC Youth Risk Behavior Survey 2007. Available at: www.cdc.gov/Features/RiskBehavior. Accessed on August 18, 2008.
42. Guttmacher Institute Web site. Available at: www.guttmacher.org. Accessed on August 17, 2008.
43. D'Alfonso A, Iovenitti P, Carta G. The adolescent and the gynecologist: our experience. Clin Exp Obstet Gynecol 2003;30(1):47–50.
44. Physiology of puberty. In: Emans SJ, Laufer MR, Goldstein DP, editors. Pediatric and adolescent gynecology. 5th edition. Hagerstown, MD: Lippincott Williams & Wilkins; 2004. p. 120–80.
45. Nakajima ST. Contemporary guide to contraception 2007. Newton, PA: Handbooks in Healthcare Company; 2007:163–77.
46. Curtis KM, Chrisman CE, Peterson HB. Contraception for women in selected circumstances. Obstet Gynecol 2002;99(6):1100–12.
47. Practice Committee of the American Society of Reproductive Medicine. Hormonal contraception: recent advances and controversies. Fertil Steril 2006;86(5 Suppl): S229–35.
48. Contraceptives and teens: what are the options? Contracept Technol Update 2000;21(9):109–11.
49. Mohllajee AP, Curtis KM, Martins SL, et al. Does use of hormonal contraceptives among women with thrombogenic mutations increase their risk of venous thromboembolism? A systematic review. Contraception 2006;73(2):166–78.
50. Mishell D Jr, Darney PD, Burkman RT, et al. Practice guidelines for OC selection: update. Dialogues Contracept 1997;5(4):7–20.
51. Sondheimer SJ. Oral contraceptives: mechanism of action, dosing, safety, and efficacy. Cutis 2008;81(1 Suppl):19–22.
52. Tolaymat LL, Kaunitz AM. Long-acting contraceptives in adolescents. Curr Opin Obstet Gynecol 2007;19(5):453–60.
53. Pettinato A, Emans SJ. New contraceptive methods: update 2003. Curr Opin Pediatr 2003;15(4):362–9.
54. Chacko MS. Issues concerning the use of hormonal contraception by adolescents. UpToDate. Available at: www.uptodate.com. Last updated 2-5-2008. Accessed on May 26, 2008.
55. Hughes Q, Watson M, Cole V, et al. Upregulation of protein S by progestins. J Thromb Haemost 2007;5(11):2243–9.
56. Heroux K. Contraceptive choices in medically ill adolescents. Semin Reprod Med 2003;21(4):389–98.
57. FDA Web site. Norethindrone tablets. Available at: www.fda.gov. Accessed on October 1, 2008.
58. FDA Web site. Depo SC Provera. Available at: www.fda.gov. Accessed on October 1, 2008.

59. FDA Web site. Implanon. Available at: www.fda.gov. Accessed on October 1, 2008.
60. Vieira CS, Ferriani RA, Garcia AA, et al. Use of the etonogestrel-releasing implant is associated with hypoactivation of the coagulation cascade. Hum Reprod 2007; 22(8):2196–201.
61. FDA Web site. Mirena. Available at: www.fda.gov. Accessed on October 1, 2008.
62. Morin-Papunen L, Martikainen H, McCarthy MI, et al. Comparison of metabolic and inflammatory outcomes in women who used oral contraceptives and the levonorgestrel-releasing intrauterine device in a general population. Am J Obstet Gynecol 2008;199(5):529e1–529e10.
63. Adolescent Health Care Committee for the American College of Obstetricians and Gynecologists. ACOG Committee Opinion No. 392. Intrauterine device and adolescents. Obstet Gynecol 2007;110(6):1493–5.
64. FDA Web site. Plan B. Available at: www.fda.gov. Accessed on October 1, 2008.
65. Comp PC, Zacur HA. Contraceptive choices in women with coagulation disorders. Am J Obstet Gynecol 1993;168(6 Pt 2):1990–3.
66. Monagle P, Chalmers E, Chan A, et al. Antithrombotic therapy in neonates and children: American College of Chest Physicians evidence-based clinical practice guidelines. (8th edition). Chest 2008;133(6 Suppl):887S–968S.
67. Quaas AM, Ginsburg ES. Prevention and treatment of uterine bleeding in hematologic malignancy. Eur J Obstet Gynecol Reprod Biol 2007;134(1):3–8.
68. van Ommen CH, Heijboer H, Buller HR, et al. Venous thromboembolism in childhood: a prospective two-year registry in The Netherlands. J Pediatr 2001;139(5): 676–81.
69. Martinelli I. Risk factors in venous thromboembolism. Thromb Haemost 2001; 86(1):395–403.
70. Wilkerson WR, Sane DC. Aging and thrombosis. Semin Thromb Hemost 2002; 28(6):555–68.
71. Nordstrom M, Lindblad B, Bergqvist D, et al. A prospective study of the incidence of deep-vein thrombosis within a defined urban population. J Intern Med 1992; 232(2):155–60.
72. Heit JA, Kobbervig CE, James AH, et al. Trends in the incidence of venous thromboembolism during pregnancy or postpartum: a 30-year population-based study. Ann Intern Med 2005;143(10):697–706.
73. Goodnight SH, Hathaway WE. Disorders of hemostasis and thrombosis. Columbus, OH: McGraw-Hill, Inc; 2001.
74. Speroff L, Darney PD. A clinical guide for contraception. Hagerstown, PA: Lippincoot Williams & Wilkins; 2005.
75. Vandenbroucke JP, Koster T, Briet E, et al. Increased risk of venous thrombosis in oral-contraceptive users who are carriers of factor V Leiden mutation. Lancet 1994;344(8935):1453–7.
76. Bloemenkamp KW, Helmerhorst FM, Rosendaal FR, et al. Venous thrombosis, oral contraceptives and high factor VIII levels. Thromb Haemost 1999;82(3):1024–7.

Adolescent Endometriosis

KEYWORDS
• Adolescent • Endometriosis • Pelvic pain • Management

The presence of endometrial glands and stroma outside the uterus, typically in the pelvis, is known as endometriosis. An adolescent with this diagnosis usually presents with chronic pelvic pain, and she and her family are anxious for an explanation of her symptoms. Traditionally, endometriosis had been thought to occur only rarely in adolescence, but with an increasing awareness of the disease among the medical community, it is being diagnosed more frequently. An outline of the disease and the issues surrounding its diagnosis and management in adolescents is the focus of this article.

INCIDENCE AND PATHOPHYSIOLOGY

The prevalence of endometriosis varies depending on the population studied; therefore, it has been difficult to establish firm rates for adolescents. Indeed, studies reporting the presence of endometriosis in adolescents undergoing laparoscopy for pelvic pain vary. Goldstein and colleagues[1] reported a 47% incidence of disease in adolescent girls undergoing laparoscopy for chronic pelvic pain, whereas Laufer and colleagues[2] have reported a finding of endometriosis at the time of surgery in 67% of adolescents who have pain refractory to simple medical treatments like nonsteroidal anti-inflammatory agents (NSAIDS) or oral contraceptive pills (OCPs).

In terms of economic burden, Gao and colleagues[3] have produced some data highlighting the importance of endometriosis among adolescents. These researchers assessed the economic burden of endometriosis and concluded that as endometriosis-related hospital length of stay steadily declined from 1993 to 2002, per-patient cost increased 61%. In addition, these researchers found that adolescents (aged 10–17 years) had endometriosis-related hospitalizations and female patients 23 years of age or younger constituted greater than 20% of endometriosis-related outpatient visits.[3]

Department of Obstetrics and Gynecology, Women's and Children's Hospital, Keck School of Medicine of the University of Southern California, 1240 North Mission Road, L919, Los Angeles, CA 90033, USA
E-mail address: templeman_c@ccnt.usc.edu

Obstet Gynecol Clin N Am 36 (2009) 177–185
doi:10.1016/j.ogc.2008.12.005
0889-8545/08/$ – see front matter © 2009 Elsevier Inc. All rights reserved.

obgyn.theclinics.com

PATHOPHYSIOLOGY HIGHLIGHTS: GENETICS, EPIDEMIOLOGY, INFLAMMATORY

The pathogenesis of endometriosis remains an enigma, and, as a result, no single theory can explain the development of endometriosis in all patients. Retrograde menstruation with implantation in the peritoneal cavity was suggested as a possible cause for endometriosis by Sampson[4] some 60 years age and seems to be particularly important in adolescents with obstructive Müllerian anomalies.[5] Retrograde menstruation is found in most women at the time of menstruation; therefore, why some women develop endometriosis and others do not is a focus of intense interest.

There are specific defects in the endometrium of women who have endometriosis that include a decrease in endometrial cell apoptosis[6] and sensitivity to progesterone, resulting in increased matrix metalloproteinase activity.[7] The effect of these defects is an increase in the number of cells with invasive capacity that are refluxed through the fallopian tubes and into the peritoneal cavity. In addition, neoangiogenesis, as the result of cytokine and vascular endothelial growth factor secretion, may play an important role in the establishment of endometriosis.[8] Another focus of research is in the area of environmental toxins and oxidative stress. In particular, dioxin has been implicated in the pathophysiology of endometriosis.[9]

Investigation into the genetics of endometriosis is being undertaken at several centers.[10] This focus includes linkage analysis for sibling pairs in which first-degree relatives of patients who have surgically confirmed endometriosis are evaluated. These data have demonstrated a 6.9% relative risk for the disease in comparison with controls.[11] In addition, microarray[12] and epigenetic evaluation of DNA[13] are techniques aimed at determining important genes in pivotal molecular pathways that may be associated with the development of endometriosis.

The finding of predominantly smooth muscle endometriotic lesions in the rectovaginal septum[14] of some women has led to the theory of embryonic Müllerian rests[15] as an cause for endometriosis. This theory is also supported by the finding of endometriosis in the pelvis of premenarcheal girls.[16] Still other patients develop endometriosis in surgical site wounds, such as caesarean section wounds or episiotomy sites. Because hematogenous and lymphatic spread to a single site is unlikely, this has led to the unintentional surgical transplantation theory of endometriosis.

Endometriosis lesions themselves seem to have a developmental pathway. Koninckx and colleagues[17] have found that the typical lesions of endometriosis—black and white scarred areas, along with endometriomas—seem to increase with age. This is consistent with other researchers who have found that red flame-like and atypical clear vesicular lesions are more prominent in younger aged patients.[18] It is these findings that have led to the suggestion that endometriosis is a progressive disease. Sutton and colleagues[19] have produced some evidence about the natural history of endometriosis. In their randomized placebo-controlled trial evaluating the laparoscopic treatment of endometriosis, these investigators demonstrated that equal numbers of placebo patients had disease that progressed, regressed, and remained static at second-look laparoscopy.

Koninckx and colleagues[17] also found that the only significant correlate with pain symptoms was the depth of endometriosis invasion. This would suggest that the more superficial red and atypical lesions present in adolescents should not be painful. It has become clear, however, that there are alternative mechanisms for the production of pain in endometriosis and that red lesions, in particular, are extremely active in the synthesis of prostaglandins,[20] which are likely to be important in pain symptomatology. In addition, several other mechanisms may be important in the production of pain in patients who have endometriosis, and these include cytokine production, bleeding within the implant itself, and stimulation of neural tissue within the lesion[21] and within the endometrium of patients who have endometriosis.[22]

PRESENTATION AND DIAGNOSIS

Dysmenorrhea in adolescents may be primary or secondary to endometriosis. The true prevalence of primary dysmenorrhea is difficult to assess because many girls do not seek medical attention, with one study revealing 98% of adolescents using nonpharmacologic means to address their symptoms.[23] Dysmenorrhea is reported to have a significant impact on school absenteeism and quality of life in white adolescents, with recent reports confirming a similar pattern among African-American and Hispanic girls.[23]

Endometriosis should be considered in girls who do not respond to simple NSAIDS and OCPs, because two thirds of girls who are investigated with laparoscopy in this clinical setting have been found to have endometriosis.[2]

Recent data from the Endometriosis Association suggest that patients who have symptoms suggestive of endometriosis as an adolescent wait longer to be surgically diagnosed than those women who are first symptomatic as adults.[24] In addition, girls who saw a physician other than a gynecologist have a longer time to definitive diagnosis.[24] Some of this delay may be explained by the diversity of symptoms that patients who have endometriosis experience, in addition to the fact that laparoscopy is required for a definitive diagnosis.

A detailed history and physical examination are critical in the assessment of adolescents presenting with pain symptomatology. If appropriate, a pelvic examination for signs of uterosacral nodularity and levator tenderness may point to the diagnosis of endometriosis; however, in virginal patients, this examination is likely to be omitted. External genital inspection with labial traction and rectoabdominal examination should be considered if there is suspicion of an obstructive anomaly. Abdominal wall assessment for signs of muscle injury and trigger points is helpful because this indicates that physical therapy is likely to be useful in the management of pain symptoms.[25] Imaging with pelvic ultrasound is useful to exclude the possibility of an endometrioma and to confirm the presence of a uterine anomaly. Tumor markers, such as Ca125, are unlikely to be helpful in adolescents because such patients have early-stage disease and rarely have endometriomas.

MANAGEMENT STRATEGIES

The history and physical examination should help the treating physician develop a firm idea about the likely cause of the pain symptomatology. Often, what began as pain secondary to endometriosis has progressed to involve a component of musculoskeletal pain with associated depression and anxiety.[26] Therefore, it is important to recognize that for treatment to be effective, the managing physician must seek and address all these issues, if present.

The treatment algorithms used to manage adolescents are based on research performed in adults. Typically, medical management is used initially, although surgical intervention may be required if a Müllerian anomaly is suspected or the endometriosis is of advanced stage. If the adolescent has persistent pain despite intervention with medical therapy, she should be offered laparoscopy for a definitive diagnosis. Empiric gonadotropin-releasing hormone (GnRH) agonist therapy has been used in adults with chronic pelvic pain and a suspected diagnosis of endometriosis. This approach may be considered in adolescents, with special consideration given to patient age.

In the absence of a clinically useful marker, however, the challenge is in distinguishing which patients may have progressive disease and which patients have disease that may remain the same or even regress. Clinically, however, the physician is often confronted with an adolescent in chronic pain; therefore, intervention to relieve symptoms becomes a priority.

Medical Therapy

NSAIDs are often the first-line medication used to treat dysmenorrhea, and many adolescents have used these at the time of presentation. The American College of Obstetrics and Gynecology (ACOG) has issued a statement supporting the empiric use of NSAIDS for dysmenorrhea.[27]

These drugs act through inhibition of the cyclooxygenase (COX) enzyme pathway, which is responsible for the production of prostaglandins and leukotrienes. Some drugs in this family may also act through promotion of prostaglandin E_2, a vasodilator. In placebo-controlled trials, NSAIDS have been found to decrease menstrual loss and improve primary dysmenorrhea significantly.[28] In endometriotic lesions, there is a positive feedback loop between prostaglandins and estrogen production through aromatase production. In addition, COX-2 inhibitors have been found in mouse endometriosis models to decrease the size and microvessel density within endometriosis lesions.[29]

Other medical treatments for endometriosis are aimed at suppressing steroid hormonal production from the hypothalamus or ovary. This results in atrophy of the endometrial implants, at least while the patient is taking the medication. OCPs are used empirically to treat primary dysmenorrhea and dysmenorrhea secondary to endometriosis,[30] and despite the paucity of randomized trials demonstrating effectiveness, the ACOG also supports the use of OCPs in this setting.[27] Perhaps the major reason why OCPs are so commonly used as first-line therapy in this age group is their relatively low incidence of side effects and the ease with which they can be stopped should the patient wish to change medications. In addition, a trial of OCPs after or concurrent with NSAIDS is helpful in assessing the likelihood that the adolescent has endometriosis. Laufer and colleagues[2] demonstrated that 67% of adolescents who had persistent cyclic or noncyclic pain despite OCP use were found to have endometriosis at the time of laparoscopy.

Progestins have been shown to be effective in reducing pain symptoms in patients who have endometriosis.[31] Possible mechanisms for this include down-regulation of estrogen receptors and a reduction in matrix metalloproteinases in endometriosis tissue,[32] with the added benefit of amenorrhea, particularly with the depot injections and medicated intrauterine device (IUD) delivery systems.[33] Depot medroxyprogesterone acetate is a monthly injection that has been used in adolescents who have endometriosis as a method of treating pain symptoms, with the added benefit of being an effective contraceptive. Recently, a subcutaneous monthly formulation has been introduced that has comparable efficacy to the intramuscular injection but has less impact on bone mineralization.[34] Although the medicated IUD is not approved by the US Food and Drug Administration for the treatment of endometriosis, a Cochrane review suggested that this system does reduce painful periods in women who have had surgery for endometriosis; however, this review was based on one small study, and these researchers also comment on the need for further well-designed randomized controlled trials (RCTs) in this setting.[35] Of note, the ACOG, in a technical bulletin, supports the use of IUDs in the adolescent population.[36] Newer drugs available in experimental protocols in adults include aromatase inhibitors;[37] however, there are no data on the use of these medications in adolescents.

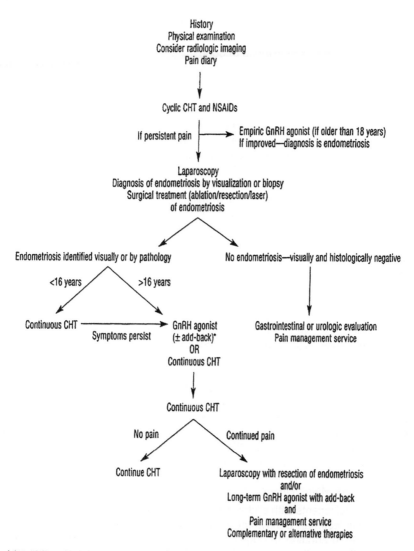

History
Physical examination
Consider radiologic imaging
Pain diary

Cyclic CHT and NSAIDs

If persistent pain → Empiric GnRH agonist (if older than 18 years)
If improved—diagnosis is endometriosis

Laparoscopy
Diagnosis of endometriosis by visualization or biopsy
Surgical treatment (ablation/resection/laser)
of endometriosis

Endometriosis identified visually or by pathology

No endometriosis—visually and histologically negative

<16 years / >16 years

Continuous CHT → GnRH agonist
Symptoms persist (± add-back)*
OR
Continuous CHT

Gastrointestinal or urologic evaluation
Pain management service

Continuous CHT

No pain / Continued pain

Continue CHT

Laparoscopy with resection of endometriosis
and/or
Long-term GnRH agonist with add-back
and
Pain management service
Complementary or alternative therapies

Abbreviations: NSAIDs, nonsteroidal antiinflammatory drugs; CHT, combination hormone therapy (oral contraceptive pills, estrogen/progestin patch, estrogen/progestin vaginal ring, norethindrone acetate, medroxyprogesterone acetate); GnRH, gonadotropin-releasing hormone.
*Add-back indicates use of estrogen and progestin or norethindrone acetate alone.

Fig. 1. Protocol for evaluation and treatment of adolescent pelvic pain and endometriosis. (*Modified from* Bandera CA, Brown LR, Laufer MR. Adolescents and endometriosis. Clin Consult Obstet Gynecol 1995;7:206; with permission.).

GnRH agonists have been shown to be effective in reducing pain associated with endometriosis.[38] They are effective by suppressing the hypothalamic pituitary axis, which results in a hypoestrogenic environment and side effects like hot flushes and mood changes. Empiric use of GnRH analogues has been advocated for adults with chronic pain, but they should not be used in adolescents younger than 18 years of age because of detrimental effects on bone density.[27] They may be used in adolescents as young as 16 years of age who have known endometriosis and are refractory to other medical therapies, with some special considerations. These include the use of add-back therapy, typically norethisterone acetate (5 mg/d), vitamin D, and calcium, along with appropriate monitoring of bone mineral density by means of age-matched z scores at least every 2 years.[27,39] These measures are aimed at maximizing the effect of GnRH analogues and minimizing the side effects.

Laparoscopic surgery remains the "gold standard" for the diagnosis of endometriosis. This is typically performed in adolescents who have pain symptoms refractory to medical treatment or if there is concern about a Müllerian anomaly. In looking for endometriosis in adolescents at the time of surgery, it is important to be aware that the disease is most commonly located in the cul-de-sac and is atypical in appearance.[40] Two RCTs in adults have established a relation between surgical intervention and reduction of pain in patients who have endometriosis. Sutton and colleagues[19] demonstrated a significant reduction in pain, lasting up to 6 months, in patients who underwent resection of their disease when compared with those who had diagnostic laparoscopy alone. Interestingly, these results were poorer for stage I disease than for stage III disease. Abbott and colleagues[41] confirmed these results and included quality-of-life measures, which were also improved at 6 months of follow-up. Whether such intervention changes the natural history of the disease or improves future reproductive potential in adolescents is unknown. In terms of long-term follow-up, Abbott and colleagues[42] have shown that the improvement in pain may last up to 5 years but that the risk for further intervention is higher with younger age and less aggressive surgical measures. Nerve ablation techniques, including presacral neurectomy and uterine nerve ablation techniques, have not been studied in the adolescent population.

Pre- and postoperative hormonal suppression generally have not been shown to be of benefit in terms of decreasing the number of patients with symptom recurrence over time.[43] There is a paucity of randomized trials in this area, however, and further research is needed. Recently, there has been a report of a significant reduction in endometrioma recurrence at 36 months in patients who take the OCP after surgery compared with those who do not.[44] Further studies, particularly RCTs, are required to confirm this finding, however. **Fig. 1** presents a protocol developed by the ACOG for the management of chronic pelvic pain and endometriosis in adolescents.[27]

Complimentary Management

In treating adolescents with endometriosis, it is important to realize than chronic pain is often multifactorial. Behavioral modification techniques, such as relaxation and biofeedback, in addition to cognitive therapy aimed at improving coping skills can be helpful. Physical therapy may also be helpful in patients in whom musculoskeletal conditions of the abdominal wall and pelvic floor are contributing to their symptoms.[45] Wayne and colleagues[46] have reported on a small RCT using Japanese acupuncture. A total of 18 patients were enrolled, and 14 completed the study treatments over 8 weeks. Pain was reduced in the treatment group, but there was no statistically significant difference between the groups after 4 weeks. Larger trials in this area are needed.

SUMMARY

The natural history of endometriosis remains largely unknown; therefore, it is difficult to determine whether early intervention in adolescents enhances future fertility or improves long-term disease outcome. The most immediate issue is a young woman in pain and a physician who needs to make a diagnosis and manage the symptoms. Laparoscopy remains the gold standard for establishing the diagnosis, and long-term control of symptoms in adolescents requires medical management, often in combination with complimentary therapies. Current research focused on the pathophysiology of endometriosis is likely to add to our understanding of the natural history of the disease, allowing future studies to better assess therapeutic outcomes in adolescents.

REFERENCES

1. Goldstein DP, De Cholnoky C, Emans SJ. Adolescent endometriosis. J Adolesc Health Care 1980;1(1):37–41.
2. Laufer MR, Goitein L, Bush M, et al. Prevalence of endometriosis in adolescent girls with chronic pelvic pain not responding to conventional therapy. J Pediatr Adolesc Gynecol 1997;10(4):199–202.
3. Gao X, Outley J, Botteman M, et al. Economic burden of endometriosis. Fertil Steril 2006;86(6):1561–72.
4. Sampson J. The development of the implantation theory for the origin of peritoneal endometriosis. Am J Obstet Gynecol 1940;40:549–57.
5. Sanfilippo JS, Wakim NG, Schikler KN, et al. Endometriosis in association with uterine anomaly. Am J Obstet Gynecol 1986;154(1):39–43.
6. Harada T, Kaponis A, Iwabe T, et al. Apoptosis in human endometrium and endometriosis. Hum Reprod Update 2004;10(1):29–38.
7. Osteen KG, Yeaman GR, Bruner-Tran KL. Matrix metalloproteinases and endometriosis. Semin Reprod Med 2003;21(2):155–64.
8. Di Carlo C, Bonifacio M, Tommaselli GA, et al. Metalloproteinases, vascular endothelial growth factor, and angiopoietin 1 and 2 in eutopic and ectopic endometrium. Fertil Steril 2008 Jul 19.
9. Bruner-Tran KL, Yeaman GR, Crispens MA, et al. Dioxin may promote inflammation-related development of endometriosis. Fertil Steril 2008;89(5 Suppl): 1287–98.
10. Montgomery GW, Nyholt DR, Zhao ZZ, et al. The search for genes contributing to endometriosis risk. Hum Reprod Update 2008;14(5):447–57.
11. Simpson JL, Elias S, Malinak LR, et al. Heritable aspects of endometriosis. I. Genetic studies. Am J Obstet Gynecol 1980;137(3):327–31.
12. Mettler L, Salmassi A, Schollmeyer T, et al. Comparison of c-DNA microarray analysis of gene expression between eutopic endometrium and ectopic endometrium (endometriosis). J Assist Reprod Genet 2007;24(6):249–58.
13. Wu Y, Halverson G, Basir Z, et al. Aberrant methylation at HOXA10 may be responsible for its aberrant expression in the endometrium of patients with endometriosis. Am J Obstet Gynecol 2005;193(2):371–80.
14. Nisolle M, Donnez J. Peritoneal endometriosis, ovarian endometriosis, and adenomyotic nodules of the rectovaginal septum are three different entities. Fertil Steril 1997;68(4):585–96.
15. Batt RE, Smith RA. Embryologic theory of histogenesis of endometriosis in peritoneal pockets. Obstet Gynecol Clin North Am 1989;16(1):15–28.
16. Marsh EE, Laufer MR. Endometriosis in premenarcheal girls who do not have an associated obstructive anomaly. Fertil Steril 2005;83(3):758–60.
17. Koninckx PR, Meuleman C, Demeyere S, et al. Suggestive evidence that pelvic endometriosis is a progressive disease, whereas deeply infiltrating endometriosis is associated with pelvic pain. Fertil Steril 1991;55(4):759–65.
18. Davis GD, Thillet E, Lindemann J. Clinical characteristics of adolescent endometriosis. J Adolesc Health 1993;14(5):362–8.

19. Sutton CJ, Ewen SP, Whitelaw N, et al. Prospective, randomized, double-blind, controlled trial of laser laparoscopy in the treatment of pelvic pain associated with minimal, mild, and moderate endometriosis. Fertil Steril 1994;62(4):696–700.

20. Wu MH, Shoji Y, Chuang PC, et al. Endometriosis: disease pathophysiology and the role of prostaglandins. Expert Rev Mol Med 2007;9(2):1–20.

21. Tokushige N, Markham R, Russell P, et al. Nerve fibres in peritoneal endometriosis. Hum Reprod 2006;21(11):3001–7.

22. Tokushige N, Markham R, Russell P, et al. Different types of small nerve fibers in eutopic endometrium and myometrium in women with endometriosis. Fertil Steril 2007;88(4):795–803.

23. Harel Z. Dysmenorrhea in adolescents and young adults: etiology and management. J Pediatr Adolesc Gynecol 2006;19(6):363–71.

24. Greene R, Stratton P, Cleary SD, et al. Diagnostic experience among 4,334 women reporting surgically diagnosed endometriosis. Fertil Steril 2008 Mar 24.

25. Schroeder B, Sanfilippo JS, Hertweck SP. Musculoskeletal pelvic pain in a pediatric and adolescent gynecology practice. J Pediatr Adolesc Gynecol 2000; 13(2):90.

26. Sinaii N, Cleary SD, Younes N, et al. Treatment utilization for endometriosis symptoms: a cross-sectional survey study of lifetime experience. Fertil Steril 2007; 87(6):1277–86.

27. ACOG Committee Opinion No. 310, April 2005. Endometriosis in adolescents. Obstet Gynecol 2005;105(4):921–7.

28. Roy SN, Bhattacharya S. Benefits and risks of pharmacological agents used for the treatment of menorrhagia. Drug Saf 2004;27(2):75–90.

29. Ozawa Y, Murakami T, Tamura M, et al. A selective cyclooxygenase-2 inhibitor suppresses the growth of endometriosis xenografts via antiangiogenic activity in severe combined immunodeficiency mice. Fertil Steril 2006;86(4 Suppl):1146–51.

30. Davis L, Kennedy SS, Moore J, et al. Modern combined oral contraceptives for pain associated with endometriosis. Cochrane Database Syst Rev 2007;(3): CD001019.

31. Prentice A, Deary AJ, Bland E. Progestagens and anti-progestagens for pain associated with endometriosis. Cochrane Database Syst Rev 2000;(2): CD002122.

32. Rodgers AK, Falcone T. Treatment strategies for endometriosis. Expert Opin Pharmacother 2008;9(2):243–55.

33. Vercellini P, Frontino G, De Giorgi O, et al. Comparison of a levonorgestrel-releasing intrauterine device versus expectant management after conservative surgery for symptomatic endometriosis: a pilot study. Fertil Steril 2003;80(2):305–9.

34. Schlaff WD, Carson SA, Luciano A, et al. Subcutaneous injection of depot medroxyprogesterone acetate compared with leuprolide acetate in the treatment of endometriosis-associated pain. Fertil Steril 2006;85(2):314–25.

35. Abou-Setta AM, Al-Inany HG, Farquhar CM. Levonorgestrel-releasing intrauterine device (LNG-IUD) for symptomatic endometriosis following surgery. Cochrane Database Syst Rev 2006;(4):CD005072.

36. ACOG Committee Opinion No. 392, December 2007. Intrauterine device and adolescents. Obstet Gynecol 2007;110(6):1493–5.

37. ACOG Committee Opinion. Aromatase inhibitors in gynecologic practice. Obstet Gynecol 2008;112(2 Pt 1):405–7.

38. Dlugi AM, Miller JD, Knittle J. Lupron depot (leuprolide acetate for depot suspension) in the treatment of endometriosis: a randomized, placebo-controlled, double-blind study. Lupron Study Group. Fertil Steril 1990;54(3):419–27.

39. Laufer MR. Current approaches to optimizing the treatment of endometriosis in adolescents. Gynecol Obstet Invest 2008;66(Suppl 1):19–27.
40. Laufer MR. Identification of clear vesicular lesions of atypical endometriosis: a new technique. Fertil Steril 1997;68(4):739–40.
41. Abbott J, Hawe J, Hunter D, et al. Laparoscopic excision of endometriosis: a randomized, placebo-controlled trial. Fertil Steril 2004;82(4):878–84.
42. Abbott JA, Hawe J, Clayton RD, et al. The effects and effectiveness of laparoscopic excision of endometriosis: a prospective study with 2–5 year follow-up. Hum Reprod 2003;18(9):1922–7.
43. Yap C, Furness S, Farquhar C. Pre and post operative medical therapy for endometriosis surgery. Cochrane Database Syst Rev 2004;(3):CD003678.
44. Vercellini P, Somigliana E, Daguati R, et al. Postoperative oral contraceptive exposure and risk of endometrioma recurrence. Am J Obstet Gynecol 2008; 198(5):504 e1–e5.
45. Greco CD. Management of adolescent chronic pelvic pain from endometriosis: a pain center perspective. J Pediatr Adolesc Gynecol 2003;16(3 Suppl):S17–9.
46. Wayne PM, Kerr CE, Schnyer RN, et al. Japanese-style acupuncture for endometriosis-related pelvic pain in adolescents and young women: results of a randomized sham-controlled trial. J Pediatr Adolesc Gynecol 2008;21(5):247–57.

Postscript:

The following article is an addition to
Colposcopy, Cervical Screening, and HPV,
the December 2008 issue of *Obstetrics and
Gynecology Clinics of North America*
(Volume 35, Issue 4)

The Epidemiology of Anal Human Papillomavirus and Related Neoplasia

Joel M. Palefsky, MD[a,b,c,]*, Mary Rubin, PhD, NP[b,d]

KEYWORDS

- Anal cytology • Human papillomavirus (HPV)
- High resolution anoscopy (HRA) • Geriatric • Management

The relationship between cervical cancer and human papillomavirus (HPV) is well known. Cervical cancer remains one of the most common cancers among women worldwide, resulting in approximately 275,000 deaths per year globally.[1] In developed countries the incidence of cervical cancer has been reduced through screening for the cervical cancer precursor, high-grade cervical intraepithelial neoplasia (CIN), and removal of the lesion before it progresses to cancer. The advent of an effective vaccine against HPV 16 and HPV 18, which together account for approximately 70% of cervical cancers, offers another new approach to reducing the incidence of cervical cancer.

In addition to cervical cancer, several other cancers are known to be associated with HPV, and the HPV vaccine has focused new attention on the role that HPV vaccination may play in their prevention. These include cancers of the penis, oropharynx, vulva, vagina, and anus.[2] Among these, cancers of the oropharynx[3] and anus stand out for their increasing incidence.[4] Both of these cancers occur among men and women. Unlike oral cancer, anal cancer in the general population is more common

This work was supported by the National Cancer Institute (R01 CA 88739 and R01 CA 085178), NIH/NCRR UCSF-CTSI Grant Number UL1 RR02413,1 and the American Cancer Society (Grant SPRSG-03-242-01).

This article was originally planned to appear in the December 2008 issue of Obstetrics and Gynecology Clinics of North America.

[a] Division of Infectious Disease, Department of Medicine, University of California, Box 0126, Room M1203, San Francisco, CA 94143, USA

[b] Anal Neoplasia Clinic, University of California Helen Diller Family Comprehensive Cancer Center, San Francisco, CA, USA

[c] Clinical and Translational Research School of Medicine, CA, USA

[d] School of Nursing, University of California, San Francisco, CA, USA

* Corresponding author. Division of Infectious disease, Department of Medicine, University of California, Box 0126, Room M1203, San Francisco, CA 94143.

E-mail address: joel.palefsky@ucsf.edu (J. M. Palefsky).

among women than among men. However, the epidemiology of anal cancer is particularly distinctive in that the risk is particularly high in certain risk groups, including those with HIV-related and transplant-related immunosuppression. Like cervical cancer, anal cancer is preceded by a series of precancerous changes, ie, anal intraepithelial neoplasia, raising the possibility that like cervical cancer, anal can be prevented. Further, given the known risk factors for anal cancer, prevention efforts could be targeted to high-risk groups, providing a unique example of a screening program targeted to high-risk individuals. This article describes the epidemiology of anal HPV infection, anal intraepithelial neoplasia (AIN), and anal cancer among men and women, as well as current efforts to prevent anal cancers.

EPIDEMIOLOGY OF ANAL CANCER

The incidence of anal cancer in the population continues to grow.[4] In contrast, the incidence of cervical cancer has steadily declined over the past 40 years. According to data from the American Cancer Society, an estimated 5070 new cases will occur in 2008, including 3050 women and 2020 men, and 690 persons will die of anal cancer.[5] This is in comparison to 11,070 new cases of cervical cancer with 3870 deaths estimated to occur in 2008.

The incidence of anal cancer is relatively uncommon in the general population. Between 1973 and 1979, rates of anal cancer were lower for men than for women (1.06 per 100,000 compared with 1.39 per 100,000). However, between 1994 and 2000 rates were similar for men and women (2.04 per 100,000 and 2.06 per 100,000 respectively) and increased for both genders.[6]

Risk factors for anal cancer include a history of smoking, history of condyloma (reflecting exposure to HPV), and history of anal intercourse, reflecting acquisition of HPV in the anal canal.[7,8] Given these risk factors, it is not surprising that a history of having sex with men is an important risk factor for anal cancer among men.[7,9] Before the AIDS epidemic in 1982, the incidence of anal cancer among men who have sex with men (MSM) was estimated to be between 12.5 and 36.9 per 100,000, a figure that is nearly as high as the incidence of cervical cancer in the general population of women before the introduction of cervical cytology screening.

The onset of the HIV epidemic heralded two successive eras of increased risk of anal cancer among MSM. The first corresponds to the years before the advent of highly active antiretroviral (ART) therapy for HIV when HIV-positive men and women were immunosuppressed and usually died of an HIV-related complication. Despite their relatively short lifespan after onset of HIV-related immunosuppression, the incidence of anal cancer among HIV-positive MSM was estimated to be double that of HIV-negative MSM.[10–12] One study matching cancer databases to AIDS databases, the relative risk of developing anal cancer among HIV-positive men with a history of homosexual contact was 59.5.[13] In that same report, the relative risk for anal cancer was 6.8 (2.7–14.0) in HIV-positive women compared with the general population of women.

In the general population of San Francisco, the incidence of anal cancer increased in men aged 40 to 64 from 3.7 in 1973 to 1978 to 20.6 per 100,000 in 1996 to 1999.[14] These data likely reflecting the large proportion of MSM and the large number of HIV-positive men living in San Francisco, because similar increases were not demonstrated in any other counties in California.

The second era corresponds to the widespread availability of ART, with increased lifespan among HIV-positive men and women. Although one study did not show an increase in the incidence of anal cancer in the post-ART era among HIV-positive

MSM,[15] three recent studies did show an increase, with an annual incidence rate of 75/100,000 137/100,000, and 78/100,00 respectively.[13,16,17] These numbers may reflect the presence of a longer lifespan among at-risk individuals, allowing anal cancer precursors more time to progress to cancer in the absence of systematic programs to screen and treat these lesions.

Other groups at increased risk include patients who are chronically immunosuppressed because of causes other than HIV, including taking medications to treat autoimmune disorders and other illnesses, as well as organ transplant recipients.[18–20]

Women with a history of vulvar cancer, high-grade vulvar intraepithelial neoplasia,[21] and cervical cancer[22] are also at increased risk, presumably because of increased risk of exposure to HPV in the anal region.

EPIDEMIOLOGY OF ANAL HUMAN PAPILLOMAVIRUS INFECTION

There is biologic similarity between the cervix and the anus with respect to the preferred location of HPV infection; the transformation zone of the cervix is the target area for HPV where there is transition between two types of epithelium. In the cervix this is where the squamous epithelium on the exocervix meets the columnar epithelium on the endocervical canal. In the anus, this is where the squamous epithelium of the anus meets the columnar epithelium of the rectum.

In contrast to the age-related prevalence of cervical HPV infection in women, which declines after the age of 30 years,[23] anal HPV in HIV-negative MSM remains high (50% to 60%) and is constant throughout life.[24] Although this may reflect differences between the biology of the anal canal and the cervix, it more likely is a result of the acquisition of new HPV types from a higher number of new sexual partners over time among MSM compared with women. Among HIV-positive men, anal HPV infection is nearly universal.[25,26] The primary risk factors for anal HPV infection are lower CD4+ level, and among HIV-negative men risk factors included history of receptive anal intercourse and higher number of sexual partners.[24]

A somewhat surprising finding in recent years is that in some populations of women, the prevalence of anal HPV is actually higher than the prevalence of cervical HPV infection. This was shown in the Women's Interagency HIV Study among HIV-positive women and women at high risk of HIV infection, as well as other similar populations.[27–29] Anal HPV infection was also found to be as common as cervical HPV infection in a population of healthy Hawaiian women.[30] Overall, the distribution of HPV types in the anal canal is similar to that of the cervix, but individual women do not necessarily have concurrent infection with same HPV types. Risk factors among women include HIV positivity, lower CD4+ level, cervical HPV infection, and younger age.[28] Together these data indicate that anal HPV infection is more common than has been appreciated in the past. The clinical consequences of anal HPV infection in women include the development of anal cancer and potentially spread of HPV to the cervix. It is also clear that the anus must be less biologically susceptible to cancer development than the cervix since the incidence of anal cancer per anal HPV infection is likely lower than that of cervical cancer per cervical HPV infection.

EPIDEMIOLOGY OF ANAL INTRAEPITHELIAL NEOPLASIA

The histopathologic classification of AIN 1, 2, and 3 corresponds to CIN 1, 2, and 3. Well-understood cervical cytology and histology classifications are also used for anal disease, although in the anus, squamous intraepithelial lesions (SIL) are often called anal intraepithelial neoplasia (AIN) grades I, II, and III. Low-grade AIN includes AIN 1 and condyloma whereas high-grade AIN includes AIN 2 and AIN 3. Although there are no large population-based studies showing direct progression of an AIN 2–3 lesion to anal cancer, several studies of smaller groups of patients demonstrate the oncogenic potential of AIN 2–3.[31–33] Among HIV-negative MSM, the age-related prevalence of abnormal cytology mirrors that of anal HPV infection in that the age-related prevalence is flat between the ages of 25 and 60 years. In one study, 18% to 23% of MSM had AIN on anal cytology after the age of 20 with 5% to 10% having AIN 2–3. These numbers underestimate the true prevalence of AIN because, like cervical cytology, anal cytology is relatively insensitive.[34]

The prevalence of AIN is higher among HIV-positive MSM than among HIV-negative MSM.[35,36] In one study performed after the introduction of ART, the prevalence of high-grade AIN was over 50% among HIV-positive MSM.[35] Additionally, the incidence of AIN 2–3 is higher among HIV-positive MSM compared with HIV-negative MSM.[37,38]

Data have now been accumulating regarding the effect of ART on the natural history of AIN, and the evidence to date suggests that there is limited or no benefit for reduction of high-grade disease and cancer. In studies examining CIN, ART seems to have little or no effect on regression of CIN 2–3.[39] None of the studies show that HPV is eradicated from the cervix; there is neither a regression nor a lower incidence of high-grade AIN.[23]

There are relatively few data on the prevalence and incidence of AIN in women. In one of the earliest studies, abnormal anal cytology was found in 26% of HIV-positive women and 8% of high-risk HIV-negative women.[26] Risk factors among HIV-positive women included anal intercourse and abnormal cervical cytology, consistent with the relationship between anal and cervical HPV infection. In a more recent, larger study, AIN was found in 21% of HIV-positive women and 6% of high-risk HIV-negative women.[40] Among HIV-infected women, risk factors for AIN 1/condyloma were younger age, history of receptive anal intercourse, anal HPV, and cervical HPV infection. In multivariable analyses among HIV-infected women, the only significant risk factor for AIN 2–3 was anal HPV infection. The same HPV types associated with high grade disease in the cervix are found in association with high-grade AIN, with HPV 16 responsible for most high-grade AIN as well as anal cancer.[41]

SCREENING FOR ANAL INTRAEPITHELIAL NEOPLASIA AND ANAL CANCER

It is clear that patients who are HIV-positive and other immunosuppressed individuals are at increased risk to develop anal cancer, as are MSM and HIV-negative women with a history of anal intercourse and/or other HPV-related anogenital malignancies. Given the high prevalence and incidence of anal HPV infection and high-grade AIN in these populations, as well as the demonstrated potential of high-grade AIN (HG-AIN) to progress to anal cancer, the authors and others have suggested that these groups be considered for screening to identify and treat HG-AIN. United States Public Health Service and Infectious Disease Society of America guidelines have not recommended routine screening because studies to demonstrate that treatment of high-grade AIN prevents cancer have not yet been done. Instead, they cite expert opinion to indicate that some experts in the field believe that screening may be warranted.[42] Other professional societies, such as the New York State Department of Public Health recommend routine anal cytology screening for HIV-positive men and women (http://www.hivguidelines.org/GuideLine.aspx?PageID=257&GuideLineID=22#V.%20ANAL%20DYSPLASIA%20AND%20CANCER).[43]

Before establishing an anal cytology screening program, the authors recommend that each of the following components be in place: (1) clinicians trained to perform anal cytology; (2) clinicians trained to perform high-resolution anoscopy (HRA) and

HRA-guided anal biopsy; (3) pathologists trained to interpret anal cytology and pathology; (4) clinicians trained to treat AIN in the office; and (5) anal surgeons trained to treat AIN in the operating room and complications of anal diagnostic and treatment procedures. Anal cytology screening has been shown to be cost effective among both HIV-positive and HIV-negative MSM; studies have not yet been done in women or other risk groups.[44,45]

It is also important to understand the role of digital rectal examinations (DRE). DRE is a test that clinicians, even those without any special training, should consider for all at-risk patients, at least annually. The purpose of DRE is to feel for masses consistent with cancer, and DRE is thus considered to be an anal cancer screening test. Conversely, anal cytology and HRA-guided biopsy are primarily aimed at detecting AIN, and are thus focused instead on prevention of anal cancer; the latter should be performed only by trained clinicians. The authors therefore recommend that people at increased risk of anal cancer have regular and careful DRE, and, in settings where the infrastructure described above is in place, anal cytology screening and HRA. Patients with any symptoms or abnormalities suspicious for cancer, including otherwise unexplained anal pain or bleeding, rapid growth of a lesion, and inguinal adenopathy, should be referred to clinicians experienced in managing anorectal problems for assessment and biopsy.

The anus is composed of squamous epithelium. The rectum or colon is columnar epithelium. The anal canal is mucosa lined and the anal margin is epidermal. The proximal end of the anal canal begins at the junction of the levator ani muscle and external anal sphincter and extends to the anal verge. It is 2 to 4 cm in length, and is shorter in women compared with men. The dentate line is approximately equivalent to the original squamocolumnar junction (SCJ) in colposcopic terminology and is considered to be a "fixed" anatomic zone, whereas the anal transformation zone (AnTZ) is dynamic and undergoing squamous metaplasia. The AnTZ is the current SCJ. The anal margin begins at the verge and represents the transition from mucosal to epidermal epithelium and extends to the perianal skin. By consensus, perianal skin is considered to extend approximately 5 cm from the anal margin. Areas for screening include the SCJ, AnTZ, anal canal, verge, margin, and perianal skin. Thorough evaluation with HRA for warts and perianal intraepithelial neoplasia is also recommended.

Screening procedures used for the cervix, including cytology and colposcopy, have been modified for screening of AIN. Sensitivity and specificity of anal cytology are similar to cervical cytology and liquid-based cytology has been shown to improve quality of samples.[46] Colposcopy of the anal canal is called HRA. Colposcopy techniques, including use of Lugol's solution, and terminology have been validated for anal canal disease.[47]

ANAL SCREENING ALGORITHMS

Different screening algorithms may be used. The one used at the University of California San Francisco Anal Neoplasia Clinic is shown in **Fig. 1**. In settings where there is a sufficient number of trained anoscopists, high-risk patients could be considered for direct referral to HRA instead of undergoing anal cytology screening, given their very high risk of AIN. Although there are still a limited number of centers with trained individuals who perform HRA, it is becoming more routine in many areas of the country for those high-risk individuals with abnormal anal cytology to undergo HRA. Some primary care clinicians who care for immunocompromised patients refer patients with a history of genital warts, irrespective of abnormal cytology.

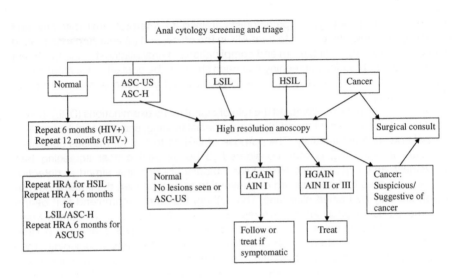

Fig. 1. Algorithm for anal cytology and high-resolution anoscopy.

The role of HPV testing is not yet clear; given the high prevalence of anal HPV infection in high-risk populations, it is unlikely that anal HPV testing will add significant positive predictive value when used alone or in conjunction with cervical cytology. It is possible that anal HPV testing might provide negative predictive value if the HPV test is negative, and in low-risk populations, it is possible that a positive anal HPV test might provide useful positive predictive value. Further research is needed in each of these areas.

PERFORMING ANAL CYTOLOGY

These features of the anal canal lend themselves well to securing an anal cytology specimen. The steps to securing an adequate sample are as follows:

1. The anal cytology specimen should be performed before any other procedures to provide the highest yield of cells.
2. There must be no lubrication before obtaining a cytology sample because the lubricant may interfere with the processing and interpretation of the sample.
3. Gently separate the buttocks; the patient can hold their right cheek to facilitate view.
4. Insert a moistened Dacron swab as far into the anus as possible, approximately 3 to 4 cm, to ensure sampling of cells from the AnTZ. The swab should be inserted until it reaches the wall of the rectum. If initial resistance is encountered, change position of swab and re-insert.

5. Remove swab in a circular motion to sample cells from all aspects of the anal canal. Apply pressure so that the swab bends while slowly removing it. Count slowly to 10 as you remove it.
6. Preserve quickly on slides or in liquid medium. Fewer cells exfoliate from the anal canal than the cervix and it is easier to get air-dried artifacts.

PERFORMING A HIGH-RESOLUTION ANOSCOPY

1. Obtain relevant history including current anal symptoms such as pruritis, bleeding, and pain. Determine prior history of anal or perianal condyloma and whether treatments were surgical or office-based. Determine prior history of any anal abnormalities such as fissures, fistula, abscesses, or hemorrhoids requiring intervention. Determine any prior treatments that may have caused scarring or other alterations in the normal anal mucosa such as abscess lancing, fistula repairs, or hemorrhoidectomies.
2. Consent patient with explanation of procedures to be performed.
3. Assist the patient into one of the following positions:
   - Left Lateral
   - Lithotomy can be used if also performing cervical examination but most women prefer to switch to left lateral for the HRA
   - Prone (if overhead colposcope is available)

   In the left lateral and prone positions, patients should be as close to the bottom edge of the table as possible to facilitate focusing the colposcope.
4. Be clear and consistent in describing location of lesions and the position used. The "anal clock" is different than the "gynecologic clock." The coccyx is 12:00, regardless of the position used to examine the patient. When referring patients for follow-up to anal surgeons it is helpful to use anatomic descriptors (posterior, anterior, left or right lateral) in place of or in addition to the "clock" positions.
5. Obtain cytology specimen if needed (new patients or those referred with abnormal cytology specimens >3 months old).
6. Lubricate the anal canal with KY jelly mixed with 1% to 5% lidocaine.
7. Perform DRE: palpate for warts, masses, ulcerations, fissures, and focal areas of discomfort or pain. The presence of hard and fixed lesions should increase the index of suspicion for cancer because these are not the usual presentation of hemorrhoids and warts.
8. Insert anoscope, remove obturator, and insert Q-tip wrapped in gauze, which has been soaked in 3% acetic acid. Remove anoscope leaving the Q-tip wrapped gauze pad inside. Soak for 1 to 2 minutes.
9. Remove gauze and re-insert anoscope.
10. Observe through colposcope while slowly removing the anoscope until the anal transformation zone (AnTZ) comes into focus.
11. Continue to apply acetic acid with scopettes or Q-tips during the examination. Using Q-tips to manipulate folds, hemorrhoids, or prolapsing mucosa as well as adjusting the anoscope will help to view all aspects of the AnTZ. In most cases, the entire AnTZ should be seen and the examination will be considered satisfactory. Continue withdrawing the anoscope until the entire canal has been observed.
12. Biopsies
    - Biopsies are directed at areas thought to represent the highest grade of abnormality.
    - Anal biopsies should be smaller than those typically taken of the cervix using forceps no larger than 2 to 3 mm.

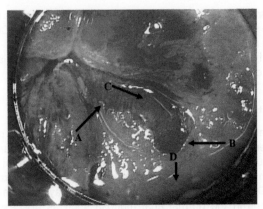

Fig. 2. Normal squamocolumnar junction (*arrows A and B*); columnar epithelium of the colon (*arrow C*); squamous epithelium of the anus (*arrow D*); no lesions seen.

- Internal biopsies do not require anesthesia. External biopsies require injecting a small amount of 1% lidocaine with epinephrine buffered with sodium bicarbonate (2 mL $NaHCO_3$: 10 mL lidocaine) similar to biopsies of the vulva. The injection can be preceded by numbing topically with lidocaine gel or spray.
- Monsel's solution or silver nitrate is used for hemostasis, although the pressure of the anal walls will generally stop bleeding for internal biopsies.

HRA can reveal the wide range of cellular and vascular changes associated with cytologic abnormality. **Figs. 2 to 10** demonstrate changes from normal to cancer.

TREATMENT MODALITIES

Once AIN has been diagnosed with HRA and biopsy, treatment planning begins. With low-grade AIN the choices range from follow-up without treatment at 6-month intervals to chemical treatment of warts and flat lesions with bichloroacetic acid or trichloroacetic acid (TCA). This is effective for small lesions, typically limited in number but requires multiple applications. External condyloma may also be treated with imiquimod, podophyllotoxin, and 15% sinecatechins ointment (green tea extract).

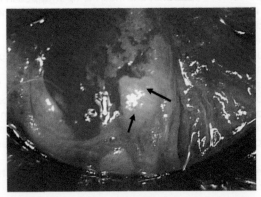

Fig. 3. Low-grade AIN with acetowhite epithelium from 6 o'clock to 9 o'clock at the squamocolumnar.

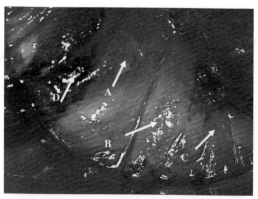

Fig. 4. LGAIN with areas of partial Lugol's staining (*arrow A*) or no staining (*arrows B* and *C*); Lugol's staining consistent with normal anal tissue (*arrow D*).

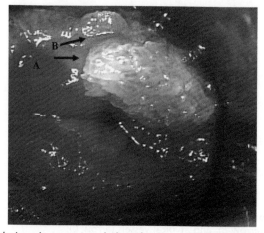

Fig. 5. Focal warty lesions (*arrows A* and *B*) at the squamocolumnar junction.

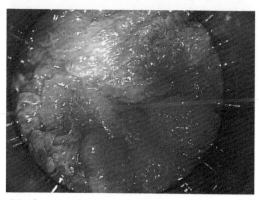

Fig. 6. Warty lesions 360 degrees obscuring the squamocolumnar junction.

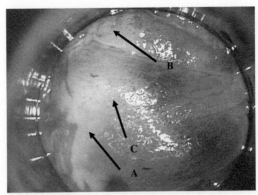

Fig. 7. Large high-grade AIN lesion acetowhite epithelium (*arrows A* and *B*), punctation (*arrow C*).

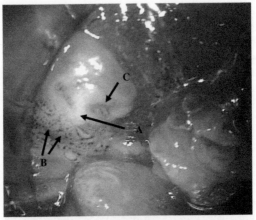

Fig. 8. Early invasion: nodular lesion with acetowhite epithelium background (*arrow A*), coarse punctation (*arrow B*), and atypical vessels (*arrow C*).

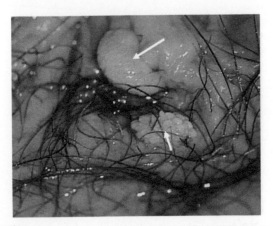

Fig. 9. Peri-anal warts.

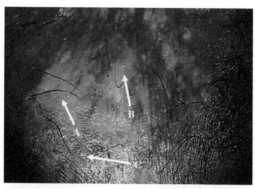

Fig. 10. Peri-anal high-grade anal intraepithelial neoplasia: partially denuded epithelium (*arrow A*), acetowhite epithelium (*arrow B*), and hyperpigmented epithelium (*arrow C*).

None of these products are approved for intra-anal use. Cryotherapy is used primarily for external disease and like TCA often requires more than one treatment.

Infrared coagulation (IRC) can be used for intra-anal or peri-anal low-grade AIN or high-grade AIN. Symptoms and extent of the disease help to dictate which treatment might be most appropriate and effective. Recent studies show that about two thirds of HIV-positive patients with high-grade AIN can be successfully treated after 1 year of follow-up.[29,48] Electrocautery and laser therapy are also options for intra-anal disease. Surgery is reserved for patients undergoing examination under anesthesia where biopsies to rule out cancer are not possible in the office, and to treat extensive AIN. Recent surgical data show improved outcomes compared with earlier surgical experience.[49]

SUMMARY

With the advent of the HPV vaccine, increased attention is being paid to cancers associated with HPV in addition to cervical cancer. Because of its strong association with HPV 16, the vaccines currently approved for use to prevent cervical cancer may well prevent anal cancer as well; however, results from studies to determine their efficacy to prevent anal HPV infection and AIN are not yet available. Further, if these vaccines do work to prevent anal HPV infection and disease, it will be necessary to reexamine vaccination strategies, because vaccination of boys will be necessary to prevent spread of HPV among high-risk groups such as MSM.

Regardless of whether these vaccines prevent anal HPV infection and AIN, they are designed to be preventative and will likely not help individuals who already have anal HPV infection and AIN owing to HPV types in the vaccine. For these individuals, screening and treatment of high-grade AIN may be the only way to prevent development of anal cancer, but studies to demonstrate the efficacy of this approach have not yet been done. A critical question is how to best care for at-risk men and women until all of the study results are available. The approach of the authors is to screen and treat high-risk individuals with high-grade AIN until those results are available, based on the assumption that the cervical model of prevention is valid. However, there is divergence of opinion on the best approach at this time and not all centers have the infrastructure to screen and treat appropriately; in these settings, at a minimum, clinicians should be vigilant for anal cancer and perform routine visual inspection and DRE. This is especially true for clinicians caring for men and women immunosuppressed because of HIV or other causes; men who have sex with men; and women with a history of cervical or vulvar cancer.

ACKNOWLEDGMENTS

The authors gratefully acknowledge the support and contributions from Dr. J. Michael Berry and Dr. Naomi Jay.

REFERENCES

1. Schiffman M, Castle PE, Jeronimo J, et al. Human papillomavirus and cervical cancer. Lancet 2007;370:890–907.
2. Human papillomavirus. IARC Monogr Eval Carcinog Risks Hum 2007;90:1–36.
3. Chaturvedi AK, Engels EA, Anderson WF, et al. Incidence trends for human papillomavirus-related and -unrelated oral squamous cell carcinomas in the United States. J Clin Oncol 2008;26:612–9.
4. Joseph D, Miller J, Wu X, et al. Understanding the burden of human papillomavirus-associated anal cancers in the US. Cancer 2008;113:2892–900.
5. American Cancer Society. Available at: http://www.cancer.org/docroot/CRI/content/CRI_2_4_1X_What_are_the_key_statistics_for_Anal_Cancer_47.asp?sitearea=. Accessed November 28, 2008.
6. Johnson LG, Madeleine MM, Newcomer LM, et al. Anal cancer incidence and survival: the surveillance, epidemiology and end results experience 1973-2000. Cancer 2004;101:281–8.
7. Daling JR, Madeleine MM, Johnson LG, et al. Human papillomavirus, smoking, and sexual practices in the etiology of anal cancer. Cancer 2004;101:270–80.
8. Holly EA, Whittemore AS, Aston DA, et al. Anal cancer incidence: genital warts, anal fissure or fistula, hemorrhoids, and smoking. J Natl Cancer Inst 1989;81:1726–31.
9. Daling JR, Weiss NS, Hislop TG, et al. Sexual practices, sexually transmitted diseases, and the incidence of anal cancer. N Engl J Med 1987;317:973–7.
10. Frisch M, Biggar RJ, Engels EA, et al. Association of cancer with AIDS-related immunosuppression in adults. JAMA 2001;285:1736–45.
11. Frisch M, Biggar RJ, Goedert JJ. Human papillomavirus-associated cancers in patients with human immunodeficiency virus infection and acquired immunodeficiency syndrome. J Natl Cancer Inst 2000;92:1500–10.
12. Goedert JJ, Cote TR, Virgo P, et al. Spectrum of AIDS-associated malignant disorders. Lancet 1998;351:1833–9.
13. Patel P, Hanson DL, Sullivan PS, et al. Incidence of types of cancer among HIV-infected persons compared with the general population in the United States, 1992-2003. Ann Intern Med 2008;148:728–36.
14. Cress RD, Holly EA. Incidence of anal cancer in California: increased incidence among men in San Francisco, 1973–1999. Prev Med 2003;36:555–60.
15. Engels EA, Biggar RJ, Hall HI, et al. Cancer risk in people infected with human immunodeficiency virus in the United States. Int J Cancer 2008;123:187–94.
16. D'Souza G, Wiley DJ, Li X, et al. Incidence and epidemiology of anal cancer in the multicenter AIDS Cohort Study. J Acquir Immune Defic Syndr 2008;48:491–9.
17. Piketty C, Selinger-Leneman H, Grabar S, et al. Marked increase in the incidence of invasive anal cancer among HIV-infected patients despite treatment with combination antiretroviral therapy. AIDS 2008;22:1203–11.
18. Adami J, Gabel H, Lindelof B, et al. Cancer risk following organ transplantation: a nationwide cohort study in Sweden. Br J Cancer 2003;89:1221–7.

19. Ogunbiyi OA, Scholefield JH, Raftery AT, et al. Prevalence of anal human papillomavirus infection and intraepithelial neoplasia in renal allograft recipients. Br J Surg 1994;81:365–7.

20. Patel HS, Silver AR, Northover JM. Anal cancer in renal transplant patients. Int J Colorectal Dis 2005;22:1–5.

21. Ogunbiyi OA, Scholefield JH, Robertson G, et al. Anal human papillomavirus infection and squamous neoplasia in patients with invasive vulvar cancer. Obstet Gynecol 1994;83:212–6.

22. Melbye M, Sprogel P. Aetiological parallel between anal cancer and cervical cancer. Lancet 1991;338:657–9.

23. Schiffman MH. Recent progress in defining the epidemiology of human papillomavirus infection and cervical neoplasia. J Natl Cancer Inst 1992;84:394–8.

24. Chin-Hong PV, Vittinghoff E, Cranston RD, et al. Age-related prevalence of anal cancer precursors in homosexual men: the EXPLORE study. J Natl Cancer Inst 2005;97:896–905.

25. Critchlow CW, Holmes KK, Wood R, et al. Association of human immunodeficiency virus and anal human papillomavirus infection among homosexual men. Arch Intern Med 1992;152:1673–6.

26. Palefsky JM, Holly EA, Ralston ML, et al. Prevalence and risk factors for human papillomavirus infection of the anal canal in human immunodeficiency virus (HIV)-positive and HIV-negative homosexual men. J Infect Dis 1998;177:361–7.

27. Melbye M, Smith E, Wohlfahrt J, et al. Anal and cervical abnormality in women—prediction by human papillomavirus tests. Int J Cancer 1996;68:559–64.

28. Palefsky JM, Holly EA, Ralston ML, et al. Prevalence and risk factors for anal human papillomavirus infection in human immunodeficiency virus (HIV)-positive and high-risk HIV-negative women. J Infect Dis 2001;183:383–91.

29. Williams AB, Darragh TM, Vranizan K, et al. Anal and cervical human papillomavirus infection and risk of anal and cervical epithelial abnormalities in human immunodeficiency virus-infected women. Obstet Gynecol 1994;83:205–11.

30. Hernandez BY, McDuffie K, Zhu X, et al. Anal human papillomavirus infection in women and its relationship with cervical infection. Cancer Epidemiol Biomarkers Prev 2005;14:2550–6.

31. Rickert RR, Brodkin RH, Hutter RV. Bowen's disease. CA Cancer J Clin 1977;27:160–6.

32. Scholefield JH, Castle MT, Watson NF. Malignant transformation of high-grade anal intraepithelial neoplasia. Br J Surg 2005;92:1133–6.

33. Watson AJ, Smith BB, Whitehead MR, et al. Malignant progression of anal intraepithelial neoplasia. ANZ J Surg 2006;76:715–7.

34. Palefsky JM, Holly EA, Hogeboom CJ, et al. Anal cytology as a screening tool for anal squamous intraepithelial lesions. J Acquir Immune Defic Syndr 1997;14:415–22.

35. Palefsky JM, Holly EA, Efird JT, et al. Anal intraepithelial neoplasia in the highly active antiretroviral therapy era among HIV-positive men who have sex with men. AIDS 2005;19:1407–14.

36. Palefsky JM, Holly EA, Ralston ML, et al. Anal squamous intraepithelial lesions in HIV-positive and HIV-negative homosexual and bisexual men: prevalence and risk factors. J Acquir Immune Defic Syndr Hum Retrovirol 1998;17:320–6.

37. Critchlow CW, Surawicz CM, Holmes KK, et al. Prospective study of high grade anal squamous intraepithelial neoplasia in a cohort of homosexual men: influence of HIV infection, immunosuppression and human papillomavirus infection. AIDS 1995;9:1255–62.

38. Palefsky JM, Holly EA, Ralston ML, et al. High incidence of anal high-grade squamous intraepithelial lesions among HIV-positive and HIV-negative homosexual/bisexual men. AIDS 1998;12:495–503.
39. Heard I, Palefsky JM, Kazatchkine MD. The impact of HIV antiviral therapy on human papillomavirus (HPV) infections and HPV-related diseases. Antivir Ther 2004;9:13–22.
40. Hessol N, Holly E, Efird J, et al. Anal intraepithelial neoplasia in a multisite study of HIV-infected and high-risk HIV-uninfected women. AIDS 2009;23:59–70.
41. Frisch M, Fenger C, van den Brule AJ, et al. Variants of squamous cell carcinoma of the anal canal and perianal skin and their relation to human papillomaviruses. Cancer Res 1999;59:753–7.
42. Guidelines for prevention and treatment of opportunistic infections in HIV-infected adults and adolescents recommendations from CDC, the National Institutes of Health, and the HIV Medicine Association of the Infectious Diseases Society of America. MMWR Recomm Rep 2008;57.
43. New York State Department of Public Health. Available at: http://www.hivguidelines.org/GuideLine.aspx?PageID=257&GuideLineID=22#V.%20ANAL%20DYSPLASIA%20AND%20CANCER. Accessed November 27, 2008.
44. Goldie SJ, Kuntz KM, Weinstein MC, et al. Cost-effectiveness of screening for anal squamous intraepithelial lesions and anal cancer in human immunodeficiency virus-negative homosexual and bisexual men. Am J Med 2000;108:634–41.
45. Goldie SJ, Kuntz KM, Weinstein MC, et al. The clinical effectiveness and cost-effectiveness of screening for anal squamous intraepithelial lesions in homosexual and bisexual HIV-positive men. JAMA 1999;281:1822–9.
46. Darragh TM, Jay N, Tupkelewicz BA, et al. Comparison of conventional cytologic smears and ThinPrep preparations from the anal canal. Acta Cytol 1997;41:1167–70.
47. Jay N, Holly EA, Berry M, et al. Colposcopic correlates of anal squamous intraepithelial lesions. Dis Colon Rectum 1997;40:919–28.
48. Goldstone SE, Hundert JS, Huyett JW. Infrared coagulator ablation of high-grade anal squamous intraepithelial lesions in HIV-negative males who have sex with males. Dis Colon Rectum 2007;50:565–75.
49. Chang GJ, Berry JM, Jay N, et al. Surgical treatment of high-grade anal squamous intraepithelial lesions: a prospective study. Dis Colon Rectum 2002;45:453–8.

Index

Note: Page numbers of article titles are in **boldface** type.

Obstet Gynecol Clin N Am 36 (2009) 201–212
doi:10.1016/S0889-8545(09)00018-7
0889-8545/09/$ – see front matter © 2009 Elsevier Inc. All rights reserved.

obgyn.theclinics.com

Moving?

Make sure your subscription moves with you!

To notify us of your new address, find your **Clinics Account Number** (located on your mailing label above your name), and contact customer service at:

E-mail: elspcs@elsevier.com

800-654-2452 (subscribers in the U.S. & Canada)
314-453-7041 (subscribers outside of the U.S. & Canada)

Fax number: 314-523-5170

Elsevier Periodicals Customer Service
11830 Westline Industrial Drive
St. Louis, MO 63146

*To ensure uninterrupted delivery of your subscription, please notify us at least 4 weeks in advance of move.

ELSEVIER

Printed and bound by CPI Group (UK) Ltd, Croydon, CR0 4YY

14/10/2024

01773706-0001